THERAPY IN PRACTICE SERIES

Edited by Jo Campling

This series of books is aimed at 'therapists' concerned with rehabilitation in a very broad sense. The intended audience particularly includes occupational therapists, physiotherapists and speech therapists, but many titles will also be of interest to nurses, psychologists, medical staff, social workers, teachers or volunteer workers. Some volumes are interdisciplinary, others are aimed at one particular profession. All titles will be comprehensive but concise, and practical but with due reference to relevant theory and evidence. They are not research monographs but focus on professional practice, and will be of value to both students and qualified personnel.

Brain Injury Rehabilitation

A neurofunctional approach

Gordon Muir Giles
Director
Occupational Therapy
The Guardian Foundation
Berkeley
California
USA

and

Jo Clark-Wilson
Head Injury Clinical Management Services
Ticehurst House Hospital
East Sussex
UK

CHAPMAN & HALL
London · Glasgow · New York · Tokyo · Melbourne · Madras

Published by Chapman & Hall, 2—6 Boundary Row, London SE1 8HN

Chapman & Hall, 2—6 Boundary Row, London SE1 8HN, UK

Blackie Academic & Professional, Wester Cleddens Road, Bishopbriggs, Glasgow G64 2NZ, UK

Chapman & Hall GmbH, Pappelallee 3, 69469 Weinheim, Germany

Chapman & Hall USA, 115 Fifth Avenue, New York, NY 10003, USA

Chapman & Hall Japan, ITP-Japan, Kyowa Building, 3F, 2-2-1 Hirakawacho, Chiyoda-ku, Tokyo 102, Japan

Chapman & Hall Australia, 102 Dodds Street, South Melbourne, Victoria 3205, Australia

Chapman & Hall India, R. Seshadri, 32 Second Main Road, CIT East, Madras 600 035, India

Distributed in the USA and Canada by Singular Publishing Group Inc., 4284 41st Street, San Diego, California 92105

First edition 1993
Reprinted 1995

© 1993 Gordon Muir Giles and Jo Clark-Wilson

Typeset in 10/12pt Times by Intype, London
Printed and bound by Ipswich Book Company, Ipswich, Suffolk

ISBN   0 412 33520 4   1 56593 052 5 (USA)

A catalogue record for this book is available from the British Library

Contents

Preface

The true extent of the human tragedy is hard to appreciate from the statistics but each year more than 800 000 people suffer traumatic brain injury in the United States and 200 000 in the United Kingdom. Ninety percent of victims survive the injury and of these a quarter or more will have significant residual complaints. Brain injury may affect all areas of human life. Psychiatric and personality as well as cognitive and behavioural changes are common. Many of those with residual impairment are under 30 years old and will live a normal life span. Growing numbers of such individuals are living in institutions or in the community dependent upon family or state support. Individuals with brain injury therefore represent a significant charge on public and private resources.

In addition to the effect on the brain-injured person the repercussions of brain trauma on family members may be substantial. In some cases the change of roles from equal partner to 'attendant' may cause severe anxiety. Families burdens may increase with time. For some the additional work of caring for the survivor may become progressively more exhausting. There is evidence that some survivors of brain injury experience behavioural and psychosocial deterioration over time (Chapter 1). Patient and family satisfaction should be weighted in determining the rehabilitation outcome. In some cases we have observed that patients and their families reach an emotionally satisfactory outcome despite severe handicap. The influence of pre-morbid factors, type of injury environmental factors and therapeutic intervention in achieving this type of outcome have not been sufficiently elucidated. It is possible that the chances of achieving an emotionally satisfactory outcome may be reduced by the financial trauma on the family. The actual financial cost after injury may be staggering but changes in family structure and lifestyle may be more marked. In a study by McMordie and Barker (1988), almost a quarter of wives reported that they had to go to work after their husband's brain injury. Nearly a tenth of spouses declared bankruptcy. Family income is often markedly reduced.

Adequate planning and resource provision is complicated by the inability to predict an individual's therapeutic outcome or future needs. Considerable research effort has examined patient prognosis but this research has been performed primarily by neurosurgeons and their co-workers who are concerned with determining prognosis immediately following the insult. We might be better able to predict ultimate outcome by analysing factors evident at six months or one year. For example, if at one year following trauma we could predict those most likely to return to work, given appropriate rehabilitation services, it would be helpful in allocating resources. In addition researchers should examine prognosis using functionally and ecologically sound outcome measures.

Most research into brain injury has been academic and has not attempted to answer clinical needs. For example, to evaluate the effects of brain injury on an intact nervous system, researchers have excluded patients with a previous history of brain trauma, learning disability, mood disorder, substance abuse or mental retardation. Unfortunately, excluding these patients makes the results non-productive for real clinical practice. In a series of patients treated at a Transitional Living Centre for brain-injured adults, 51% of patients had one of the just mentioned complicating factors while 19% had two or more (Giles, 1989, unpublished data).

There is increasing understanding of the need for cost effective rehabilitation services (Cole *et al.*, 1985). One way to provide for these needs is to have the patient's progression in treatment centres parallel their reduced need for medical supervision. As they no longer need medical care they move out of the hospital, as they no longer need residential services they become out-patients and so on. This movement in turn reflects the change from being a passive recipient of care to being an autonomous agent.

Intervention must address a behaviour of real clinical importance. The difference between 40% adequate street crossing before intervention and 60% after intervention may be statistically stable and significant: however, the lethal outcome likely to be associated with even the reduced level of unsafe street crossing results in this type of change being clinically irrelevant. A certain degree of social relativity has to be accepted: social skills are an obvious area which have a high degree of social relativity. For example, it is important to consider what level of a specific (noxious) behaviour family, friends or care staff will tolerate. Despite the relativity of some behaviours, the criteria for others remain more fixed, at or very close to zero, e.g. severe aggression. This issue is discussed again in Chapter 6.

Clinicians should be prepared to evaluate and treat a wide range of behaviours in patients with brain injury. If therapists are working in trans-disciplinary teams they must be willing to go beyond their areas of training to perform activities which they might have thought were in the domain of other disciplines. Professionals bring their own areas of expertise, but also much that is general to being a 'therapist', to the treatment of the brain injured. It is for this reason that, while this text is directed towards occupational therapists, much of what is said applies to all those who work in the rehabilitation of this population.

Rehabilitation staff require a high level of expertise in order to meet the needs of the brain-injured population adequately. Staff require commitment and the ability to monitor and govern their own emotional reactions to personally confronting clients. Staff who wish to have their interventions or moral worth validated by clients may not have this need met. Subtle social and behavioural deficits may be disregarded by team members who would find confronting these disorders personally threatening. It is essential to foster close working relationships and team support. Development of a close team prevents staff being divided by patient or family members. We will frequently return in this text to the difficulties experienced by staff in working with the brain-injured population. Poorly trained staff may regard patients as being wilful or unmotivated towards recovery. These views can be held even when staff are aware of the behavioural sequelae of brain injury and the frequent difficulties patients have in sustaining effort and in initiating behaviour. A partial explanation for this phenomenon comes from attribution theory. Observers tend to attribute behaviour in others (particularly aberrant behaviour which violates normative expectations) to personality factors under the individual's control, though they attribute such behaviour in themselves to environmental factors (Hamilton, 1979). Attribution of inappropriate or socially unacceptable behaviour to factors under the individual's control may be accentuated when the behaviour causes anxiety in the observer. Staff may then seek confirming evidence for the hypotheses. Given the complex sequelae on brain trauma, it is often possible to find evidence of unusually good performance to justify regarding inferior performance as lack of effort or 'moral weakness'. This type of interpretation may also rely on a belief in an intact pre-injury version of the person hidden inside the brain-injured individual.

THE NEUROFUNCTIONAL APPROACH

The neurofunctional approach provides a new frame of reference in occupational therapy. Although it does advocate a theoretical stance the theory which underlies it is applied theory. The aim of the frame of reference is to maximize functional independence and psychosocial adaptation. Central to the approach are the following.

1. Consideration of the neuropsychiatric and neuropsychological limitations to new learning resulting from damage to the central nervous system (Giles and Fussey, 1988). These limitations are considered in the development of functional treatment programmes. Emphasis is placed on the assessment process.
2. Functional activities which are used to address deficits and to enhance plastic changes in the central nervous system learning. The approach is 'bottom-up' not 'top-down' (Chapter 2).
3. Specific techniques which are advocated for use in the rehabilitation of individuals with neurofunctional deficits. These are based on the scientific principles of applied behavioural analysis and treatment.

The central features of the neurofunctional approach are elaborated throughout this text. The neurofunctional approach represents a group of procedures of proven efficacy. While some critics have referred to some of our methods as 'commonplace' (Heacock *et al.*, 1989) it is our view that the vast majority of brain-injured clients do not receive adequate rehabilitation services. Therapists have a professional obligation to ensure that clients are provided with the most effective treatment that can be provided. In an effort to deliniate a framework for future research and intervention we provide treatment guidelines. Our discussion borrows from that of Houtin *et al.* (1988).

ETHICAL ISSUES IN REHABILITATION

In the acute care settings, ethical issues frequently centre on when to withhold treatment. In the rehabilitation stage issues often revolve around who is provided with services and there is debate regarding the value systems which contribute to making that determination (Berrol, 1986). Again unlike acute medical intervention (which despite attacks continues to use the medical model), rehabilitation concerns not only the trauma but also the environment. The environment may exacerbate disability or produce handicaps which are not inherently part of the condition (Chapters 2 and 6). The model advocated in this book places the patient firmly within an environmental context; this is, however, not without ethical ramifications. In the medical model the patient is viewed as the passive recipient of treatment: the patient is not encouraged to take responsibility other than in a very limited sense (i.e. complying with treatment recommendations). Rehabilitation on the other hand requires the patient to take an active part in managing his or her own life. The aim of treatment is not to cure the effects of the trauma but to establish emotional well-being, and develop functional capacities and societal reintegration.

This situation produces frequent opportunities for disagreement about the aims of therapy. For example a rehabilitation team may see the patient's primary aims as the development of skills for independent living while family members see the overriding aim as independent ambulation. Disagreements may not be limited to those between the family and treatment staff but may involve government agencies, health service administrators and third party payors. For example health insurance companies may regard attempts to help a traumatically brain injured client return to work as 'not medically necessary' and therefore not reimbursable. It is common for the treatment team to have different aims, at least initially, from those of the patients. This situation is particularly complicated in the case of individuals with acquired brain injury. Initially the likely

outcome of rehabilitation may be unclear – patients may have
unrealistic aims. The terms 'independence' and 'quality of life'
are often used with little effort to establish what they mean to
the patient and family. These problems may be minimized by
the early establishment and maintenance of open lines of communication with the family and patient. They should not only
be informed about team decisions but should be given clear and
concise justification for courses of action. Patient and family
members should understand the structure of authority in the
rehabilitation setting and how decisions are made. The team
should present a consistent treatment philosophy and be able
to communicate the aims of treatment clearly. Though authority
in decision making is often distributed in the team, an efficient
and explicit channel of communication should be established
with the family. As noted by Caplan *et al*. (1987), achieving
accommodation between patients, families, friends and pro-
viders as to what constitutes the appropriate ends of rehabilitation and acceptable quality of life is one of the most arduous
tasks facing rehabilitation professionals.

A THERAPEUTIC ENVIRONMENT

Clients have a right to expect a therapeutic environment which
provides safety, an adequate level of comfort and positive social
interaction. Staff should be competent, caring and provide social
support to the client. The therapeutic environment should foster
an appropriate level of functional independence. The environment should be the least restrictive possible, and provide
maximum access to preferred activities. As a client progresses,
the 'least restrictive' rule suggests that he or she progress
through treatment settings consistent with safety and treatment
needs. Within the context of a therapeutic environment the
client should be adequately assessed and constraints imposed
on the individual by his or her neurological disorder considered.
Assessment should be functionally oriented.

TRAINING IN FUNCTIONAL SKILLS

The aim of the neurofunctional approach is to help individuals
function in both their current environment and other environments which they are likely to experience. Functional skills

training involves assisting clients to develop personal, domestic and community activities of daily living, skilled social behaviours and work skills. Functional skills training may also include the reduction of behaviours which may be dangerous or socially unacceptable (e.g. aggressive behaviours directed toward the self or others).

Intervention programmes are designed on the basis of assessments performed by qualified professionals and should include ongoing assessment of efficacy. It may, during an intervention programme, be appropriate to expose the individual to some discomfort or risk. This needs to be carefully monitored and risk kept to the minimum consistent with the patients progress. Examples of discomfort include a time out programme for physical aggression, whereas an example of risk taking involves teaching a client to cross the street (Houten *et al.* 1988). Procedures should only be implemented when they are incorporated into a total treatment plan specific to the individual. This plan should be functionally established on the basis of existing capacities but should not limit the client's progress.

TREATMENT EFFICACY

An individual has a right to the most effective procedure available and wherever possible interventions should be of scientifically proven efficacy. The treatment chosen should be the most valid, the least restrictive available and applied only if a clinically significant behavioural change is a reasonable expectation. A less restrictive treatment should not be selected if it will take much longer to work or if other procedures are more effective.

FOCUS AND OBJECTIVES

The central focus of this book is traumatic brain injury. Patients with related diagnoses are discussed when their treatment is of particular interest and where symptom complexes are similar to those which follow traumatic brain injury. Other disorders discussed include infections such as herpes simplex, encephalitis, anoxia and damage of vascular origin such as aneurysms.

There is little written in the rehabilitation literature to assist therapists work with patients with these diagnoses. Treatment principles are often similar however. We believe the approaches advocated here are applicable to many therapeutic disciplines. Both authors being occupational therapists, however, we acknowledge a certain degree of bias. We have attempted to develop an interdisciplinary approach relevant to all therapeutic disciplines.

This text is intended for practicing therapists, educators and students. Since it is practice oriented, the reader should be able to take much of the material and apply it directly to work with clients. This text does not provide the reader with sufficient training to perform applied behavioural analysis and further training should be undertaken. Therapists do not prescribe medication but they should be able to advise physicians about the likely effect of medications on the areas of patient functioning of concern to the therapist. A brief discussion of pharmacological therapy is therefore included in this text. Further reading is available in Silverstone and Turner (1988) and Gualtieri (1988). In addition we have included discussion of brain injury prevention. Those in rehabilitation have a special duty to advocate increased safety awareness and the adoption of safe practices in the general population such as the use of crash helmet laws and the introduction of passive restraining devices (e.g airbags) in automobiles.

After reading this book, the reader will understand

1. the causes and consequences of severe brain injury;
2. theories of recovery of function and current intervention models;
3. the principles of neurofunctional assessment and treatment.

Within the neurofunctional approach the therapist will be able to

i. understand neurofunctional assessment methods with brain-injured individuals;
ii. appreciate the constraints placed on human learning by brain injury;
iii. establish functional treatment programmes focusing on acute symptoms, neuropsychiatric and neuropsychological disorders, motor relearning and interpersonal skills,
iv. apply the neurofunctional approach in community and work settings;

v. work with the patient's family and social support systems to maximize function in real world contexts.

We welcome comments from students, teachers or practitioners which will help us improve either the content or the presentation of this text.

ACKNOWLEDGEMENTS

We wish to thank all those who have helped us in writing this book in America and the United Kingdom. In America, Aracelli Antonio of Bay Area Recovery centers; Jill Kneeter, Program Director; Ann Dill, Clinical Director; and Mike Shore, Director of Neuropsychology; all of Transitions Berkeley; Fernando Miranda MD FAAN. Liz Allen and Mary Beth Badke MS of the University of Wisconsin: Harry Hatzichristidis, Jay and all at Ground Zero. In the United Kingdom we also wish to thank Alec Tredre, and Mike Oddy, Ticehurst House Head Injury Rehabilitation Unit; Martyn Rose, Kemsley Unit; Anne Gent, Grafton Manor and Amanda Davis, Harrowlands.

Errors of fact or interpretation are however the sole responsibility of the authors. In addition we wish to thank the following journals which have kindly allowed us to reprint material we have reported previously: *The American Journal of Occupational Therapy, Archives of Physical Medicine and Rehabilitation, Brain Injury, The British Journal of Occupational Therapy* and *The Journal of Clinical and Experimental Neuropsychology.*

1

The nature and consequences of brain injury

Despite continuing medical advances, traumatic brain injury remains a significant cause of death and disability. Approximately 50% of those who survive in coma for six hours or more die by the end of six months (Jennett *et al.*, 1977). Baxt and Moody (1987a) followed the medical course of 545 patients with major trauma both with and without severe brain injury (Glasgow Coma Score of 8 or less). All patients were treated continuously by one US medical service from the site of injury until hospital discharge. One hundred and four patients with major multi-system trauma had severe brain injury and 441 patients with major multi-system trauma were without severe brain injury. The mortality of the brain injury group was 30.8% whereas the mortality of the group without major central nervous system (CNS) trauma was 0.9%. Many of the brain injured group appear to have sustained injuries so severe, they were unable to be saved. In contrast, most of the patients who sustained major injury without CNS damage responded to energetic medical management. Appropriate airway management, volume replacement, operative intervention and intensive care were key elements of emergency medical care. Unfortunately, severe non-CNS injury may complicate the management of the patient with brain trauma. Recent reports suggest that although there has been a decline in fatality from secondary ischaemic lesions, they remain a significant cause of death (Baethmann, 1987). The presence of associated major system injury continues to play a significant role in secondary brain trauma.

The annual incidence of brain injury in the United States has been estimated at between 180 and 294 per 100 000 population (Annegers *et al*, 1980; Fife *et al*, 1986; Kraus *et al*, 1984). Variation in the reported incidence may be due to different data collection methods and the diversity of the populations studied. Fife *et al.* (1986) analysed hospital admission data for all those with brain injury in Rhode Island over a two-year period. The authors found admissions of 152 per 100 000 population with incidence peaking in three age groups. The first peak occurred in early childhood (1–2), the second in late adolescents and early adulthood (15–25) and the third in the elderly (65 and older). The incidence in males exceeded that in females in every age group except the oldest. The incidence from all causes increased with declining income and with rising population density suggesting that those most at risk for brain trauma are low income inner city dwellers. People with below average incomes are considerably more likely to be victims of assault and are slightly more prone than those in higher income groups to falls. There is little variation in the incidence of motor vehicle accidents between high and low income groups.

Johnson and Gleave (1987) estimated the incidence of traumatic brain injury in Great Britain by identifying all those in a known population (Cambridge). In one year there were 160 traumatic brain injury survivors per 100 000 population. At the two-year follow up 0.38 per 100 000 were in need of continuing care, and 0.75 per 100 000 were unemployed and in need of outpatient treatment. Figures exclude those 65 and older, are from a predominantly rural population and may therefore result in an underestimate if applied to the general population. Figures are comparable to those obtained in population studies in the USA.

The majority of studies which have estimated incidence of brain injury have been limited to hospital admission data. This method of data collection results in an underestimate of the incidence of brain injury since not all mild or moderate injuries result in hospital admissions. A US study by Fife (1987) indicates that those hospitalized represent only 18% of all those medically attended following brain trauma. These figures are of particular interest due to the growing evidence of disabling symptoms potentially following mild brain trauma (Rimel *et al.*, 1981; Binder, 1986). In the same study, Fife (1987) showed that the likelihood of hospitalization varied depending on age, circumstances of injury and family income. Those with work or motor vehicle related brain injuries were most likely to be hospitalized whereas children, the elderly, or those with low incomes were less likely to be admitted to hospital. Because an individual is not admitted to the hospital does not imply that they are not in need of services.

Alberico *et al.* (1987) described the cause of injury in a series of 330 severely brain-injured patients in the USA. 66% of adults and 92% of paediatric injuries were motor vehicle related either as a passenger, a pedestrian or while riding a bicycle. Of non-motor vehicle related injuries in adults 2% occurred at work, 9% were assaults and 17% occurred in the home. Five percent were classified as other. In children 5% of injuries were classified as domestic and 3% as other. In a British consecutive series of 151 fatal non-missile brain injuries reported by Adams *et al.* (1980) 123 were males and 28 females, 46% were road traffic accidents, 43% were falls, 9% were assaults and 2% were crush injuries.

RISK FACTORS

Alcohol

Alcohol use and abuse is frequently associated with brain trauma. Recent reports indicate that 42 – 58% of patients are intoxicated at the time of hospital admission, figures which do not vary significantly between the USA and Great Britain (Rutherford, 1977; Brismar *et al.*, 1983). As many as 40% may have a history of alcohol dependency and 25% report having used narcotics (Brismar, *et al.*, 1983).

As blood alcohol levels increase, psychomotor performance deteriorates and the probability of being involved in a serious automobile crash increases (Fell, 1977). Brain injury as a result of assaultive behaviour frequently involves alcohol or drugs in either the aggressor the victim or both. The use of alcohol or illegal drugs may result in decreased social inhibition and judgement and an increased tendency to express emotions (Reilly *et al.*, 1986). Hillbom and Holm (1986) examined the extent to which traumatic brain injuries contribute to the intellectual impairments found in alcoholics. Findings indicated that the incidence of brain injury may be two to four times higher in the alcoholics than in the general population. Not surprisingly, the alcoholics with brain injuries demonstrated more neuropsychological impairment than either control group or alcoholics without brain injuries. Recognition of the dual diagnosis can lead to an appropriate dual rehabilitation effort.

Not only may intoxication increase the risk of injury, it may also lead to more severe injury from a comparable insult. Experimental studies with animals indicate that ethanol potentiates the damage resulting from traumatic brain injury. Minor brain injury may have more severe consequences in those who are intoxicated (Flamm *et al.*, 1977). Luna *et al.* (1984) studied the effect of acute alcohol intoxication on the recovery of brain injured motorcylists. An intoxicated motorcyclist involved in a motor vehicle accident is considerably more likely to have a severe brain injury than his sober counterpart. In addition the intoxicated rider is twice as likely to die of an apparently comparable brain injury than a sober rider. Waller *et al.* (1985) analysed 1000 000 crashes and found that when injury related variables such as seat-belt usage, vehicular deformation, mode of crash, speed, driver age and vehicle weight are controlled for, the intoxicated driver is still more likely to incur serious injury or death than his sober counterpart. In four studies in the USA (reported by Fell, 1977), 39–75% of drivers responsible for crashes had been drinking alcohol or had a combination of alcohol and other drugs in their system just prior to the crash. Brookes *et al.* (1989) found that as habitual alcohol use increased, outcome from brain injury deteriorated. To have a short period of post-traumatic amnesia (PTA) and to have drunk heavily led to a worse outcome than that found in patients with a considerably longer PTA who had drunk lightly or not at all. It remains unclear from this research however whether the effect in these patients is from an acute or chronic toxic effect (Brookes *et al.*, 1989).

Early development and school history

Poor school adjustment may be a risk factor for traumatic brain injury (Fahy *et al.*, 1967; Fuld and Fisher, 1977). Haas *et al.* (1987) examined pre-morbid prevalence of poor academic performance in individuals who later suffered severe brain injury. Parameters used to indicate unusually low scholastic achievement included failure in two or more academic subjects, a diagnosis of learning disability or school dropout. Haas and co workers found that 50% of severely brain-injured patients demonstrated poor pre-morbid academic performance, suggesting an increased risk for severe brain injury. This increased risk could represent an expression of a primary neurological impairment leading to distractability, limited attention span, lowered frustration tolerance or impulsivity or a secondary process related to social difficulties. Those with poor academic adjustment may be given to more rebellious, egocentric and sociopathic behaviour as well as an increased rate of substance abuse (Haas *et al.*, 1987). Individuals demonstrating poor social skills often attempt to compensate for these by taking alcohol. Clinicians are familiar with patients who demonstrate poor school adjustment and/or academic development disorder. Intensive education intervention in these high risk groups is recommended (Haas *et al.*, 1987).

C. T. S., aged 34, (coma duration 13 days) was injured in a single-driver motor vehicle accident. His father was a physician and his mother a lawyer. He had severe learning difficulties in school and had taken remedial classes. He had been socially isolated at school and had few friends. C. T. S. had been regarded as the black sheep of the family. He had had multiple short-lived heterosexual relationships and acknowledged alcohol and drug use, significant enough to interfere with work. The patient had been out drinking alone. While driving home he lost control of his car and struck a lamppost.

Personality type

Individuals who experience severe brain injury may not represent a random distribution of personality types (Rose, 1988). Type 'A' personalities whose behaviour pattern is characterized by excessive competitiveness, hostility and time urgency may be at greater risk for traumatic brain injury (Suls and Sanders, 1988). Type 'A' are more likely to die from violence or from accidents than type 'B's (who have lower levels of hostility and competitiveness) (Zyzanski, 1978). Type 'A' bus drivers had more accidents than type 'B' bus drivers (Evans *et al.*, 1987a). The male drivers most responsible for fatal or serious accidents, regardless of age or alcohol involvement, display personality traits such as belligerence, verbal expansiveness and impulsivity and significantly differ from the norm in these respects (Fell, 1977). A study using family report on personality type and its relationship to brain trauma would further elucidate the relationship between personality type and severe brain injury. Others have suggested a relationship between brain injury and accident proneness (a concept which is itself under dispute). While this notion is appealing, direct evidence is negligible (Sims, 1985).

Sporting activity

Numerous studies have found that professional and amateur boxers have significant and lasting neurological deficits as a result of repeated mild brain trauma (Casson et al., 1984; Ross et al., 1983). Research by Levin et al. (1987b) suggests that the neuropsychological impairments found in this group are not due to pre-morbid impairment and that the damage typically occurs late in the boxer's career. Off road motorcyclying has a high incidence of injury. A recent patient series (Wilson-MacDonald et al., 1987) found that 23 of 155 individuals treated after an off-road motorcycle accident sustained brain injury but none had a severe injury. All but three were wearing helmets. Those involved in the sport should continue to emphasize the importance of safety equipment.

Many sporting activities carry significantly increased risk when appropriate safety procedures are not followed. For example, of 36 fatal snowmobile accidents in Sweden between 1973 and 1984, 30 drivers were under the influence of alcohol (Eriksson and Bjornstig, 1982). One of the most widespread causes of injury among young people is bicycling. Bicycling injuries have been estimated to account for 19–20% of all head injuries in children (Ivan et al., 1983; O'Rooke et al., 1987) and up to 7% of injuries in the general population (Kraus et al., 1987). In a controlled study of 235 persons with brain injuries following bicycling accidents, who sought emergency care at one of five hospitals in Seattle, Washington, 7% were wearing helmets (Thompson et al., 1989). Of the 99 bicyclists with severe brain injury only 4% were wearing helmets. Using regression analysis the authors calculated that riders with helmets had an 85% reduction in their risk of head injury (including facial injuries) and an 88% reduction in the risk of brain injury. There were marked age variations between those wearing and not wearing helmets. Individuals over 25 were substantially more likely to wear helmets than younger people. The authors conclude that bicycle helmets are an effective means of preventing injury and support helmet use among children.

MECHANISMS OF BRAIN INJURY

Various methods are used to classify traumatic brain injury. We will discuss brain injury under the headings 'Open versus closed brain trauma', 'Focal versus diffuse brain trauma' and 'Primary versus secondary brain trauma'.

Open versus closed brain trauma

Brain injuries are categorized as open or closed (or penetrating versus blunt) depending on whether the skull and the meninges have been breached leaving the brain exposed. The majority of non-combat brain injuries are closed brain injuries. Open brain injury can be caused by gunshot wounds, traffic accidents and industrial accidents and although not as frequently encountered as closed brain trauma, individuals with open brain injuries are regularly treated in acute rehabilitation units. Whether closed and open brain injury should be regarded as completely different conditions in terms of deficit constellation and rehabilitation outcome is a matter of debate (Teuber, 1969). Benton (1979) suggests that the modal post-traumatic behavioural pictures are different.

Focal versus diffuse brain injury

Focal brain injury

Focal damage includes cerebral contusions and various types of secondary brain damage (Adams *et al.*, 1983). Typically contusions occur at the poles and on the inferior surfaces of the frontal and temporal lobes. Recent evidence has led to a re-evaluation of the belief that contusions are most severe in the region of the brain directly opposite the point of impact (contra coup) since individuals with either frontal or occipital injuries typically have their most severe contusions at the frontal lobes

(Adams *et al.*, 1980a). Contusions are usually more severe in patients with skull fracture than in those without fracture.

Intracranial haematoma is a common complication of non-missile brain injury (Adams *et al.*, 1980b). Haematoma may be either extradural or subdural. Risk factors for extradural haematomas in those with mild to moderate injury are skull fracture, clouding of consciousness or focal neurological dysfunction. Patients with large or expanding lesions show uniformly good outcome when surgical evacuation is performed early (Servadei *et al.*, 1988). Subdural haematomas are collections of blood under the dura and are frequently associated with poor outcome. Patients with basal ganglia haematoma are typically more severely injured and have a poorer prognosis than patients with other intracranial haematomas (Macpherson *et al.*, 1986). Herniation is a result of differential pressures in the compartments of the brain. These compartments are formed by the falx cerebri and the tentorium cerebelli. Mass changes may lead to pressures forcing parts of the brain to be compressed against, or herniate through, the gaps in these structures. Herniation is associated with poor outcome.

Diffuse brain injury

Diffuse brain injury may be divided into four types. Three types of diffuse brain injury; diffuse axonal injury, hypoxic damage and diffuse brain swelling are frequently encountered in patients who survive traumatic brain injury. The fourth type consists of multiple small haemorrhages and is virtually restricted to patients who die soon after injury (Adams *et al.*, 1983).

Some degree of diffuse axonal injury is probably present in all cases of closed brain injury severe enough to result in loss of consciousness. Those with severe diffuse axonal injury are less likely to have skull fractures, cerebral contusions and intracranial haematomas. Diffuse axonal injury is the result of mech anical stress on axons. Computer tomography scans may fail to reveal this type of damage. Animal studies suggest that the more severe the diffuse axonal injury, the more protracted the duration of coma and the worse the outcome (Gennarelli *et al.*, 1982). There may be a continuum of axonal trauma. Some axons may be damaged and have impaired functioning but retain the ability to repair themselves. Mechanisms for axonal repair are activated in both physically disrupted and non-disrupted axons but are ineffective in the latter (Gennarelli *et al.*, 1986). Severity of the clinical syndrome depends on the location of the damaged axons and the ratio of damaged to intact axons. Severe axonal injury is a common cause of the persistent vegetative state (Jennett and Plum, 1972; Adams *et al.*, 1980b).

Hypoxic brain damage is common following traumatic brain injury. In a series of 151 consecutive fatal brain injuries 65 suffered hypoxic brain damage (Adams *et al.*, 1980b). Arterial boundary zones are particularly susceptible, but hypoxia may occur throughout the cortex. Hypoxic damage is associated with raised intracranial pressure and is frequently discovered in patients who remain in a persistent vegetative state or who are severely disabled after injury (Graham *et al.*, 1983). Even patients with severe hypoxic injury may have an unremarkable CT scan.

> S.T., a 50-year-old school teacher (coma 3 days), was first seen for consultation six weeks after injury. The patient was in a semi-secure psychiatric unit at an acute care hospital. S.T. was fully ambulatory, profoundly amnestic, dysphasic, agitated and occasionally combative. The pattern and severity of ST's symptomatology was unusual considering the duration of the coma. However, S.T. had incurred multiple system injury with a pneumothorax and flail chest, probably resulting in anoxic brain damage. Although the patient continued to have profound memory deficits 18 months post-injury, he eventually made an adequate functional recovery to live with his wife in the community and go into his local neighbourhood independently.

Brain swelling may occur in all or part of the brain after brain injury. The term brain swelling is more accurate than 'cerebral oedema' since vasodilation may produce swelling without an increase in water volume. Swelling almost always surrounds an area of focal damage and has been attributed to changes in the vascular system (Plum and Posner, 1980, pp 93–94). Diffuse bilateral brain swelling appears to occur most frequently in younger patients, particularly those under 18.

Those in motor vehicle related accidents have a high proportion of diffuse injuries (63%) while those in work, assault, domestic or other categories are more likely to have mass lesions (Alberico *et al.*, 1987). When the incidence of mass lesions in the adult and paediatric groups is compared, 46% of adults and only 24% of children had mass lesions. Since mass lesions are associated with significantly poorer outcome this may partially account for the more favourable outcome reported in children.

Primary versus secondary brain injury

Primary damage is the result of forces exerted on the brain at the time of injury. Secondary damage refers to changes compromising brain function which result from the brain's reaction to trauma or other system failure. The original or primary injury – which may appear trivial – may initiate secondary processes which lead to severe and at times fatal damage. Meticulous medical management in the early stages of treatment both increases the chances of survival and improves outcome (Becker *et al.*, 1977). A reduction in mortality of trauma victims was reported following modernization of the brain injury service in San Diego County (Klauber *et al.*, 1985), and similar reductions have been reported in other regions (Ornato *et al.*, 1985; West *et al.*, 1983). Since primary injury is a constant, the reduced mortality is a result of the intervention and minimization of the effects of secondary injury. The introduction of airmedical emergency services have also been shown to reduce mortality, (Baxt and Moody, 1987b). In 128 patients treated by land support and 104 treated by rotocraft there was a mortality rate of 40% and 31% respectively. The most striking reduction was in patients with a Glasgow Coma Scale (GCS) of 4 whereas there was little effect on the unfavourable outcome of those with a GCS score of 3.

Improvements in medical treatment in the 1980s can be traced to increasingly rapid detection of treatable complications. Some secondary processes can be ameliorated whereas others are only now being understood. Miller *et al.* (1988) and Servadei *et al.* (1988) have reported earlier detection and better survival rates in individuals with extradural haematomas. These lesions can expand rapidly and lead to severe brain damage or death hours or days following the original injury. Causes of secondary damage which are being increasingly appreciated include brain swelling and impaired cerebral perfusion. These are now actively treated in the intensive care setting using a range of pharmacological agents. It is now known that delayed hippocampal injury occurs in humans after cardiopulmonary arrest. The fact that certain types of insult cause neuronal death hours or days following the initial insult suggests that as yet unknown techniques may be capable of interrupting the process (Petito *et al.*, 1987).

Neurological complications and the possibility of secondary brain injury are not necessarily confined to acute hospitalization. In a series of patients provided with CT scans in an acute rehabilitation setting 21% were found to require neurosurgical intervention for ventricular enlargement, subdural haematoma, or cerebral abscess (Cope *et al.*, 1988). Neurological complications may also be overlooked in patients with other types of trauma. Davidoff *et al.* (1985) found that 42% of all spinal cord injury patients reported loss of consciousness or post traumatic amnesia (PTA) or both. Although these injuries are often mild to moderate, the sequelae may be significant given the demands for both new learning and emotional adjustment placed on spinal cord injury patients. Interestingly, rehabilitation services were unlikely to assess the consequences of these brain injuries.

EPILEPSY

Post traumatic epilepsy (PTE) may emerge months or years following brain trauma and is more common after severe brain injury. Five percent of those hospitalized with traumatic brain injury suffer the disorder but as many as 10% of the severely injured do so. Epilepsy after trauma may be divided into early or late. In adults, early epilepsy (within seven days of injury) occurs most often in conjunction with one of the following risk factors: depressed fracture, intracranial haematoma or severe injury. In 60% of cases the first and often only seizure occurs within 20 hours and in half of these within the first hour (Jennett, 1983).

More than half of those who develop late epilepsy (occurring more than seven days after injury) have their first seizure within a year of injury (Jennett, 1983). The principal risk factors for late epilepsy are a depressed fracture, an acute intracranial haematoma and early epilepsy. Late epilepsy may take various forms, often occurring in different forms in the same person.

Approximately half of those with late epilepsy experience grand mal seizures and about a fifth have temporal lobe seizures. The majority of post-traumatic epilepsies involve partial seizures (Pellock, 1989). The nature of partial seizures are such that they may not be recognized as epileptiform in nature and include absences and automatisms. There is some evidence that those with PTE may have poorer functional outcomes than patients without PTE. Armstrong and co-workers (1990) found that both PTE and non-PTE groups improved their level of functioning during a course of acute rehabilitation. However the PTE group functioned at a lower level and required more nursing care at discharge than the non-PTE group. The degree to which the difference can be ascribed to antiepileptic medication is unclear (Armstrong *et al.*, 1990).

There is no consensus as to the advisability of prophylactic treatment for PTE with anti-seizure medications. Pellock (1989) points out that prophylactic treatment is often initiated before any seizures occur and questions this practice on the grounds that no studies clearly indicate that prophylaxis prevents PTE; PTE rarely causes death unless status epilepticus develops and is prolonged; adverse cognitive, behavioural and quality-of-life effects may be marked and there is risk of drug sensitivity. As well as being attacked on the grounds of efficacy, the prophylaxis has been attacked on the grounds that it is applied capriciously. Soroker *et al.* (1989) found that prophylactic treatment is not instituted in 40% of patients who belong to a widely accepted high risk group but is initiated in about 30% of patients who, on accepted criteria, would be considered at minimal risk.

EARLY ASSESSMENT

Detailed discussion of early assessment procedures is reserved for Chapter 8. Here assessment is discussed briefly to provide a context for the discussion of predictors of outcome which follows. The rapid assessment of trauma severity is important for a number of reasons. Severity of injury influences early management and is an indicator of prognosis. Techniques are increasingly available which allow the visualization of damage to the brain (computerized tomography, magnetic resonance imaging) and this has led to considerable reduction in mortality and morbidity in patients with some types of injury (Miller *et al.*, 1988; Servadei *et al.*, 1988). It is now widely accepted that all patients with severe brain injury should have a CT scan. Diffuse axonal shearing may not be distinguishable, necessitating estimation of the severity of this type of injury on other indicators.

Initially patients are examined for level of responsiveness. Later duration of alteration of consciousness can be used to infer the degree of diffuse axonal shearing. The Glasgow Coma Scale (Teasdale and Jennett, 1974) has gained wide acceptance in many centres as a method of assessing severity of injury. The best responses in the three categories of motor response, verbal response and eye opening are assigned a numerical value which are summed to produce a Glasgow Coma Scale score (Chapter 8). A severe injury may be defined as a GCS of 8 or less, a score of 9–12 indicates brain injury of moderate severity and of 13–15 a mild brain injury. Duration of coma may be used as an indicator of severity of injury, 0–20 minutes indicating mild injury, 20 minutes to one hour indicating moderate injury and one hour and above indicating severe injury. Duration of post-traumatic amnesia cannot be used in initial assessment but remains a useful indicator. Russell's criteria are used most often and are provided in Table 8.2 (Russell and Smith, 1961).

Unfortunately many of the early predictors of outcome – GCS, duration of coma – are not recorded in the acute hospital and are unavailable at the post-acute care setting. In order to use early factors to predict outcome it is necessary to rate degree of recovery. Statistical procedures may then be used to relate severity of injury of a large group of patients to severity of outcome. In the acute stage there are a number of factors which are powerful predictors of death or persistent vegetative state (PSV) or survival and recovery. In the next section, factors which influence outcome will be discussed. To conclude this section, two frequently used outcome scales will be described. Assessment in the acute stage of recovery will be discussed further in Chapter 8.

The Glasgow Outcome Scale (GOS) is a five-point scale with the categories of death, persistent vegetative state, severe disability, moderate disability and good recovery (Jennett and Bond, 1975). The authors developed the scale in order to provide a reliable method to compare the outcome of alternative methods of patient management. It is a great improvement over the ill-defined outcome measures used prior to its introduction. Of the five categories of the GOS the categories of death and PVS are self-explanatory. Severe disability is defined as conscious but disabled, moderate disability as disabled but independent (independent in daily life activities, able to use public transport and attend sheltered work). The final category of good recovery is somewhat unclear – it is defined as a resumption of normal life, but return to work is excluded as a criterion. A more comprehensive outcome scale has been devised by Livingstone and Livingstone (1985). The Glasgow Assessment Schedule (GAS) is a comprehensive rating scale which includes subscales for the assessment of physical, psychological, social, personality and activities of daily living deficits and could be used to note trends in recovery and responses to intervention.

PREDICTORS OF OUTCOME

Type of injury

The nature of the injury is a predictor of outcome and the type of focal injury can be a particularly powerful prognostic indicator. Gennarelli *et al.* (1982) found that patients with subdural haematoma have a poor outcome and a 61% rate of mortality. Good recovery or moderate disability in patients with a subdural haematoma is associated with surgery within 2.5 hours (Seelig *et al.*, 1981). Death was associated with surgery which occurred 4.5 hours or longer following injury. Patients with epidural haematomas had only a 20% rate of mortality and good outcome or moderate disability occurred in 63% of patients.

Uzzell and co-workers (1987) examined outcome at six months in 117 severely traumatically brain injured patients (Glasgow coma score of 6 or less after 6 hours) whose computerised tomographic (CT) examinations demonstrated diffuse axonal injury (DAI), diffuse swellings (DS) or focal injuries (excluding extra cerebral collections). Neuropsychological sequelae were determined from two examinations of 30 of the conscious survivors in the year following injury. Outcome differences as rated by the GOS varied with type of lesion. DS and focal injuries resulted in a greater number of favourable outcomes (good recovery). Mortality rate was higher after DAI. Neuropsychological outcomes also vary according to the type of injury, with differences among the three CT lesion categories. Differences were found in measures of learning and memory but there were no significant differences in measures of intelligence and visuomotor functions. Ratings of memory, learning and visuomotor speed were higher after DS but improved less. Greater improvement occurred in memory, learning and visuomotor speed after DAI even though the full extent and duration of this improvement was unknown. After focal injuries only visuomotor speed improved. The authors suggest that the improvement in the DAI survivors may be because axons are damaged (and initially non-functioning) but not destroyed, increasing the potential for later recovery.

Eye movement

An eye movement scale is included in the GCS (see Table 1). Mueller-Jensen and co-workers (1987) analysed the oculocephalic and oculovestibular reflex in 81 patients with coma from various causes. Sixty-seven percent of patients with preserved oculocephalic and oculovestibular reflex had good outcome. Ninety-two percent of patients with abolished eye reflex movements died. The combination of absent oculocephalic and oculovestibular reflex and abolished pupillary light reflexes allowed prediction of negative outcome in 100% of cases.

Age

Age is a predictor of outcome. Patients in the paediatric age range (1–19) more frequently have a better outcome following severe brain injury than adults and with the exceptions of those aged 1–4, are less likely to die. As age increases so does risk of mortality and there is a corresponding decrease in the likelihood of good outcome. In the series of Alberico *et al.* (1987) 55% of the paediatric population achieved good outcome as opposed to only 30% of the adults. Percentage mortality was also lower in the paediatric population, 24% as opposed to 51% in adults.

Heiskanen and Sipponen (1970) showed that the mortality rate for those patients aged 60 and above is twice that of those aged 20 or below. The work of Teuber (1975) indicates that even small variations in age affected recovery from penetrating brain injury. Individuals aged 17–20 fared significantly better on some parameters than those 21–25 and considerably better than those 26 and over (Teuber, 1975). Wilson and co-workers (1987) found that none of those aged 65 or older who had GCS scores of 3–12 (moderate or severe injury) survived. All patients with mild injuries survived. Seventy-two percent of survivors experienced a change in functional status. Whilst only a small proportion of patients required additional help with activities of daily living, many had changed living situations, had more family visits or made increased use of statutory services. As well as a predictor of general outcome, age is also a predictor of return to work. In a study by Brooks *et al.* (1987) increased age did not become a factor until the age of 45, but from 45 years of age, the older the individual, the lower their chances of returning to work.

Subjective predictors of outcome

Rao and co-workers (1988) assessed the ability of physicians to predict outcome of severe brain injury using a variety of subjective measures. The physicians were asked to generate a list of factors which, based on their experience and past clinical judgements, they considered predictive of outcome but were subjective in nature. Physicians thought abstraction, attention, denial, concentration, patient desire for rehabilitation, family support and realism might be predictive. The functional performance and discharge outcomes of patients were measured using items from the functional evaluation system (FES). None of the subjective measures were found to be related to outcome. Only objective measures of coma duration and age were related to outcome variables. This result is important because many clinicians report using criteria to indicate outcome that are not traditionally quantifiable. Results are consistent with a growing amount of research with other populations indicating the unreliability of predictions made by treatment staff using unsubstantiated measures. Considerable evidence from both the fields of psychology and medicine indicate that formal or mechanical methods of prediction surpass in accuracy those which rely on clinician judgement (Kleinmuntz, 1984). Attempts to account for this phenomena have pointed to the following three factors. First, clinicians tend not to think probablistically; second, they attempt to collect and process an excessive amount of data;

and third, they tend to be misled by subjectively preferred or irrelevant features of a problem (Elstein *et al.*, 1978).

Severity of injury

Brooks (1984) reviewed evidence relating to severity of injury and cognitive changes. Brooks showed that patient's functioning deteriorated in the areas of IQ score, memory and language functioning as duration of PTA increased. Type of symptomatology may also be related to duration of post-traumatic amnesia. Individuals with mild brain injuries most frequently complain of difficulties with concentration, fatigue, headache, dislike of loud noises and irritability. This constellation of difficulties have been labelled 'intolerances'. These problems do occur in the severely brain-injured population but are more likely to be found in those who do not have marked cognitive, behavioural or other types of functional deficits (Van Zomeren and Van Den Burg, 1985).

Mild injury

There is growing support for the notion that organically based impairment in function can result from 'mild' brain trauma (sometimes referred to as the post-concussive syndrome). Gross deficits in memory and intelligence are not found following uncomplicated minor brain trauma but deficits in the rate of information processing and reaction time have been found. Yarnell and Rossie (1988) have described a group of patients who experienced whiplash injury. Triage occurred at an emergency room and all patients were then seen at an outpatient neurology clinic. Alcohol was not a pertinent factor in any of the patients under study. Twenty-seven patients were seen 12 months or more post injury and all had continuing sequelae. Imaging techniques did not demonstrate pathology, however subjective symptoms described included multiple somatic, affective and cognitive dysfunction. Neuropsychological tests did demonstrate impairment such as disorders of vigilance, selective attention, memory, mental endurance and mental flexibility. Edna and Cappelen (1987) followed up 485 mildly brain-injured subjects (GCS scores of 13–15 in 88% of males and 90% of females) to examine frequency and risk factors for post-concussional

symptoms. Follow up was 3–5 years (mean 4.0 years), 51% had
no complaints and 22% had more than three new complaints.
Most obvious parameters such as level of consciousness on
admission, duration of post-traumatic amnesia and days in the
hospital were poor predictors of later complications. Sex,
repeated brain injury and skull fracture (hearing loss, tinnitus,
balance problems) were strongly predictive. Age was a risk
factor for multiple complaints.

Debate continues as to the importance of any single mild
brain trauma (Rimel *et al.*, 1981; Dikmen *et al.*, 1986; see Binder,
1986, for a review). Minor injuries are likely to be more significant when they are multiple (cumulative effect) and when they
occur in an individual who already has symptoms of neurological dysfunction (Haas *et al.*, 1987). Repeated injury is not
uncommon even in individuals who are not in 'at risk' groups
(Mclatchie *et al.*, 1987).

Moderate injury

McMillan and Gluckman (1987) examined the ability of 24 moderately brain-injured adults to process information rapidly when
compared with a matched orthopaedic control group. Moderate
brain injury was defined by duration of post-traumatic amnesia
of between one and 24 hours and all patients were seen within
seven days of injury. A range of neuropsychological tests were
used including the paced auditory serial addition test (PASAT)
in both fast and slow conditions (Gronwall, 1977). Moderate
brain injury patients performed less well on the fast (one word
per two seconds) administration of the PASAT but not on the
slow rate. This result supports the view that there are differences in information processing speed in the moderate brain
injury group when compared to those without neuropsychological trauma. The degree of task difficulty appears to be a central
variable.

Severe injury

Brooks and co-workers (1986) examined the five-year outcome
of 42 severe closed brain injury patients from a relatives' perspective. There are both advantages and disadvantages in using
relatives as interview and questionnaire respondents about a

patient (McKinlay and Brooks, 1984). Relatives' reports of their family members' problems may be biased by their own emotional reactions which may change through time (see below). Such mechanisms may involve attribution, i.e. where behaviour post-dating the injury is attributed to the injury, or sensitization where the relatives' tolerance of a behaviour decreases over time. An advantage of using relatives as a way for the clinician or researcher to gather data include the fact that the nearest relative is most likely to know the patient best. Family members can describe not only what the patient can do but what they actually do, including types of behaviour the patient only displays with close relatives. Results of the five-year follow up study indicated persisting severe deficits and in some cases findings were that the patient was more impaired than at one year (McKinlay *et al.*, 1981; Brooks *et al.*, 1986). The ten problems most frequently reported by relatives about their impaired loved one were personality change, slowness, poor memory, irritability, bad temper, tiredness, depression, rapid mood changes, tension and anxiety and threats of violence. The percentage of relatives reporting personality change in their injured family member between years one and five rose from 60% to 74% while those reporting threats of violence increased from 15% to 54%. Actual violence against relatives had also risen (reported by 20% of relatives). Some relatives were afraid of their family member. Others expressed a high state of anxiety and attempted not to provoke aggressive outbursts (Brooks *et al.*, 1986). In regard to activities of daily living, at five-year follow up six patients out of the total sample of 42 (14%) were unable to wash and dress independently. Twenty-one percent of relatives reported that their family member needed someone to look after them at home and 43% (contrasting with the 18% at one year) reported that the patient could not be left in charge of the household. Oddy (1985) examined the social adjustment of severely brain injured patients seven years after injury as a follow up to an earlier study conducted two years after injury (Oddy *et al.*, 1978). The subjects for the study were drawn from a rehabilitation centre and all had PTA in excess of seven days. There were no changes in the patients' physical or cognitive status and personality problems were still commonly reported. The less disabled had continued to make progress in returning to their former level of vocational and social activity. Those patients who had been working at two years continued to do so at seven; four of these subjects had returned to their former occupations. A number of the employed had frequent job changes and in some their present position appeared precarious. None of those unemployed at two years were employed at seven years. Unfortunately those who could not work also had a dearth of other interests and leisure activities. Although reported by some, boredom seemed less of a problem than might have been expected, as many of the patients appeared content to lead relatively inactive lives. Social isolation, on the other hand, which was evident at two years continued and was severe among those who were unemployed. About half of those studied had only very limited contacts with friends, 60% had no girl or boyfriends. This was often seen by both patients and relatives as a major problem. In a number of cases, girlfriends who had maintained friendship with the patient during the first two years following injury subsequently curtailed contact.

Thomsen (1984) studied the late outcome of 40 patients 10–15 years after very severe closed brain injuries. None of the subjects had a PTA of less than one month and in 27 cases PTA exceeded three months. Although physical impairment, speech disorder and memory impairment remained severe in many cases, the psychosocial sequelae presented the most severe problems. Permanent changes in personality were reported in two-thirds of the patients and interestingly was reported with particular frequency in the youngest patients. The worst overall outcome was in patients with frontal or brain stem injury or both. Long-term improvement in functional status continued but 12 patients continued to have difficulty with self cares. Half the patients who could not be left alone at two-years follow up became independent during the following years. Four patients showed aggressive behaviour. The author also noted that impairment in daily living skills were most associated with personality and cognitive problems rather than physical incapacity. Thomsen (1984) also discusses differing reactions of spouses and parents to the subjects' disabilities, the former expressing very realistic appraisals of their loved one's problems while parents had more unrealistic views of the children's abilities.

Other factors

A range of factors influence the outcome of traumatic brain injury. The specific contribution of some factors is unknown and probably varies from individual to individual. They can be conceptualized under three headings: severity and type of injury, endowment (e.g. learning disorders, genetic components of intelligence, genetic risk for psychiatric disturbance) and environmental resources (e.g. socioeconomic status, life history and available social support). Factors relating to severity of injury, age and some aspects of endowment have been discussed in this chapter. The influences of environmental and personality resources are discussed in Chapter 2. Here it is important to note the dangers of treating traumatic brain injury as an isolated phenomena strictly within the medical model. At the extreme, the interaction of brain injury and environmental factors is demonstrated by the work of Lewis *et al.* 1986, 1988. They examined the neuropsychiatric, psychoeducational and family characteristics of juveniles condemned to death and of a general sample of death row inmates. The life histories of these individuals appeared to predispose them to psychiatric disturbance. For example, 12 of the 14 juveniles studied had been brutally physically abused and five had been sodomized by relatives. All of the subjects in the adult sample and most of the adolescents had significant cerebral trauma, often as a result of multiple injuries. History of brain trauma was confirmed by current neurological deficits (e.g. Babinski sign), skull indentation or hospital records in all but eight of the total group ($N=29$). In none of the cases had this information been brought to the attention of the court as a factor known to reduce the individual's ability to control his behaviour (Lewis *et al.*, 1986, 1988). This is noteworthy given that poor impulse control and disinhibition are widely recognized consequences of brain injury (Bach-y-Rita *et al.*, 1978; Spellacy, 1978). It should be noted that it is not possible to ascribe any specific cause to the subject's dysfunctional behaviour. Genetic abnormalities, developmental disorders and extremely abnormal parental behaviour as well as brain trauma are probable contributory factors (Bach-y-Rita *et al.*, 1978).

THE PSYCHIATRIC AND SOCIAL EFFECT OF BRAIN INJURY ON RELATIVES

Recently workers have examined the effect of severe brain injury on family members both as an indirect way of assessing the patient's level of functioning and as an important factor in itself. Livingstone *et al.* (1985a) interviewed female relatives of minor and severe brain injury victims. Relatives were seen at home three months after their family member's injury. The severe group consisted of patients with a PTA in excess of 48 hours and the mild group had PTA under one hour. The relatives of the severely injured patients suffered significant psychiatric morbidity compared to the relatives of the patients with minor brain injury. Relatives of the severely injured perceive themselves as suffering a much higher level of burden than relatives of the mildly injured. They also showed poorer functioning in social roles associated with the home. Evidence pointing to a difference in reaction between mothers and spouses is less clear but there is a suggestion that wives are more severely handicapped psychosocially compared to control wives than mothers compared to their controls.

In a further study the same authors (Livingstone *et al.*, 1985b) followed the social and psychiatric outcome of the same patients' relatives up to a year post injury. Relatives' social functioning estimated at 6 and 12 months was considerably worse than at three months. Marital functioning is particularly affected. Wives' perceived burden became most marked at six months and continued to 12 months, whereas mothers showed a modest decrease in perceived burden. However comparison of wives' and mothers' perceived burden at three, six and 12 months showed no statistically significant difference. Measures of relative's outcome were frequently associated with measures of patient outcome with the level of complaint voiced by the patient emerging as the single most predictive factor. The relatives of brain injured patients in this study were found to have significant psychiatric difficulty throughout the year following injury, with over 30% of relatives reporting levels of anxiety likely to have clinical significance.

One area which has received little attention is the psychological pressure on families of patients in prolonged coma. Stern *et al.* (1988) describe two families who reported suicidal thoughts

and who subsequently demonstrated marked anger or assaultive behaviour towards staff. In both cases the patients' were in
a persistent vegetative state and the authors present the parents'
difficulties in terms of a double bind. They are unable to give
up hope and continue with their own lives when the patients'
condition is essentially unchanged, even though their loved
one's prognosis is becoming increasingly poor. Hostility
directed towards the staff can be viewed as a partial resolution
by projection of these conflicts. The position of the staff may be
particularly vulnerable as the nature of the parents' projections
arouses self doubt in staff as to their own professional adequacy
(Stern *et al.*, 1988). This association of overt hostility with a
barely hidden conflict has been demonstrated by the family of
a patient treated by one of the authors where family members
insisted there was nothing wrong with their son, and that the
facility where he was being treated would be sued if they did
not cure him.

ADDITIONAL DIAGNOSTIC CATEGORIES DISCUSSED IN THIS
TEXT

Herpes simplex encephalitis (HSE)

Herpes simplex type 1 is the most common primary infective
cause of acute necrotizing encephalitis in temperate climates.
The virus has a destructive effect on temporal and frontal lobe
structures and may result in a range of behavioural abnormalities and cognitive deficits. The selective destruction of certain
structures has been explained by the proximity of those structures to the entry of the virus into the encephalon via the
olfactory pathways or the meningeal branches of the trigeminal
nerve. More recently, Damasio and Hoesen (1985) have argued
persuasively for a special affinity between the herpes simplex
type 1 virus and the limbic cortices. These structures have a
particular neurological structure less complex than that of the
neocortex. The destructive action of the virus follows the brain's
architecture very closely.

During the onset of acute viral encephalitis, the patient becomes pyrexial and may have headache, seizures and olfactory,
gustatory or auditory hallucinations. The patient's level of consciousness gradually deteriorates until they lapse into coma.

For a discussion of medical considerations at this stage, the reader is referred to Plum and Posner, 1980, pp. 263–267). Improved treatment of the condition has led to an increased survival rate. This has led inevitably to the wider presentation of the residual problems associated with the condition. The behavioural consequences of herpes simplex encephalitis have been likened to the Kluver-Bucy syndrome first described by Kluver and Bucy in 1937 as the result of bilateral temporal lobe lesions in monkeys (Kluver and Bucy, 1939). Descriptions of HSE survivors symptomatology includes impairments of intellectual function, most frequently of severe memory impairment, hyperorality, and behaviour disorders including sexual disinhibition and aggression (Greenwood *et al*. 1983). Remarkably little has been published on the rehabilitation of these patients. None the less our own group has demonstrated that intensive rehabilitation efforts can result in meaningful functional gains (Giles and Clark-Wilson, 1988a, 1988b; Giles and Morgan, 1989).

Other causes of acquired brain injury

Anoxic damage is most frequently the result of cardiorespiratory arrest but may also be caused by carbon monoxide poisoning, metabolic hypoglycaemia and asphyxiation from various causes, e.g. attempted suicide from hanging. Anoxic brain damage is frequently encountered by therapists, particularly those in tertiary care settings. While the most frequently encountered symptom complexes have been described, rehabilitation in general and the role of the occupational therapist in particular has been largely ignored. There does seem to be an association between duration of coma and functional outcome. Bates and co-workers (1977) in a multi-centre co-operative study followed 310 patients with non-traumatic coma for up to one year. Patients whose comas were believed to be secondary to sedative drugs or alcohol were excluded as almost all patients with coma of this origin make a full recovery with adequate supportive therapy. The most common cause of coma was diffuse hypoxia/ischaemia. The chance of regaining independence was greater in patients who, by one day, obeyed commands or moved limbs appropriately in response to noxious stimuli or who produced orienting eye movements, normal responses to oculocephalic or oculovestibular stimulation, or had normal muscle tone. Conversely, the chance of regaining any independent existence declined in patients who, after one day, had either extensor responses of the limbs, failed to move in response to noxious stimuli or who lacked the other positive indicators mentioned above.

SUMMARY

Brain injury is a significant cause of death and prolonged disability in the USA and Great Britain. The nature of the injury and its type and severity influence prognosis. Therapists should understand how different types of injury affect the type of symptom complex and influence outcome. Factors in the individuals' lives before injury may both predispose them to injury and complicate the recovery process and community reintegration. Alcohol abuse is one of the most significant of these factors but other social and personality factors may also be important. Many patients are only marginally independent in the community before injury, a fact which complicates their ability to establish a viable independent lifestyle after injury. Therapists cannot attempt to predict outcomes based on social variables. Social and personality factors can however assist our treatment and placement decisions.

Viral and anoxic causes of brain damage are reviewed briefly. These patients are frequently seen in rehabilitation departments but factors which affect their rehabilitation are rarely discussed. The symptom complexes are different but the principles of treatment are the same and are discussed throughout the text.

2

Theories of recovery following brain injury

Predicting the extent of recovery in an individual after brain injury is problematic due to the many variables involved. Therapists who work with patients in the acute care or acute rehabilitation settings may overvalue the role of therapy in promoting the patient's improvement. In the months immediately following medical rescue, natural recovery is undoubtedly the factor most responsible for the brain-injured patient's progress. None the less, we believe that there are good reasons for providing energetic treatment in the early stages of recovery. Whether preference should be given to any one of the competing techniques available to guide the therapists is open to question. In the later stages of recovery we advocate a specific model – the neurofunctional approach. This chapter will discuss theories of recovery, the likely effects of intervention and the theoretical rationale for the differing types of treatment (more concrete discussion of intervention strategies will be provided in the ensuing chapters).

NEURAL PLASTICITY UNDERLYING RECOVERY OF FUNCTION

Theories which ascribe recovery to changes in structure or function (reorganization) in the brain are theories of neural plasticity. These hypothesized changes can be divided into restitution and substitution. The term restitution implies changes in activity, or the regrowth of damaged neurones, whereas the term substitution implies reorganization of undamaged portions of the brain to subserve functions previously performed by damaged brain tissue.

Restitution

1. Diaschisis

Diaschisis is a hypothesized suspension of function as a reaction of surviving neurones to destruction of remote but related neurones (Monakow 1914). After an unspecified period neurones, the functioning of which has been depressed, recover their ability to function. Evidence for the existence of diaschisis (though not for its involvement in recovery of function) has come from studies of cerebellar blood flow in relation to space-occupying lesions on the contralateral side of the brain. This 'crossed cerebellar diaschisis' has been reported by Baron *et al.* (1980) and others (Fukuyama *et al.*, 1986; Pantano *et al.*, 1968) and is thought to be the result of damage to fibres descending from the cerebral cortex to the cerebellum. Damage at one site in the brain could have remote effects in many other areas though so far only crossed-cerebellar diaschisis has been convincingly demonstrated. Whether or not diaschisis has a significant role in recovery of function after brain injury remains a matter of debate (Finger and Stein, 1982). It has been argued that diaschisis should not be considered a form of plasticity since it was envisaged by Monakow as a depression of function which gradually resolves and which does not involve any 're-wiring' of the system (Teuber, 1975) or re-routing of neuronal transmission.

2. Denervation supersensitivity

The theory of denervation supersensitivity – which also may not be considered a true theory of plasticity – suggests that, when the number of dendrites impinging on an intact neurone is reduced, it becomes more sensitive to those which remain (Cannon and Rosenblueth, 1949). Denervation supersensitivity has received some experimental support (Glick and Greenstein, 1973), but the duration of the process is unclear. Denervation supersensitivity on its own cannot account for recovery of function since it presupposes sparing of some capacity in a given system and is therefore probably best considered in conjunction with redundancy theories discussed below.

3. Regeneration

Functional regeneration of severed axons in man occurs only in the peripheral nervous system (Schoenfeld and Hamilton, 1977). To be effective a viable axon would have to reconnect to its previous target cells or cells serving a similar function to those with which it was previously connected. There is little evidence that this type of re-connection occurs in the human CNS. However this is an area of considerable interest. If the conditions necessary for regeneration in the CNS were to become known, then it may be possible to produce them via pharmacological intervention (Laurence and Stein, 1978), see Chapter 15.

4. Collateral sprouting

Collateral sprouting (or reactive synaptogenesis) concerns non-lesioned neurones which, it is suggested, take over the site of a synaptic junction no longer occupied by a lesioned cell. Collateral sprouting may underlie some recovery of brain function but its effect is probably limited.

Substitution

In this section we discuss theories of sparing of function of compensation. Theories of substitution do not imply changes in the 'hard wiring' of the brain but may suggest that alternative brain systems are used.

1. Redundancy

The theory of redundancy suggests that there was, prior to injury, functional capacity in the brain which was surplus to requirement. Although theories of equipotential do not accord with our current knowledge, there are studies which indicate that recovery can be subserved by a very small percentage of surviving neurones if circumstances are favourable (Bach-y-Rita, 1980). Various cognitive and motor functions may have differing amounts of redundancy and it is clear that in some of these systems devastating results can be produced by very small lesions. Phylogenenetically newer functions may be subserved by smaller brain areas (Giles and Fussey, 1988).

2. Unmasking

Unmasking of hidden connections or neuronal system has been proposed as a possible mechanism of recovery of brain function. Unmasking has been defined by Bach-y-Rita (1980) as 'calling on anatomically established synapses when the usually dominant system fails'. Unfortunately the evidence for unmasking, which is clear in animals, has not indicated that it subserves recovery of function.

3. Neurological substitution

Neurological substitution is the theory most closely related to a rehabilitation strategy which could be deliberately pursued by occupational therapists – that of the neurological reorganization model. This theory suggests that brain systems can change function and that the brain can re-establish a lost function in an undamaged area of the brain. Miller (1985) has highlighted some of the difficulties involved in determining the possible role of neurological substitution in the recovery of function. For neurological substitution to be clearly responsible for recovery of function it would be necessary to demonstrate that: a part of the brain not previously involved in a function becomes involved; the part of the brain subserving the role now never had the role in the past; the function is not simply being performed by use of substitute strategies. These factors have not been adequately taken into account in most work claiming to demonstrate neurological substitution (Miller, 1985).

4. Behavioural compensation

Behavioural compensation is not a theory of neural plasticity but suggests that the individual, employing undamaged brain systems, adopts the use of strategies that were not used prior to injury. The use of this type of compensation has been demonstrated in both animals and man.

There is increasing evidence that changes in the CNS take place normally as a response to change in both the internal and external environment. Changes in dendritic arborization may be a normal process in man and may partially subserve new learning. Learning may also be subserved by changes in neurochemical activity within and between cells (Black *et al.*, 1988). As Laurence and Stein (1978) point out, these changes do not represent alterations in the rules of how the brain operates. While it is possible that there is a limited time during the recovery process during which rehabilitation may be effective (a 'window effect') and that this may occur during 'spontaneous' recovery, there is no direct evidence to support this notion (Teuber 1975). As we have pointed out elsewhere, the efficacy of available rehabilitation techniques in manipulating factors which are thought to underlie recovery techniques is severely limited (Giles and Fussey, 1988). Recovery of function probably does not depend on any individual factor. The full effects of retraining, the best time to intervene, the areas most responsive to intervention and so on will not be known until the mechanisms underlying recovery are more fully understood.

POSSIBLE ACUTE AND SEMI-ACUTE TREATMENT EFFECTS

Preventing complications

For the patient in an intensive care unit, a range of passive motion exercises, splinting (to prevent soft tissue contraction), serial casting and positioning are all designed to prevent complications affecting the subsequent recovery of the motor system. In addition, therapists may attempt to prevent the learning of poor motor patterns and the development of behaviour problems. It is difficult to demonstrate that particular interventions in the acute stage of recovery prevent complications in the later stages (although, for example, the basic scientific research on the reaction of skeletal muscle to prolonged shortening is persuasive).

The curve of recovery

Most individuals with brain injury get better. It is generally accepted from the analysis of group data that most patients recover rapidly early on and that this process gradually slows as time from injury increases (Bond, 1975; Brooks, 1972, 1975). This general view, however, requires considerable qualification. Evidence cited is from group data and does not establish that there is a 'Law of Recovery' to which each individual recovery conforms. It is unlikely that all subjects experience a similar recovery curve. The recovery curve does not remain uniform across the domains of cognitive function, behavioural control, and motor skills. For example, an individual may make rapid physical gains but remain amnesic. Memory function provides another example of non-linear progression, there being a more marked change around the time of the resolution of post-traumatic amnesia (PTA). Other individuals may make a rapid recovery in most areas but remain severely functionally compromised by inadequate behavioural control.

Early multi-national data comparing outcomes of treatment protocols used at different centres of excellence in neurological care revealed similar results (Jennett *et al.*, 1977). The lack of outcome variability was interpreted as supporting the view that there is a rigid and unmodifiable natural history of recovery. Bond (1975) examined the recovery of patients with severe brain injury by serial administration of the Wechsler Adult Intelligence Scale (WAIS). He found that return of function was rapid in the first six months following injury and slowed considerably after that time. Recovery was most rapid and slowed earliest in the less severely injured (PTA 3–6 weeks). In the more severely injured, recovery was still at its most rapid in the first six months but improvement continued until it reached maximum at 24 months. Recovery on the verbal components of the test occurred earlier than on the performance components. Performance components include the integration of multiple perceptual tasks and manual dexterity. Although these findings are important, their influence was probably too pervasive and the usefulness of the WAIS in this type of study has been challenged (Mackworth *et al.*, 1982). The WAIS and other intelligence tests are only poorly related to real-world function among the neurologically impaired. Furthermore, functions tapped by intelligence tests may be less susceptible to therapy than other types of behaviours. The effect of therapy is not addressed. It has been suggested that most complex mental functions take longer than six months to recover and this is linked to the protracted nature of recovery from memory impairments. The WAIS shows more rapid improvement because of the relatively light demands placed on memory by both the verbal and performance components of this battery (Mackworth *et al.*, 1982).

More recently there have been attempts to track a recovery curve in real functional skills. Panikoff (1983) describes the course of recovery of functional skills of 80 severely head injured adults. The 78 patients for whom duration of coma could be ascertained were divided into two groups depending on period in coma (i.e. coma of 14 days or less and coma of 15 days or more). All patients were rated in basic activities of daily living (feeding, grooming, bed mobility), wheelchair mobility, dressing, functional transfers, basic hand skills, community skills, kitchen skills and the Jebsen hand function test. Rating occurred at 2-, 4-, 6-, 12- and 24-month intervals. All of the subtests were itemized to give impairment ratings between zero and four. All the impairment ratings for the long coma group (LCG) were higher and more variable than for the short coma group (SCG). The SCG were less disabled initially and recovered more rapidly than the LCG. Improvement continued on the majority of sub-tests in both groups throughout the 24-month period. Improvement was considerably less marked in the 12–24 month period than in the 6 – 12 month period. While this study is a noteworthy first step in describing the return of functional skills, the results are likely to be distorted by the data collection methods. The percentage of individuals for whom data was actually available at any one time is rarely over 60%. So although it can be concluded from the data that groups of patients improved throughout the 24 month period it is not possible to state that any individual did so. This paper does not address treatment efficacy.

In some cognitive domains progress may cease early and in others continued improvement may be seen for years in the same individual. This variability in the shape of the recovery curve for each individual means that while it is reasonable to state that continued rapid recovery is expected, it is not possible, even with serial test administration to predict with a high degree of certainty the actual recovery slope. Also, as will be noted below, long term deterioration from the highest point achieved is common in some domains (e.g. behavioural control).

The shape of the recovery curve might also be affected by

age, previous brain injury, alcohol and drug abuse, or other neurological damage as well as the nature of the brain damage. The Santa Clara Valley Medical Center study (1982) examined the recovery curve after severe brain injury. Findings indicated that the process of recovery takes longer for those with more severe injuries. Patients with comas of 14 days or less had steeper recovery curves than those in coma for longer than 14 days. Some functions were shown to return faster than others, for example, physical recovery occurred faster than functions depending on memory. Complex sequential processes returned later than simple functions. There was also evidence that recovery during the first 12 months was linear and only began slowing after that period. Dikmen and co-workers (1987) examined the relationship of severity of brain injury and memory function, as measured by the Wechsler Memory Scale and the selective reminding task, at one month and one year post injury. The authors found, as might be expected, that the degree of impairment at both one month and one year was predicted by the severity of injury. Persistent memory impairment was associated with coma of more than one day and this association was more pronounced for those in a coma for seven days or more. Those who originally had the most severe deficits improved the most by one year but remained the most impaired.

D.W. (23 years old) was involved in a motorcycle accident when a motorist performed an illegal U-turn in front of him. D.W. was in a coma for three months and remained hospitalized in an acute hospital for two years. During this time he remained dependent in all basic self-care activities, except self-feeding. He had been non-weight bearing for so long that his lower legs and ankles had decalcified. Although he possessed an electric wheelchair, he was unable to use it in the community because he had not developed skills for mobilization. On admission to a transitional living centre he was provided with a programme of progressive weight bearing to promote lower extremity recalcification, gait training and an intensive programme of behaviourally oriented functional skills training covering personal, domestic and community skills. On discharge from the programme five months later, the patient was independent in indoor ambulation with a walker and was able to walk outside for short distances. He was independent in washing and dressing, light meal preparation and was shopping, going to restaurants and doing his own laundry. A suitably adapted home was purchased for him and he was able to achieve independence in community living though he continued to need help with long-term planning. D.W. redeveloped the majority of his independence in functional skills over 24 months post-injury. Independence in community living was achieved at 32 months. The course of improvement of D.W. shows that some patients demonstrate a non-standard slope of recovery.

Stimulation to maximize recovery

The most direct route to stimulating recovery might be via some pharmacological agent, but none have so far proved effective. Therapists have attempted to stimulate patients into accelerated recovery (Ylvisaker, 1985: Soderback and Normell, 1986a, 1986b). In the acute stage, coma stimulation is viewed as an essential component of treatment by many therapists. In later stages of acute recovery occupational therapists have attempted to stimulate patients by the use of tasks of graded difficulty. Hierarchies in various cognitive, behavioural and physical domains have been constructed and therapists attempt to 'move' patients through these. It has been suggested that the earlier patients can be exposed to this type of acute rehabilitation the greater the recovery (Cope and Hall, 1982). This type of intervention could have an effect both on the rapidity of improvement and on its overall extent. Alternatively, it could alter the slope of recovery but not the ultimate level of outcome. Of course it could also have neither effect. These possibilities are expressed graphically in Figure 2.1. Accelerated improvement – whether or not it has durable effects – could result in the patient leaving the hospital earlier and suffering fewer medical and psychological complications as a result. There would, of course, be considerable cost savings.

Animal models suggest that there is considerable effect of early physical intervention. Delayed motor rehabilitation in monkeys resulted in more rapid improvement later but their ultimate level of recovery, in comparison with the early

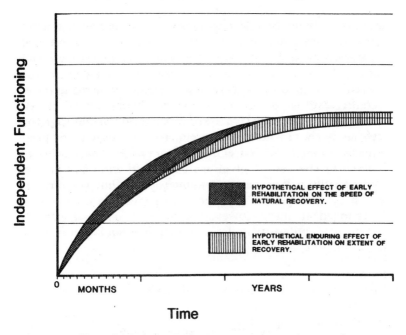

Figure 2.1 Hypothetical slope of recovery across patients and domains of impairment. The shaded area represents hypothetical effects of therapy.

'rehabilitation' group, was never achieved (Black *et al.*, 1975). There have been no results directly supporting a comparable effect for cognitive functions. Attempts to study the benefits of early intervention with controlled trials on human subjects (Cope and Hall, 1982) have been so complicated by methodological difficulties that results have been uninterpretable (Giles and Fussey, 1988).

Shaw *et al.* (1985) describe two patients who became disruptive in a nursing home setting and who were transferred to a rehabilitation centre. When given appropriate training, the improvement of these two patients was so rapid that it suggests that some stimulation is necessary to ensure that patients function at the level permitted by their neurological recovery.

There is no evidence that one specific form of interaction has a greater effect at this early stage on potentiating recovery than another. Patients may be discharged from treatment too early, at a point where their true abilities are not known. For example, both acute agitation and PTA are known to hamper learning (Levin *et al.*, 1988), and patients may be discharged as 'plateaued' who are only experiencing a temporary hiatus in recovery. In cases of profound injury, psychiatric disorders and adjustment issues may be masked by behavioural and cognitive deficits. In those who make a rapid recovery, psychiatric problems, depression, anxiety and significant relationship problems may occur after the stage of acute delirium and often emerge in the second half of the post-traumatic year. Only when recovery in the acute stage is slowing can patients begin to adjust to changed abilities. However, stress may occur as patients recognize that they can do less and that their families treat them differently (Lezak, 1987).

POST-ACUTE TREATMENT

Prevention of complications

Prevention of complications in the post-acute setting includes relapse prevention. There is increasing evidence that the traumatically brain injured often deteriorate (Brooks *et al.*, 1986). This deterioration is particularly marked in the area of behavioural control and in addition to this, the TBI population suffer increasing social isolation. We discuss factors which may be associated with relapse and preventative measures in Chapter 13.

Systems approaches to post-acute treatments

Though used in some centres as a continuation of early intervention, the general stimulation model is widely regarded as being less effective in the post-acute treatment of brain-injured patients and alternative methods have been developed. Cognitive rehabilitation therapists have attempted to devise methods to enable patients to practice specific cognitive skills. Others have developed unit-based approaches utilizing specific methodologies or rationales for therapy. These unit-based approaches are often predicated on the idea that a specific constellation of deficits is of special significance. Specialized units have addressed emotional disorders (Prigatano, 1986), behavioural disturbance (Eames and Wood, 1985a), social isolation (Ben-Yishay *et al.*, 1978) and work skills. Three basic rationales for post-acute treatment are identifiable in the literature.

The mental exercise model

The mental exercise model suggests that the practice of a mental faculty, such as memory, will lead to improved function. Some cognitive training techniques are based on the idea that a specific computer programme or technique can impact a cognitive faculty and that gradually increasing demands, coupled with the patient's gradually improving performance on the task, demonstrate cognitive gains translatable into real world function. While this approach has been widely used it has been unsupported by well designed studies (these issues are discussed further in Chapters 4 and 10).

Soderback and Normell (1986a) describe a method of rehabilitation of the brain injured which they call intellectual function training (IFT), the aim of which is to provide cognitive retraining. A set of training materials comprising 900 pages is divided into sections loosely based on the factorial studies of intelligence of Thurstone and Thurstone (1941) (visual perceptual ability, spatial ability, memory ability and logical ability). The material is used in an individualized daily one-hour session carried out over a period of 2 – 4 months. A training programme is designed for each client and the materials are used in order of difficulty (Soderback and Normell, 1986a). In a subsequent paper results of the training programme were evaluated (Soderback and Normell, 1986b). Significant differences were found between the non-randomly assigned treatment and control group. Unfortunately, the test materials for evaluation were very similar to the training materials. The authors point out that the patients' improvement appears to be on the same pencil and paper tasks that they had been practicing and that the ability of patients to transfer strategies learned on paper and pencil tasks to activities of practical significance for daily life was questionable. Soderback and Normell's approach provides an example of the practice of activities which involve the use of cognitive skills. It is not clear whether the practice is related to cognitive skills or to 'tasks', which are often poorly related to the patient's needs in the real world. The practice of a task which involves the cognitive faculty does not mean that the faculty is being developed.

The neurological reorganization model

The neurological reorganization model hypothesises that treatment may stimulate the rearrangement of mental processes so that performance on a task can be achieved through by-passing a damaged faculty. In this theoretical model, any behaviour can be disrupted by an injury which interrupts any part of its functional system. The chain can be broken by interrupting any link, therefore the role of rehabilitation is to mend the break in the chain at the point at which it has been broken. The theory further suggests that there may be multiple functional systems responsible for specific skills and an injury that interrupts only one functional system may not result in a functional deficit, since a substitute functional system could still produce the behaviour. Therefore, rehabilitation may teach the patient to use an alternative (intact) functional system (Powell, 1981).

Both the mental exercise model and the neurological reorganization model view real-world performance as based on a range of underlying component skills. For example, being able to arrive on time to a doctor's appointment involves remembering the appointment, planning and problem solving about how to get to the doctor's office, being able to initiate the behaviour in advance and so on. These views are unremarkable. Specialists in rehabilitation have, based upon these views, attempted to address fundamental cognitive skills on the grounds that improvement in these areas will result in improved functioning in all behaviours which rely on these skills. This set of concepts is represented schematically in Figure 2.2.

Unfortunately, the attempts to redress skill deficits such as memory as a basic cognitive function have been largely ineffective (Wood and Fussey, 1987; Fussey and Giles, 1988; Chapter 10). As a result of this orientation, less 'fundamental' skills have been largely ignored as a focus of therapy.

A SCHEMATIC REPRESENTATION OF LEVELS OF
THERAPEUTIC INTERVENTION

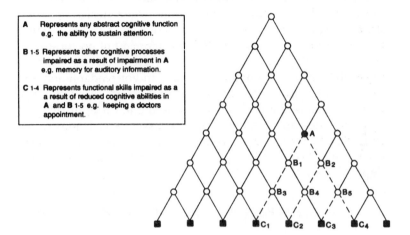

A   Represents any abstract cognitive function
     e.g. the ability to sustain attention.

B 1-5 Represents other cognitive processes
      impaired as a result of impairment in A
      e.g. memory for auditory information.

C 1-4 Represents functional skills impaired as a
      a result of reduced cognitive abilities in
      A and B 1-5 e.g. keeping a doctors
      appointment.

Figure 2.2 A hierarchical pyramid with functional skills at the bottom and cognitive skills higher up. Therapeutic intervention close to the apex represents an attempt to address a general skill (e.g. memory) with a concomitantly wide-ranging impact on function skills lower down. The lower in the pyramid the intervention, the more limited its hypothetical effect on functional skills.

The neurofunctional model

The last model to be discussed here (and that which is advocated in this book – see particularly Chapters 6,7,9 10, 11 and 12) is a neurofunctional approach based on training and experience in recovery of function. The model builds on some of the unit-based approaches described above, but it is not as limited in its application. It is influenced by these unit-based approaches, in that it stresses control of the patient's total learning environment. Unlike the unit-based models, it is not restricted to patients with one type of disorder or one level of severity in disturbance of function. Rather than the 'top down' models described above, it is a 'bottom up' model in which the aim and method of rehabilitation is the development of real functional skills. Central to the intervention is an understanding of the neuropsychiatric, neuropsychological and neurophysiological limits placed on the individuals by the brain trauma. Some of these may be addressed by neuropharmacological interventions but all need to be taken into account when designing intervention programmes. Training in concrete tasks and experience in real-world settings leads to the development of practical competencies. Following Anderson (1989) we prefer to describe these changes as learning, adjustment and/or readaptation and reserve the term recovery for spontaneous recovery. The manipulation of the environment is central to the approach and has been demonstrated to improve psychosocial adjustment (Prigatano, 1986) and produce adaptive behavioural change (Eames and Wood, 1985a). These issues are discussed in more depth in Chapters 11 and 12.

OTHER FACTORS AFFECTING RECOVERY

As discussed in Chapter one, a wide range of factors affect recovery from brain injury. Some of these less frequently considered can be usefully conceptualized as illness behaviour, learned helplessness and institutionalization.

Illness behaviour

In Chapter one we describe the increasing evidence that neurological damage underlies the symptoms which may be experienced following 'mild' brain injury. Seen within the medical model, an 'either or' approach has been adopted in which disease was either present or absent: the patient was either neurologically impaired or malingering. This 'either or' model may not be helpful in understanding the experience of patients after brain injury. The view that neurological disruption is involved in the production of a set of behaviours need not necessarily support a view which dismisses social, personality and environmental factors as irrelevant.

A model of illness behaviour can assist in the understanding of help-seeking behaviour (Mechanic 1986). It incorporates information on the interaction of neurological state, psychological processes, social and environmental factors. Unfortunately many rehabilitation specialists responded to the premature rejection of a neurological component in complaints following minor brain injury by flying to the opposite extreme and engaging in medical reductionism. Here all aberrant behaviour which follows a brain injury is ascribed to it. It should however be recognized that a change in behaviour attributable to one cause may later be maintained by other factors. This model applies to instances where illness occurs in the absence of injury, or in disproportion to the severity of the injury. Factors to be considered involve neurological factors (discussed in Chapter 1) and personal factors including data on current psychological state, level of distress, personality and coping style, expectations and attributions, and the interference the patients disabilities have on everyday life functioning. Consideration needs to be given to the patient's family relationships, social support and cultural background (see for example Gains, 1986) and other factors which could influence illness behaviour, including past illness experience, the accessibility of health care services, and the patient's ethnic background. Cognitive processes are central to illness behaviour and environmental events are selectively filtered depending on factors unique to the individual. Lazarus and Folkman (1984) have suggested that this process involves an assessment of the event in terms of threat and the individual's assessment of, and ability to use, coping strategies. These authors also point out that this is likely to be an ongoing dynamic process. The focus on cognitive appraisal allows a non-pejorative examination of the individual's phenomenology regarding an illness episode.

Kleinman (1980) introduced the concept of explanatory models as a useful framework to identify the meaning of a particular illness to the individual. The explanatory model of the patient, the patient's family and the treatment team may all vary. Explanatory models are often highly influenced by social and cultural values and this is particularly so in multi-cultural contexts such as Great Britain and the United States. It is important for all those involved in treating individuals from diverse cultural backgrounds to make the effort to understand these factors.

Environmental stressors are involved in an individual's response to illness (not simply their proneness to it). Environmental stressors might include specific life events, family factors (such as expressed emotion) and the degree of social support available. There is ample evidence to suggest that the amount of social support available to an individual has an important influence on reaction to illness. The mechanism by which social support has its effect however is unclear.

While the model of illness behaviour has been available for some time, it has not been applied to the brain-injured population generally. In fact, the difficulty in operationalizing the concept has contributed to its failure to be widely adopted as a model. In addition, medical personnel are reluctant to give up total control of treatment. Obviously, the nature and the depth of inquiry depends on the presenting complaints and whether there is a repetitive help-seeking behaviour, or apparently disproportionate distress or excessive complaint. When any of the factors are marked, more extensive inquiry into life circumstances is warranted. The only facilities where a true transdisciplinary team effort addresses this type of problem in the context of medical complaints are in specialized programmes such as some adolescent treatment programmes. Some attempts in this direction are currently being made in some rehabilitation units and Transitional Living Centres (TLC) for the brain injured.

Learned helplessness and institutionalization

Seligman (1975) introduced the concept of learned helplessness based on experiments relating to escape behaviour in animals. Seligman found that animals who were initally prevented from escaping from an aversive stimulus failed to attempt to escape later when they were able to do so. Individuals after brain injury may display a learned incapacity which may be treated by exposing them to repeated experience of success. Brain-injured patients may be particularly prone to developing an expectation that they will not make their own decisions and that care staff or family members will do things for them. This may be partly the result of inappropriate compensatory strategies and partly the response to the pressure of institutionalization. The brain-injured patient's particular proneness may be due to the extensive duration of recovery or as a result of the changes in the patient's cognitive ability, such as difficulties in learning new information and mental inflexibility.

THE ORGANIZATION OF REHABILITATION SERVICES

In many ways the organization of rehabilitation services dictates what services are provided. The progress from the medical model to the multidisciplinary, interdisciplinary and transdisciplinary team has followed the expansion of medical rehabilitation services to the point in the treatment continuum where the patient's medical stability is no longer the primary area of concern. The repeated attacks on the medical model mounted by workers with a psychosocial or educational perspective have failed because the medical model is extremely effective in addressing the needs of those in medical crisis. When the patient is severely medically ill, the overall management of the patient is most appropriately vested in a trained physician working with skilled nursing professionals. The important work of the therapist is adjunctive to the major task of keeping the patient alive.

The multidisciplinary team

The patient continues to require medical investigation procedures and nursing care. However, as the patient recovers and the need for life-saving medical care recedes, the physician and nursing staff are no longer able to meet the patient's complex needs. The physician typically retains overall charge of the patient's treatment. Multidisciplinary team meetings provide a focus for the exchange of information and for informing the physician of the patient's progress in what are not strictly medical domains. It may be possible to coordinate simple procedures such as transferring techniques and establish uniformity in simple behavioural interventions but the multidisciplinary team's ability to coordinate treatment is limited. Acute rehabilitation units, which frequently utilize the multidisciplinary team approach, may be staffed as distinct entities separate from other hospital departments or through their respective disciplinary departments. In the latter case, conflicting rehabilitation team and departmental demands may make a co-ordinated approach difficult to achieve.

There has been a tendency in recent years for services provided by the multidisciplinary team to become increasingly diversified with more professional disciplines represented making a coherent approach to the patient's difficulties harder to achieve. As time from injury increases the patient's need for intensive medical management recedes and learning considerations predominate. It is becoming more widely recognized that the interdisciplinary and transdisciplinary team approach is a more appropriate organization for professional intervention during this post-acute period.

The interdisciplinary/transdisciplinary team

In the post-acute stage of treatment, ongoing invasive medical procedures are no longer necessary. Rather than achieving medical stability, the task of rehabilitation is to assist the individual in eliminating maladaptive behaviours and to develop appropriate behaviours for community reintegration. The team leader is frequently not a physician but a clinician from a therapeutic discipline who has experience in working with the client population and as a programme manager. Team meetings determine goals for each client depending on the client's needs. Usually between two and four goals are selected with the active involvement of the client and the client's family. The treatment plan is designed taking into account learning principles. This team approach is described as interdisciplinary/transdisciplinary because only rarely does a client's goal fit wholly within the artificial domain of any therapeutic discipline. Instead, goals are overlapping and related to many disciplines. The primary task of an individual working in an interdiscplinary/transdisciplinary team context is to develop and carry out interventions depending on the client's needs and not the constraints of their individual disciplines. The concerns of the individual discipline are addressed but they are subordinated to the aims developed by the team.

Advantages of the interdisciplinary/transdisciplinary team

The transdisciplinary team allows for the overall co-ordination of goals. This type of intervention is essential for those who have difficulties in acquiring new information and stable patterns of behaviour. The interdisciplinary/transdisciplinary team approach allows a uniform approach to problem behaviours and interdisciplinary support. It prevents the fractionalization of services and may foster a truly functional approach to patient's problems. It is likely to be the most appropriate structure for a rehabilitation service for the post-acute treatment of individuals with severe brain injury. Post-acute patients treated in a multidisciplinary team environment are likely to be described as not being able to 'make use of treatment' meaning that their slope of spontaneous recovery has reached asymptote.

Disadvantages of the interdisciplinary/transdisciplinary team

Stepping out of role may be stressful for therapists trained in a multidisciplinary team. The approach requires a relatively high percentage of meeting time and not only must treatments be planned and coordinated, it is often necessary for the staff to practice an intervention so that it becomes automatic. Another limitation of the interdisciplinary/transdisciplinary team is the number of clients who can be treated at any one time. In a multidisciplinary team, when there are more clients than can be reasonably treated by a given number of staff, it is possible to simply add more staff. Unfortunately, this does not work in the interdisciplinary/transdisciplinary team. The major limitation is around the number of treatment programmes the therapists can learn and apply consistently. When there are 12 clients and each client has three programmes, therapists have to be able to carry out 36 programmes with efficiency. When there are 20 clients, 60 programmes have to be remembered (in our view a next to impossible task). Unfortunately, this limitation cannot be solved by splitting into teams in the same facility as clients will frequently target staff who are not on their team. There is now a general consensus that the ideal number of patients to be served by a single interdisciplinary/transdisciplinary team is 12–15.

For all the difficulties of the interdisciplinary/transdisciplinary team, we consider it the most effective team organization to serve those with severe brain injury in the post-acute period.

SUMMARY

In this chapter models of recovery of function have been examined. The mechanisms of recovery following brain trauma are poorly understood, but the more that is appreciated about how recovery takes place the greater the ability to intervene to maximize it. The course of recovery is usually described as a slope or curve. However the analysis of recovery across patients may obscure more idiosyncratic individuals' recovery patterns. The duration of recovery has been described and the idea that most recovery occurs in the first 12 months following injury needs to be qualified, as this figure was decided by looking at group neuropsychological data. Other factors may be more indicative of recovery as the early recovery projection looked at factors which are not usually considered targets of therapy (e.g. IQ). A case vignette of a patient whose primary period of functional return occurred during intensive treatment at a transitional living facility 24 months and more post injury has been reported. Finally, severity of injury should be considered when attempting to project a time course of recovery.

In discussing models of intervention, treatment periods were divided into acute, semi-acute and post-acute. Models of treatment appropriate in early treatment may not be relevant in later stages of rehabilitation. A range of possible models was discussed. Following a topic first discussed in Chapter one, personality and other cognitive factors which can affect recovery, were looked at. The application of the model of illness behaviour was used as a possible method of understanding patients whose symptom severity is inconsistent with their neurological impairment. Finally in this chapter the organization of rehabilitation services was discussed. This is an important patient care issue because the structure of a rehabilitation service dictates what it can and cannot do. In conclusion, a multidisciplinary team could be considered most appropriate for the acute care setting whereas an interdisciplinary/transdisciplinary team is more suitable for the post-acute training stage of treatment. Both organizational systems have their costs as well as benefits. In Chapters 3,4, and 5 changes in function following traumatic brain injury will be examined.

3

Physical changes following brain injury

INTRODUCTION

The type of damage to the neurophysiological and/or musculo-skeletal systems influence the most appropriate type of rehabilitation, and the patient's potential for recovery. This chapter briefly describes the sensory and motor systems, and provides an overview of the effects of damage to them.

The central and peripheral nervous systems are involved in sensation and motor behaviour. Some areas of the brain and spinal cord are primary centres for sensation and movement, whilst other areas influence the quality of input and output. After brain injury, localized damage results in specific types of sensory and motor deficits. These are discussed below in relation to Figure 3.1.

THE BRAIN, SPINAL CORD AND PERIPHERAL NERVOUS SYSTEM

Sensory

Specialized sensory receptors respond to specific sensory stimuli or are polymodal, responding to more than one type of stimulus. Superficial sensation arising from the skin receptors has four primary components, touch, pain, temperature and chemosensitivity. Subcutaneous structures are concerned with deep pain, pressure and proprioception enabling the recognition of joint movements and the position of body parts relative to one another. Sensory fibres in the muscles' spindles and tendons respond to stretch.

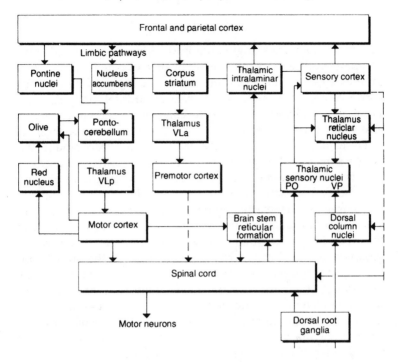

Figure 3.1 Schematic of the sensory–motor system (Laws, 1989).

Afferent impulses carried in sensory nerve fibres convey impulses directly or indirectly to motor neurones forming a reflex arc. This enables a protective withdrawal reflex action in response to pain and temperature in the ascending sensory system. Stimulation of the receptors causes impulses to pass along the first sensory neurone to the dorsal root ganglion and the spinal cord. This neurone synapses. The secondary neurone continues, crossing the midline at this level or one or two segments highers, and passing upwards to the thalamus as the spinothalamic tract. Discriminative and proprioceptive information passes up the dorsal columns and dorsal spinocerebellar tracts. Information ascending in the spinoreticular tracts may influence level of consciousness. Damage to the sensory receptors or tracts leading to the spinal cord, thalamus and sensory cortex impairs the appreciation of temperature, pain, touch and proprioception (see Sensory Disturbances below).

Motor

The motor neurones originating in the spinal cord are the final common pathway in the execution of movement. Motor programmes can be initiated from brain or peripheral inputs. The cortex co-ordinates information from the frontal, occipital, temporal, parietal lobes as well as the cerebellum and basal ganglia, and sends this via the cortico-spinal and cortico-reticular spinal tracts to the spinal cord and effector organs. Movement parameters include the speed and tonal quality of movement.

Tone can be defined as the tension between the origin and the insertion of each muscle and is determined by the combined influences of the elastic properties of connective tissue and tendons of the muscles, the properties of the muscle fibre and the degree of motor unit activity in the muscle. Tone can be modified by the interneurones at the level of the spinal cord via peripheral inputs, for example, temperature, touch, as well as through the influence of higher centres. Performance of movement feeds back information which reinforces those movements, and leads to the development of motor sets. This also means that the performance of abnormal movement increases the learning of further abnormal movements.

The brain

Precentral gyrus

The precentral gyrus responds to information from all sources and allows the execution of voluntary movements and spino-cortico-spinal reflexes.

Premotor cortex

The premotor cortex is responsible for forming the idea of the motor activity before action occurs.

Reticular formation

The main spinoreticular pathways travel through the upper aspect of the reticular formation in the brainstem. This area is concerned with arousal and the activation of movement.

Thalamus and post-central gyrus

Sensory neurones maintaining their functional specificity travel from the spinal cord to the thalamus and finally to the sensory cortex (the post-central gyrus). The thalamus links subcortical motor areas with cortical premotor and motor cortex, as well as projecting areas concerned with perception, the organization of behaviour, memory and mood. The thalamus processes the basic forms of sensory input, however recognition of type and discrimination of the intensity of stimulation occur only at the cortical level.

Basal ganglia

The basal ganglia form a complex neuronal network of subcortical nuclei in the forebrain and midbrain, which have cortical connections. The basal ganglia influence the initiation and modification of motor activity. There are several well-defined areas of the basal ganglia, which include the caudate nucleus, the lentiform nucleus (comprising of the globus pallidus and putamen), the substantia nigra and the subthalamic nucleus. The basal ganglia and, particularly, the substantia nigra are implicated in the initiation and termination of movement.

Cerebellum

The cerebellum has extensive central and peripheral connections: the muscle spindles, tendons, the skin, the vestibular nuclei and the cerebral cortex. The cerebellar cortex sends information, via the cerebellar nuclei, to the thalamus, reticular formation, red nucleus and vestibular nuclei. Cerebellar influence continues downwards to motor cells in the anterior horns of the spinal cord. The cerebellum is involved in learning skilled movements and also integrates details about body posture, limb position, and motor intentions. It is thus a co-ordinating centre controlling the synergistic action of muscles during voluntary and automatic movements, including postural adjustments. The cerebellum is involved in the timing and degree of contractions or relaxations or muscles especially when a movement involves more than one part of a limb.

Frontal lobe

The frontal lobe organizes and influences motor activity, through regulating information from the basal ganglia to the premotor cortex and motor cortex. The frontal lobe is concerned with expectation of participation in a motor action, and involved in the initiation and termination of movement, motor planning, and the sequencing of motor activity. There is some evidence, described elsewhere in this text, that brain-injured individuals have anticipatory behaviour deficits – probably related to impaired frontal lobe function (Freedman *et al.*, 1987).

Parietal lobe

Information from the thalamus is relayed to the parietal cortex via the sensory cortex. The parietal cortex is involved in the conscious awareness, expectation and perception of sensory information. The hemispheres may control different aspects of movement preferentially. The left hemisphere specializes in symbolic or sequential detail, whereas the right hemisphere is more concerned with visuo-spatial interpretations.

Occipital lobe

The occipital lobe deals with visual perceptions, and translating information received visually into specific movement parameters.

Temporal lobe

The temporal lobe is involved with memory, experience and perceived ability. This information is used when setting the parameters of motor activity.

Limbic system

Emotion influences movement via limbic system connections. The frontal, parietal and temporal lobes are affected by the information from the limbic structures and other areas, such as the raphe nuclei, lateral septal nucleus and nucleus accumbens. This system influences action and inhibits ineffective behaviours. The lateral septal nucleus is concerned if the motor system is not fulfilling the required expectations and then inhibits the unsuccessful strategies. Nucleus accumbens integrates information from the limbic system concerning success or failure of goal-directed movements and modulates transmission through the globus pallidus.

MOTOR DISTURBANCES

Damage at any point in the system may result in motor deficits, such as increased reflex activity, release of inhibitory control, abnormalities of tone, incoordination, lack of initiation or termination of movement, and impairments in planning and organizing motor output. Brink *et al.*, (1980) investigated the occurrence of motor deficits in 344 patients under the age of 18 years, one year following trauma. Ten percent of those tested did not demonstrate motor impairment, but the remainder had residual motor deficits which included spasticity (38%), ataxia (39%), soft signs (3%), spinal cord injury (1%) and peripheral nerve injury (1%).

Reflex activity

Some simple motor functions are performed economically by means of reflexes. The short chain of neurones which subserve a reflex is called a reflex arc. These neurones connect a sensory receptor to an effector organ, such as muscle or gland, so that an appropriate stimulus invariably leads to a specific response. There are two main categories of reflexes: postural and protective. The postural reflexes are responses to muscle strength and vestibular stimulation, whereas protective reflexes are responses to pain and temperature. Supraspinal facilitatory and inhibitory influences from the frontal lobes and cerebellum can be developed to abolish the reflexes. In the unimpaired nervous system many early reflex behaviours are increasingly modified (inhibited) during the course of development. After brain injury, reflexes which belong to an earlier developmental period may be released and may interfere with motor functioning. Some of these are described below:

Positive supporting reaction

The positive supporting reaction is demonstrated when stimulation is given to the sole of the feet of some brain-injured persons. They display an extensor thrust with plantar flexion and inversion of the ankle, extension at the knees and extension, adduction and internal rotation of the hips.

Crossed extensor response

This pattern is similar to the positive supporting reaction, but only occurs when one limb is flexed, causing an extensor thrust in the opposite limb.

Tonic neck reflexes

The asymmetrical tonic reflex is observed when rotation of the head to one side causes extension of the upper and lower extremities on the same side, and flexion occurs in the contralateral limbs. The symmetrical tonic neck reflex may be present if backward tilting of the head causes increased extensor tone in both upper limbs and diminishes the extensor tone of the lower limbs. Forward tilting of the head produces the opposite effect.

Grasp reflex

On placement of objects within the affected hand, a grasp is elicited and spontaneous release is difficult or impossible.

T.M. injured in a traffic accident (coma duration 6 weeks), had a hemiparesis on his right side, slight ataxia and severe dysphasic deficits. On walking downstairs he needed to hold onto a rail for stabilization due to his ataxia. He could not release his right hand from the bannister without using his unaffected hand.

Startle reflex

The startle reflex occurs as a response to loud noise or fast alterations of body position. The upper limbs flex, and the head and lower limbs extend.

Rooting reflex

The rooting reflex is elicited with tactile stimulation to the face, and results in a response of the mouth opening towards the stimulus.

E.I. has a very severe brain injury (coma duration unknown) after an assault, subsequent respiratory arrest and anoxic damage. This resulted in him having a limited awareness of his surroundings, little recognition of others and no communication. He exhibited a rooting reflex on presentation of food, and on basic hygiene activities, like shaving and cleaning teeth.

Equilibrium and balance reactions

People respond to changes in equilibrium by using their arms in protective extension, stepping reactions and alterations of movements of the upper and lower limbs and trunk in order to adjust the overall position of their centre of gravity. Equilibrium and balance reactions can be assessed when a person stands upright with feet together, first with eyes open and then with eyes closed. They should be able to stand steadily without losing balance or widening their base of support.

Associated reactions

Associated reactions occur if effort expended into a particular motor activity causes another part of the body to respond to the stimulus. Effort to move the affected limb may increase activity in the nonaffected limb, or alternatively any bodily movement may increase tone in the affected limbs.

Abnormalities of tone

Spasticity

Spasticity is a pathological increase in striated muscle tone, due to excessive motor unit activity. This increased motor unit activity is considered to be an increase in the stretch reflex due to loss of presynaptic inhibitory mechanisms in the spinal cord

(Musa, 1986; Burke, 1980) and as a result of plastic reorganization of spinal cord reflexes which occurs following CNS
damage (Lance, 1980). Presynaptic inhibition is normally
exerted by higher brain centres and augmented by input from
the periphery, particularly from the proximal limb regions. This
view has been supported by evidence of supra-segmental presynaptic inhibition through the movement of proximal limb
joints (Grillner and Rossignol, 1978). Musa (1986) has proposed
that following brain damage, peripheral input may be able to
replace the input from higher centres, thus 'switching on' presynaptic mechanisms.

In spasticity, increased muscular resistance is felt both in
passive and active movement of the limbs. Gross movement
patterns are present because of hyperactivity of one group of
muscles in comparison with another. The prime movers are
unable to relax after voluntary movements (Sahrmann and
Norton, 1977). Clonus, a series of rhythmical contractions of the
muscle, may follow a rapidly applied and maintained stretch.
Finally, environmental factors, for example, temperature, emotion and positioning, influence the degree of abnormal tone.

Flaccidity

Flaccidity is the result of damage to the peripheral nerves, the
spinal cord, or the brain. In extreme cases active movement or
stabilization of affected limbs is difficult or impossible.

Ataxia

Ataxia may result from reduced proprioceptive input or damage
to the cerebellum. Loss of proprioception causes sensory ataxia
because of unawareness of position of the limbs during movement, and a resultant inability to control movements. Sensory
ataxia is more marked when the eyes are closed, because vision
can partially compensate for loss of proprioception.

Ataxia of cerebellar origin can manifest itself in several ways.
Muscles show diminished resistance to passive movements. If
a limb is suddenly displaced, it oscillates before resuming its
posture. Movements are, therefore, not accurately directed
towards their target. For example, in attempting to touch an
object an individual with cerebellar ataxia may fall short of or

overshoot the target. Actions involving more than one joint are often broken down into their component parts, which lead to jerky puppet-like movements. The combination of these two abnormal movement patterns can result in faulty corrections of already badly directed movements.

Tremor

Involuntary movements resulting from alternating contractions of opposing muscle groups are called tremor. Martinelli (1986) has classified the types of tremor into three groups: resting, kinetic and postural tremor. A resting tremor, commonly seen in Parkinson's Disease, usually diminishes with action. Tremor, as a result of cerebellar damage, consists of discontinuous muscular contractions, which cause jerky movements. Rhythmical contraction of the proximal muscles may increase the direction of the oscillations in distal parts, and in voluntary movement tremor is more pronounced at the termination of movement. Postural tremor is an oscillation of proximal muscles and is frequently observed in those with severe kinetic tremor. A fine postural or intention tremor may develop as a side-effect of medication.

Athetosis

Athetosis is characterized by slow, snakelike, writhing movements. Choreoathetosis involves rapid, explosive twisting movements, usually of the hands and fingers, but sometimes affecting the arms and legs. When the chorea is unusually violent and flinging in nature, it is called hemiballismus. Cases of paroxysmal choreoathetosis have been reported following traumatic brain injury and attacks described consist of repeated jerking or writhing movements. These can be precipitated by a variety of factors, including movement of a limb or certain joints, or emotional stress. In some cases, these attacks can be aborted or ameliorated by grasping or squeezing the involved limbs or by an effort of will. Most of the cases reported in the literature have responded to some form of anti-seizure medication (Drake *et al.*, 1986).

Dystonia

In dystonia, specific muscle groups, commonly the head, neck and trunk or limbs, become hypertonic. An asymmetry of involuntary, contracting muscles result in unusual contortions of the body, and make movements slow and laboured.

Other problems influencing movement

Weakness

A significant period of coma or the fixation of a limb due to musculoskeletal injury may result in atrophy and weakness of muscles. Weakness could also contribute to the effects of disturbances of tone (although this is difficult to demonstrate).

Rigidity

A marked resistance to movement, which can be associated with hypertonus but is unrelated to speed or direction of movement.

Intiation of movement

An inability to initiate movement may occur for a variety of reasons. Akinesia is an inability to move an affected part of the body. Arousal difficulties due to damage in the reticular nuclei, may cause difficulty in initiating activity and also reduce motor behaviour. Apraxia (Chapter 4) may permit automatic movements, but greatly limit the performance of complex goal-directed movement.

Termination of movement

Damage to the frontal lobes can result in stereotyped movements or motor perseveration. The patient repeats the movement and is unable to inhibit the activity despite its functional irrelevance.

After suffering bilateral frontal aneurysms M.C. was unable to inhibit her motor behaviour. For example, she continued peeling a potato until nothing remained. When she wrote she was unable to inhibit the action, and covered the paper in increasingly incomprehensible scribbles.

Akathisia

Akathisia refers to a compulsion to move most frequently seen as a result of anti-psychotic medication. It is associated with, but distinct from, tardive dyskinesia. Akasthesia may be associated with subjective feelings of fear or rage, and is frequently encounted as monotonous pacing behaviour, shifting weight from foot to foot and walking on the spot (Gibb and Lee, 1986).

SENSORY DISTURBANCES

Tactile sensations

Somatosensory and kinaesthetic deficits limit motor relearning and can hinder functional independence. Somatosensory and proprioceptive disturbances may result from damage to sensory nerve-endings, the spinal cord, thalamus, parietal cortex or the cerebellum. These losses affect deep or superficial sensations such as temperature, touch and pain. Pain provides a warning of possible damage to body tissue. After brain injury, altered reactions to pain may be exhibited as an increased or reduced sensitivity. Thalamic pain syndrome is an uncommon sequelae of traumatic brain injury but causes severe and intractable pain, unlikely to be relieved by drugs. Damage which reduces sensitivity to pain is commonly associated with a lack of ability to feel pressure or superficial sensations of the skin. The ability to localize touch may also be impaired. These sensory losses contribute to abnormal motor control and often results in a disuse of the involved limbs. The initiation of movement becomes slower and actions appear clumsy, less precise and inaccurate.

Proprioception

Proprioceptive sense subserves awareness of body movement and position in space. Kinaesthesia is the conscious perception of joint position. Tension and stretch of muscles are constantly monitored and changed to accommodate voluntary and involuntary movement.

CRANIAL NERVE INJURIES AND SPECIAL SENSES. FACE NERVE INJURIES

Sensory or motor deficits of the face occur after damage to cranial nerves. Damage to the trigeminal nerve (fifth cranial nerve) or facial nerve may occur following traumatic brain injury, usually unilaterally. The facial nerve (seventh cranial nerve) may be affected by fracture of the petrous bone. Both delayed and immediate facial palsy after head injury have a relatively good prognosis (Cartlidge and Shaw, 1981). Impairment causes problems in lip closure and, consequently, presents both physical discomfort and emotional distress. Resulting inability to close the eyelid may result in corneal damage and exposes the eye to risk of infection.

Vision

Sensory information from the retinae travel to the optic nerve (second cranial nerve) and on to the optic chiasma. Fibres from the temporal half of the retina continue on the lateral aspect of the chiasma into the optic tract and the remainder from the nasal halves of the retinae descussate. The optic tracts continue to the lateral geniculate bodies and impulses are relayed along the optic radiation to the occipital cortex. The uppermost fibres (from the superior quadrants of each retina) pass through the parietal lobe, whereas the lowermost fibres travel round the temporal horn of the lateral ventricle in the temporal lobe before passing to the occipital cortex.

Visual defects immediately after brain injury often resolve within the first few days; however, if vision has not returned within the first weeks after injury the prognosis is poor (Cartlidge and Shaw, 1981). Lesions in the optic nerve, frequently damaged by blows to the frontal region, produce a total loss of vision in the affected eye, whereas those in the optic chiasma are rarely symmetrical, causing unequal involvement of both visual fields. Injuries to the optic chiasma are rare however as the type of injury necessary to produce them is very severe and the patient usually dies. Damage in the optic tract results in hononymous hemianopia, the lost half of the field of vision of each eye being opposite to the side affected. Deficits resulting from damage to the optic radiation depends on the exact site of injury. A temporal lobe lesion produces a homonymous defect involving the upper quadrants of the visual fields, and damage of the anterior part of the parietal lobe causes a homonymous hemianopia affecting the lower quadrants. A lesion at the posterior part of the parietal lobe or the occipital lobe give rise to a total homonymous hemianopia.

Disorders of eye movement caused by central damage are extremely rare (Cartlidge and Shaw, 1981). Visual disturbances often occur as a result of cranial nerve damage, where lesions are most commonly partial and do not result in complete paralysis. The most frequent consequence of damage to one of these nerves is double vision due to a failure of convergence in all or part of the visual field. Damage to the oculomotor nerve (third cranial nerve) may be the result of penetrating injuries to the skull and is often associated with temporal lobe herniation. Manifestations of injury to the oculomotor nerve depend on the location and severity of damage. Pupillary reactivity to light may be disturbed, and ptosis, diplopia, external deviation of the eye and defective ocular movements could be present. The trochlear nerve (fourth cranial nerve) innervates only the superior oblique muscle, which abducts intorts and depresses the eye. Slight weakness may be experienced in downward gaze and marked difficulty may be experienced in looking down with the eye adducted. To compensate, the patient may tilt the head downward and to the opposite side to achieve normal binocular vision. An injury to the abducens nerve (sixth cranial nerve) causes diplopia, because of the inability to abduct the eye. Both the third and sixth nerves may also be injured indirectly by disorders which raise intracranial pressure or displace the brain stem.

Nystagmus is a series of involuntary, rhythmical oscillations of one or both eyes, which may occur in horizontal or vertical planes of movements or as rotations of the eye. These oscillations may be equal in speed and amplitude in both directions of movement, or movement in one direction may be faster than in the other.

The incidence of the various types of visual impairments following traumatic brain injury are not known. Canavan *et al.*,

(1980) found that sports injuries in men were the most common cause of ocular injuries, followed by road traffic accidents. In females, road traffic accidents were the most frequent cause, and in both sexes they caused the most serious injuries (Karlson, 1982). Johnston and Armstrong (1986) showed a 60% reduction in ocular injuries after the introduction of a seat-belt law in Northern Ireland.

Gianutsos *et al.* (1988) have described the need for optometric services for survivors of acquired brain injury. In a series of 55 patients treated at a post-acute rehabilitation site, 26 were referred to a rehabilitation optometrist, and all but two of these were reported to having been treated with benefit. The most frequent recommendations were occlusion, prisms, and different spectacles for short or long-sightedness. Less frequently recommended were devices such as hand-held magnifying glasses, training or suggested management techniques. Interventions were readily instituted by therapy staff.

Hearing

Hearing impairment, resulting from vestibulocochlear (eighth cranial nerve) damage, occurs frequently following severe brain trauma as the nerve is frequently torn or stretched after skull fractures. Transverse fractures usually involve a sensorineuronal hearing loss with possible existence of central auditory dysfunction (Sakai and Mateer, 1984). The auditory nerve has two components, the cochlear nerve concerned with hearing and the vestibular nerve for appreciation of the position of the head and movement in space. Total and partial hearing loss occur in 6–8% of the severely brain-injured and there is no evidence to show that hearing loss is associated with vertigo. Tinnitus is a particularly disturbing symptom which may follow even mild injury.

Smell

The olfactory nerve fibres (first cranial nerve) ascend through the cribiform plate in the uppermost part of the nasal cavity. The first cranial nerve is high susceptible to shearing against the cribiform plate as a result of lateral oscillation of the brain. Post-traumatic anosmia, therefore, is usually associated with contusion or damage to the frontal cortex (Jennett and Teasdale, 1981). Anosmia occurs in 3–10% of those with severe head injury (Cartlidge and Shaw, 1981) and can be a result of bilateral damage. Parosmia, an alteration in the sense of smell, involves recognition of the presence of odours and sometimes correctly identifying them, but the sensation is felt to be changed. Anosmia may be associated with poor outcome due to its association with severe injury and frontal lobe damage. Varney (1988) described 40 patients who developed total anosmia as a result of closed head injury. Virtually all had major vocational problems during the two or more years after being medically cleared to return to work.

Taste

Taste is mediated by receptors in the taste buds. Axons from these receptors pass in both the glossopharyngeal (ninth cranial nerve) and facial nerves to the thalamus. Impairments in the sense of taste (ageusia) are more rare than alteration in the sense of smell.

Speech

Motor disorders are equally likely to affect speech as any other parts of the body. Precise enunciation of words and the co-ordination of lips, tongue and palate requires normal muscle tone and brain damage may cause difficulties in articulation and phonation. Dysarthria is the imperfect articulation of speech, where speech becomes irregular, slurred, distorted and explosive as the volume of sound is poorly controlled. Dysphonia is the reduced volume of speech which results from disturbances of phonation, such as the weakness of respiratory movements and reduced air flow across the vocal cords or to malfunction of the vocal cords.

SUMMARY

In this chapter we have discussed the sensory and neuromuscular changes which may follow brain injury. We have briefly reviewed the functions of brain areas as they relate to the sensory and motor system. These deficits are described in isolation and detached from the individual in whom they are present, whereas in reality, individuals display a complicated interaction of sensory and motor disorders. Some disorders of motor skills are easy to recognize but others, particularly when they occur together, may be masked and lead to erroneous attributions of non-cooperation. Damage to the cranial nerves is frequently overlooked as a cause of disability. Patients with crush injuries and those with fractures to the bones of the skull are particularly at risk. In the next chapter we discuss the psychological consequences of brain injury.

4

Psychological consequences of brain injury

INTRODUCTION

The most complex human functions – which are the most difficult to quantify – are also the most vulnerable to trauma. As
the severity of injury increases, so does the likelihood that
basic functional activities will also be disrupted. In addition,
psychological disorders hamper the individual's ability to
develop methods to compensate for functional, vocational and
interpersonal skills deficits. Central to the individual's problems
is the inability to adapt to novel circumstances. The brain-
injured individual may be unable to determine what is inter-
fering with his functioning and as a result be unable to change
his behaviour to improve performance. This chapter describes
some of the psychological deficits which may affect individuals
after brain injury. An attempt is made to relate the more abstract
description of deficits to the patient's actual difficulties in functional activities. This chapter discusses the psychological sequelae of brain injury under the headings of arousal and attention,
perception, memory and information processing, language and
problem solving. Although these functions are described separately, it should be remembered that the human brain is an
integrated unit and division by cognitive function is only on a
conceptual level (Stuss and Benson, 1987). Chapter 6 considers
how the therapist determines retraining priorities based on how
the individual's deficits impact his real-life functioning. Chapter
10 discusses functional retraining for the individual with
psychological deficits.

AROUSAL AND ATTENTION

Multiple brain regions subserve attention. The reticular formation subserves arousal, frontal and limbic regions subserve the drive and affective components of attention and the sensory system provides the raw material to be processed.

Many definitions of attention have been formulated but no single definition has been uniformly accepted (Stuss and Benson, 1986). A preferred definition describes attention as a state of alertness or arousal which allows an individual to recognize information as present and focus on it (Wood, 1987). The ability to attend is influenced by many variables such as fatigue, mood and the time of day in the unimpaired nervous system. (Watts *et al.*, 1983) and these factors influence performance in everyday tasks.

Models of attention

Many models of attention have been proposed, the most popular being information processing models (Broadbent, 1958). Researchers have examined the number of items which can be attended to at any one time, the amount of information that can be learned, speed of processing, attention span and what happens when information is presented too rapidly or otherwise exceeds the individual's capacity to process it.

Broadbent's single-channel theory of selective attention proposes that the brain processes serially (one piece of information at a time). Lewis (1970) criticized this view and demonstrated that processing may occur in different modalities simultaneously. Evidence supporting parallel processing led to the multi-processor theory of attention (Allport *et al.*, 1972) Allport and co-workers (1972) suggest that the attentional demands of one sensory input do not prevent processing in other channels, but could block processing in the same sensory system. Kahneman's model (1973) summarizes many of the features of attention discussed above.

1. Some activities require more effort than others.
2. Factors such as arousal influence the total amount of processing capacity available.
3. Several activities can be carried out at the same time provided the total effort does not exceed the available capacity.

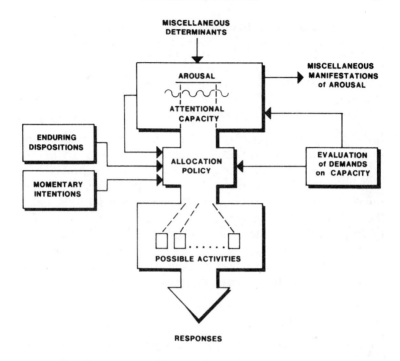

Figure 4.1 Kahneman's capacity model of attention. From *Attention and Effort* by D. Kahneman. Copyright © 1973 by Prentice Hall. Reprinted by permission.

4. There are rules or strategies by which resources are allocated to various activities, and the various stages of processing in a task.

Mechanisms of attention

Attending to new tasks requires effort. Maintenance of effort is needed to select and process information, make decisions, develop a logical sequence of action and to track performance of a task over time. Many activities are performed so frequently that they become automatic, reducing the demand on the attentional system. Even in these tasks there are critical points when failure to attend to the activity may result in 'actions not as planned' (Reason, 1979). Even mild brain injury may disrupt attentional processes. For example, selectivity of attention may be impaired so an individual's behaviour is more frequently disrupted by noise or other distractors. Mechanisms of attention, the disruption of which could interfere with functional skills, are described below.

Alertness

Immediately following trauma, the patient is unconscious and unable to attend or learn. In the early stages of recovery following the resolution of coma, the patient demonstrates little understanding of his surroundings and a high level of environmental stimulation is necessary to maintain arousal. When alert the patient's selective attention is noticeably impaired. The patient typically orients to all novel events. The patient is unable to select a specific important activity and devote attention to it. For example, a patient might become attracted to and reach for an object despite the fact that doing so will lead to a fall.

Automatic and controlled processing

Shiffrin and Schneider (1977) have described attention in terms of attention-dependent controlled processing and attention-independent automatic processing. Controlled processing is capacity limited and is required for new learning to occur. During the learning phrase of an activity the unskilled individual relies heavily on feedback about his performance on the task and consciously attends to the activity (controlled processing). This focused attention continues during the practice stage of response acquisition. Once the action is learned the individual's performance is controlled by a series of 'prearranged instruction sequences' (automatic processing) leaving the individual free to concentrate on other aspects of the same or different tasks. Automatic processing occurs without conscious control, and places only limited demands on the information processing system.

Observations of behaviour following severe brain injury suggest that many automatic skills have been impaired, forcing the patient to revert to a more conscious, controlled form of processing. To investigate the distinction between automatic and controlled processing, Levin *et al.*, (1988a) administered free recall and frequency of occurrence tasks to patients with severe head injury and a control group. In their first experiment, they found that both free recall (an effortless task) and judgement of relative frequency of occurrence (an automatic task) were impaired in 15 head-injury patients relative to the control group. In a second experiment, the authors corroborated this finding by showing that estimates of frequency were also impaired in a different group of 16 head-injured patients. Levin and co-workers (1988a) infer that cognitive tasks which individuals without cognitive impairment can perform in the absence of practice, feedback or instruction, demand conscious effortful strategies following injury. The study of Levin and co-workers (1988) suggests that for the brain-injured, focused, conscious attention is required to achieve control and safety in many activities of daily living. Shiffrin and Schneider (1977) have described what happens when the attentional system breaks down. They outline two types of failures: divided attentional deficits and focused attentional deficits.

Size and quantity estimates are performed reasonably accurately by most people automatically without actually executing the computations. An interesting example of a disrupted automatic process involved a chef who sustained a severe brain injury (coma duration four days). The patient was independent in personal and community activities of daily living, had a mild memory impairment and some difficulty in planning but was markedly impaired in the estimation of quantities. For example he would grossly over or underestimate ingredients during meal preparation resulting in considerable vocational difficulty.

Divided attentional deficit
There is a limit to the number of percepts (internal or external) that an individual can attend to at any one time. This limitation is described as a divided attentional deficit (DAD) (Schneider *et al.*, 1984). A DAD indicates a failure of the attentional system to accommodate all the information necessary for optimum task performance. This is demonstrated in gait retraining when a patient is able to ambulate with supervision, until a person walks across their visual field or says 'Good morning', whereupon they lose balance. This failure constitutes a divided attentional deficit, because the patient had insufficient attentional

capacity to walk and attend to any other information. A study by Stuss *et al.* (1989) using a complex reaction time task, confirmed the existence of DAD among brain-injured patients. Patients are slow in tasks which require consciously controlled information processing and demonstrate an inability to process multiple pieces of information rapidly. Stuss *et al.* (1988) found this to be so even in mildly concussed patients or those who would on most criteria be considered recovered.

Focused attentional deficit

A focused attentional deficit (FAD) typically occurs when an unfamiliar response is required to a stimulus, which already has an over-learned response linked to it (Schneider *et al.*, 1984). Continuous attention from the individual may be required to suppress this automatic behaviour. Stuss *et al.* (1989) developed a series of computer tasks designed to assess focused attentional deficits. The central feature of the analysis of FAD was the inability of the person after brain injury to suppress a previously learned complex level of processing when a simpler level of processing was demanded. A complex computer reaction time task which required multiple discrimination (shape, internal line orientation, colour) was followed by a task whose outward appearance was identical to this complex task but which required far less complicated discrimination. Although both patients and controls were informed of the change, the patients were less able than the control subjects to inhibit the unnecessary processing of redundant information. The work of Reason (1979) suggests that 'unplanned actions' may be extremely common. The concept of FAD depends to some extent on a Hullian notion of habit strength.

> A clear example of a FAD is a type of navigation error with which everyone is familiar. For example, driving to the doctor's office (a low frequency destination) when the route overlaps the route to work (a high frequency destination). There is a strong tendency for the more familiar behaviour (going to work) to usurp the less familiar behaviour (going to the doctor) so unintentionally the person drives to work. The automatic behaviour has to be continually suppressed or it will override the originally intended behaviour.

Individuals with brain injury may be extremely inattentive in this sense. Below, we will suggest that individuals with brain injury are also less likely to spontaneously monitor their behaviour on an ongoing basis.

Selectivity of attention

Performance of most tasks is influenced by the presence of competing attentional demands (Kewman *et al.*, 1988). The ability to selectively attend depends on discriminating task-relevant information from competing background stimuli. This ability is impaired following brain injury. For example, brain-injured individuals have more difficulty in filtering out distracting verbal information from relevant verbal information (Kewman *et al.*, 1988).

Part of the difficulty in maintaining selective attention may be due to an inability to suppress responses to novel or irrelevant stimuli. The response to a novel stimuli is called an orienting response (Solokov, 1963). As a task is practiced, novel and irrelevant stimuli become less distracting as the individual habituates to them (Lorch *et al.*, 1984). In Solokov's view (1963), habituation occurs because repeated presentation allows the individual to construct a mental representation of the irrelevant stimuli as unimportant. There is no evidence to suggest that generalization of the habituation process occurs. Therapeutically, this would suggest that there is little to be gained from attempting to teach the patient to 'attend' (i.e. habituate to distraction stimuli) in a general sense. However, it is reasonable for patients to habituate to actual distractors present in their environment (e.g. habituate to a noisy work environment).

Some individuals after brain injury have a short attention span, are unable to maintain a focus of attention and consequently passively shift their attention to extraneous stimuli when the span lapses. The reaction time studies of Stuss *et al.* (1989) suggest that the brain-injured as a group have difficulty sustaining attention. A more extensive discussion of the role of attention in the acquisition of novel behaviours is provided below.

PERCEPTION

Perceptual processes include the structuring and organization of information: recognition, identification and classification; discrimination; and the extraction of meaning from sensation. The senses: vision, hearing, touch, smell, taste and kinaesthesis, provide specific information about the environment. Perception is influenced by context and the individual's stored knowledge and expectations. Stored information is constantly being updated, evaluated and modified.

Models of perception

The analysis of perceptual processes is complex. Here some of the more interesting models of perception are mentioned. Different models emphasize different aspects of perceptual processes. The first model discussed here, the template model, assumes that an individual perceives environmental stimuli as patterns (templates) which are then matched to patterns in memory. Percepts are matched as wholes without being decomposed into parts or features. An alternative model, the pandemonium model (Selfridge, 1959) is an attempt to account for human pattern recognition via a hierarchical system of feature extraction. The pandemonium model suggests that hierarchically arranged levels interact in different aspects of the analysis. Selfridge's intriguing model suggests 'demons' (recognition node) respond to specific stimuli. Their hierarchical arrangement allows recognition of complex stimuli to be built up from recognition of a very simple stimulus feature. For example, in the recognition of the letter 'A', line and angle 'demons' pass information to more complex form 'demons' until the letter 'A' demon is reached. Movement in this model is essentially in one direction from stimulus to recognition.

Constructive models such as Neisser's (1967) analysis by synthesis model suggest that individuals use contextual information to formulate hypotheses about raw sensory data which they then test against the sensory evidence. If the information matches, it has been interpreted (perceived) correctly: if mismatched the hypothesis is reformulated and re-tested.

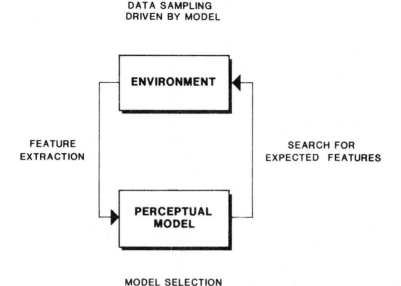

DATA SAMPLING
DRIVEN BY MODEL

ENVIRONMENT

FEATURE
EXTRACTION

SEARCH FOR
EXPECTED FEATURES

PERCEPTUAL
MODEL

MODEL SELECTION
DRIVEN BY DATA

Figure 4.2 Neisser's cyclic model of perception. From *Cognition and Reality: Principles and Implications of Cognitive Psychology* by Ulric Neisser. Copyright © 1976 by W.H. Freeman and Company. Reprinted by permission.

Perceptual deficits following brain injury

Body scheme disorders and somatic inattentions

Body scheme disorders are a group of deficits relating to the perception of one's own or other people's bodies. An individual may be considered to have a body scheme disorder if he is unable to recognize body parts or understand how they are related spatially (Semenza, 1988). Semenza (1988) studied a patient whose difficulties in spatial relations were limited to body parts and who had no difficulty in localizing single parts of other objects such as a bicycle or chair. The limited nature of the deficit supports the notion that there is a distinct conceptual semantic system for information about the body (Semenza and Goodglass, 1985; Ogden, 1985; Semenza 1988). Patients may be unable to name or touch a part of the body on command. In dressing, patients may not know where to place their clothing. (This may in part underlie the impairments sometimes described as dressing dyspraxia).

Left-right disorientation is common following brain injury and is associated with left-sided damage and aphasic disorders. Individuals may be unable to discriminate left and right when naming or touching lateralized body parts on themselves or others (reversal). However this finding should be treated cautiously as a significant proportion of right-handed adults without neurological impairment report difficulty in rapidly distinguishing between left and right sides of the body (Harris and Gitterman, 1978).

Neglect and related disorders of abnormal awareness are not well understood but may be a result of unilateral deficits in arousal and attentional mechanisms (Heilman and Valenstein, 1972; Watson *et al.*, 1974). Neglect is often multi-modal and not the result of impairment in one sensory modality. A neglect syndrome is demonstrated if patients fail to report, respond or orient to novel stimuli presented unilaterally. In mild cases, patients may be able to report stimuli once their attention is drawn to the neglected side but this 'attentional set' soon deteriorates. It may be difficult to distinguish the individual with severe visual hemi-inattention or severe somatothetic hemi-inattention from the individual with hemianopia or hemi-anesthesia (Heilman *et al.*, 1985).

Sensory extinction to simultaneous stimulation occurs when an individual is able to register (or report) a stimulus presented in isolation but unable to register this same stimulus when it occurs in conjunction with another stimulus presented to the uninvolved side. In the unusual syndrome of allesthesia, the patient responds to stimuli presented to the involved side as if it were presented to the uninvolved side.

Patients without apparent motor impairments may nonetheless fail to use an extremity. This 'hemikinesia' may occur all the time or only when the patient simultaneously uses the opposite limb (Heilman *et al.*, 1985). Patients may be unable to maintain postures or sustain movements, such as eye closure or tongue protrusion on request. This deficit has been termed motor impersistance.

Visuospatial deficits

Damage to the eye and optic nerve and the resultant visual field deficits are discussed in Chapter 3. The occipital cortex is particularly prone to damage following traumatic brain injury (see Chapter 1). Patients may lose vision in one half of the visual field (hemianopia) in a quadrant or smaller area. Evaluation by a specialist is required to determine the actual extent of the visual impairment. The functional problems arising from specific visual deficits may not be as pronounced as those resulting from severe visual neglect, as the patient is more likely to learn to compensate for the visual impairment. While there was at one time considerable enthusiasm for rehabilitation of visual field deficits (Zihl, 1981; Zihl and Cramon, 1979; 1982), the initial positive research findings have not been replicated (Balliet et al., 1985). Training in compensatory behaviour is now recognized as the most effective treatment method. Compensatory strategies should be trained in functional activities.

There have been extensive reports in the literature on the phenomenon of blindsight which may rely on subcortical mechanisms in man (Weiskrantz, 1986). In blindsight or cortical blindness the patient believes he is blind and predominantly behaves as if he is blind but appears to make some use of visual information. This may be a transient or protracted condition and is particularly associated with anoxic brain damage.

Some patients, while retaining intact visual fields, fail to attend adequately to visual information from one hemispace. Evidence is strong that each hemisphere is responsible not only for receiving stimuli from contra-lateral space but also for attending and intending in that hemispace. The idea of hemispace is complex and can be defined by body position, head position or direction of gaze. These only completely overlap when eyes and head are in the midline. In their paper 'Brain and conscious representation of outside reality', Bisiach and co-workers (1981) describe the ability of right-brain damaged patients with contralateral neglect to accurately describe the left half of recollected images. Using an appropriately counterbalanced design the authors found that patients with hemianopia and neglect were significantly poorer in describing the left half of a recollected image (the Cathedral Square in

Milan) than either controls: patients without hemianopia or neglect, or patients with hemianopia but without neglect.

The higher frequency of severe neglect following damage to the right side of the brain has been explained by asymmetry of brain function. It is proposed that the right hemisphere can activate attentional mechanisms towards either right or left hemispace. The left hemisphere can only subserve attention towards the right hemispace. This asymmetrical ability of the hemispheres to subserve attention results in left neglect occurring far more frequently than right neglect. Though this theory has generated considerable interest, it has not gone without challenge. Vilkki (1989) has demonstrated that mild hemi-inattentions may follow lesions in either hemisphere with equal frequency. Vilkki also found that the association of hemi-inattention with other cognitive deficits was dependent on the side of lesion. Only in patients with right-side damage was inattention associated with generalized cognitive and multi-modal attentional deficits (Vilkki, 1989). The incidence of mild right-sided inattention may have been underestimated by the testing procedures utilized, in which subjects point or cancel using their right hand. Hemi-inattention is reduced when the hand contralateral to the lesion is used (Joanette *et al.*, 1986).

Patients with mild hemi-spatial neglect may make reading errors or have difficulties finding objects on one side in a complex array (for example, items in a kitchen cupboard or inconspicuously placed street signs in the community). In more severe cases, patients may fail to respond to significant environmental features, or have difficulties like walking into doorways or missing half the food on a plate.

Other visuospatial deficits may result in individuals being unable to differentiate foreground from background or leave them unable to judge depths and distances. Patients may have difficulty perceiving an object in a complex array such as food items in a grocery store or socks in a drawer. The inability to judge depth may cause problems in pouring liquids or bumping into objects. Misjudging distances and speeds presents obvious difficulties for an individual attempting to cross the street.

Topographical disorientation

The terms 'topographical' and 'spatial' disorientation are used to categorize a bewildering array of symptoms. Benton (1969) discussed, under this heading, defective localization of stimuli in external space; defective memory for location; defective route finding; reading and counting disabilities (due to a deficit in correctly sequencing reading of written text); defective topographical memory; visuoconstructive disabilities; simultaneous agnosia and body scheme disorders.

Many patients are disoriented in new environments as a result of a generalized memory disorder. Some patients however have a special problem with location, out of proportion to their memory disorder. This type of topographical disorientation is frequently associated with visual deficits and right hemisphere lesions (though lesions may be bilateral). Individuals may become lost in familiar environments or have marked difficulty in learning to navigate in unfamiliar environments. Patients may be unable to describe the layout of a familiar setting, follow simple routes or to read maps. In addition, some patients may lose larger spatial or geographical concepts, for example, whether New York is on the east or west coast of the United States. It is not clear whether these should be considered as separate syndromes or different manifestations of the same underlying disorder.

Agnosia

Agnosia is the inability to derive meaning from perceptions. Debate continues as to whether many of the agnosic syndromes described in the literature are in reality primary disorders of perception rather than intact percepts stripped of meaning. Simultagnosia is impairment of the ability to interpret a visual stimulus as a whole. As a test, a subject may be asked to describe the action taking place in a picture. Some patients will be able to list the individual elements, but will be unable to interpret the central theme or event in a picture. Wolpert (1924) suggested that this deficit could reflect a modality-specific deficit in visual 'integrative apprehension', or simultaneous agnosia. Luria (1959) and Kinsbourne and Warrington (1962) suggest the disorder may be associated with left hemisphere or bilateral occipital lobe lesions, but this view remains controversial.

Prosopagnosia is the inability to recognize familiar faces (see below for an expanded definition). Patients almost always recognize faces as faces, and may be able to discriminate and match faces normally, but are unable to recognize the faces of friends or even their own face in a mirror. The disorder may range in severity from mild difficulty in recognizing infrequently encountered faces to a profound disability, where family members are not recognized. Although rare after traumatic brain injury, prosopagnosia may be seen following both penetrating and blunt brain trauma (Teuber, 1975). Patients may learn to identify people by using extra cues such as gait, dress and hair style. In some patients the condition appears to exist as part of a more fundamental problem of identifying specific objects within a class. Individuals have been reported to demonstrate difficulties in recognizing specific types of automobiles and a farmer has been reported to be unable to recognise his own cows (Lhermitte and Pillon, 1975; Bornstein *et al.*, 1969). One patient, (seen by G.M.G.), who delivered building materials as an occupation, found himself with mild difficulty in recognizing faces but with marked difficulty in distinguishing within classes of bricks and other types of building materials.

Visual object agnosia is the inability to recognize objects, although visual acuity and recognition of objects by touch remains intact. Failure to name an object even when allowed to physically manipulate the object is usually indicative of a language disorder. Visual object agnosia may be divided into two types following Lissauer's (1889) distinction between apperceptive and associative. Apperceptive visual agnosia is a deficit in the final integration of various perceptual attributes. Patients who have been reported to have apperceptive visual agnosia usually have widespread brain pathology often with marked mental deterioration. Bauer and Rubens (1985) suggest that this syndrome is most frequently a result of a constellation of deficits including attentional, perceptual, oculomotor and mnemonic deficits which differ for each patient. Lissauer's second category of associative agnosia fits more closely with the classic definition of agnosia as a 'percept stripped of meaning'. Patients with associative visual agnosia can see an object with sufficient clarity to match or draw it but do not know what the object is. The fact that patients can draw the object and not recognize it indicates that the motor system does not have the ability to cue the identification process. Patients usually find it easier to recognize real objects than pictures. The most difficulty is encountered in identifying line drawings (Bauer and Rubens, 1985). This suggested that the redundancy of information found in real situations assists in the recognition of objects. Although associative visual agnosia is frequently found in conjunction with prosopagnosia, colour agnosia and alexia it is not encountered as frequently as these conditions. Colour agnosia is the inability to recognize colours such that the patient cannot pick out the colour or name a colour on command. The patient should be able to say if two colours are the same or different. Weakness of colour perception can follow acquired brain injury and may be examined with the Ishihara plates or the Farnsworth-Munsell 100 hue test.

Somatosensory agnosia is the disruption of higher order tactile recognition in the absence of elementary somatosensory loss. A number of typologies have been proposed (Delay, 1935) but at minimum a distinction should be recognized between the ability to discriminate between objects which vary in size, weight, texture and object identification. Where basic sensation and attention is adequate but objects cannot be identified, somatasensory agnosia is likely. This disorder is most often associated with right hemisphere damage.

Auditory agnosia is an impaired ability to recognize sounds, including word and non-word sounds in the context of adequate hearing. For example, a patient may not be able to differentiate between the sound of a car engine running and the sound of a vacuum cleaner. Pure word deafness (an inability to discriminate and comprehend spoken language, but with retained ability to read, write and speak in a relatively unimpaired manner) occurs infrequently following brain injury. Amusia is the inability to appreciate various aspects of music. It is of specialist or technical interest only and rarely interferes with everyday functioning, though for some individuals it significantly affects quality of life.

Apraxia
The apraxias are disorders of skilled, purposeful movements, which cannot be accounted for by weakness; akinesia; abnormal tone; sensory loss; incomprehension of, or inattention to, commands; or non-cooperation. Apraxia is associated with left

hemisphere lesions and, as this hemisphere is also dominant for language, aphasia and apraxia frequently co-exist. The left hemisphere is predominant in the control of skilled movement. Damage to the left parietal area may result in the disruption of motor memories (Heilman *et al.*, 1975) and impairment in the learning of new motor skills. It has been suggested that the right hemisphere does have motor programmes but that these are only accessed when considerable information about an action is available (Geschwind, 1975). This would account for the fact that some patients improve their performance when shown or permitted to handle an actual functional object.

Many brain processes are involved in the production of skilled motor activity. Individuals with limb-kinetic apraxia cannot make precise movements and have particular difficulty with rapid repetitive movements such as tapping. This deficit is probably observed in functional activities as clumsiness (Heilman and Rothi, 1985). An individual with ideomotor apraxia is unable to perform a purposeful motor task on command even though he understands the idea or concept of the task. These individuals, while not able to perform actions on command, may retain kinaesthetic memory of movements and be able to carry out some well-practiced motor tasks automatically. For example, if asked to clean their teeth, the individual can describe the act and recognize it, yet be unable to pick up the toothbrush or initiate the act on command. At another time, the individual may pick up the toothbrush, put toothpaste on the brush and brush his teeth spontaneously.

The term ideational apraxia has been variously defined and continues to cause confusion. Hecaen (1968) described ideational apraxia as 'an impairment of the logical and harmonious sequence of the several elementary movements that make up a complex act, though each movement may by itself be executed correctly'. Patients with ideational apraxia cannot carry out a series of actions in the sequence required to achieve the goal. The logical sequence of single movements is not respected, objects are improperly used, or single movements in the sequence are skipped or repeated (Poeck and Lehmkuhl, 1980). Ochipa *et al.*, (1989) have presented an alternative hypothesis describing ideational apraxia as a deficit in tool selection and use. They describe a patient whose deficits could not be explained by a motor production deficit as in ideomotor apraxia because he made content errors and could not match tools with the objects upon which they should be used. The patient had severe difficulties in using 'tools' in real-life settings.

Perseveration
Perseveration is the repetition of whole or part behaviours in situations where such repetition is inappropriate or out of context. Goldberg and Bilder (1987) have noted that focal non-frontal impairments usually result in perseveration which is modality specific. Lesions to the frontal area however may result in a syndrome of perseveration which is ubiquitous, affecting every domain of cognition and behaviour. On clinical grounds, perseveration may be divided into type 'A' where the patient repeats the same elementary behaviour over and over again and 'B', where a patient can perform an initial activity without error but where subsequent activities are contaminated by this initial action. Luria suggested that a type 'A' perseveration is the result of pathology in the basal ganglia whereas a type 'B' perseveration results from impairment of the pre-frontal cortex (Luria, 1965).

MEMORY AND INFORMATION PROCESSING

Memory is intimately connected to other cognitive processes such as attention, perception, and planning. Attending to (and perceiving) the environment is essential for learning and remembering. Memory processes subserve the majority of activities.

Models of memory and information processing

Atkinson and Shiffrin (1968) proposed the Modal model of information processing. Although other models are available, the Modal model provides a basic operational theory of information processing and memory. We have found an elaboration of this model to be clinically useful. The basic components of Atkinson and Shiffrin's model are sensory buffer stores and short and long-term memory. The type of material and mode of presentation effect the probability of recall. Rate of presentation, clarity, and the organization of the material all influence whether it will be remembered. Perceptual factors, as well as the individual's beliefs about the information and its familiarity (and meaning), affect how the information is processed by the sensory buffer stores (iconic and echoic memories). Codes are used to aid information recall from these very short-term buffer stores such as, acoustic, visual, semantic and articulatory codes. Visual memories are usually richer and more extensive than those of other sensory systems.

Fisk and Schneider (1984) suggest the amount of attention allocated to a stimulus determines how well the subject is able to recognize and remember it. There is also evidence that the ability to introspectively remember unattended stimuli is poor. Nissen and Bullemer (1987) examined whether the same kind of attentional requirements exist for performance measures of learning as for introspective measures of learning. A computerized serial reaction time task was used. A light appeared at one of four locations and subjects pressed one key out of a set of four located directly below the position of the light. Learning was evaluated by measuring facilitation of performance on a repeating ten-trial stimulus sequence to which the subjects were naive. In non-neurologically impaired subjects there was considerable improvement in performance when this was the only task, however when given in a dual-task condition (a condition reducing the subject's ability to attend to the task), learning of the sequence, as assessed by verbal report and performance measures, was minimal. Patients with Korsakoff's syndrome were also able to learn the sequence in the single task condition despite their lack of awareness of the repeating pattern. Nissen and Bullemer (1987) conclude that improved performance in the task, which is dependant on procedural memory, required the subject to attend to it. Awareness of the content of what is learned is not a requirement for learning but attention to the task is.

Speed of information processing is closely linked with memory functioning. Early after brain injury, even mildly injured patients demonstrate slowed speed of information processing (McMillan and Gluckman, 1987; Van Zomeran and Deelman, 1978; Gronwall and Wrightson, 1981) as measured by tasks such as the Paced Serial Auditory Additions Task (Gronwall, 1977). Execution of simple reaction-time tasks, such as pressing a key to a stimulus, are less likely to be impaired following brain injury than is performance on activities requiring complex processing of information and decision making. A slowed rate of information processing necessitates the retention of information for an extended processing period. Cognitive processing can be conceived of as occurring within a limited cognitive 'space'. Slowed information processing means that more information is arriving into the 'space' than can be processed resulting in 'overflow' and subsequent loss of information. Additionally, the patient's inability to select the most significant element of an event results in his being overwhelmed with data.

Short-term memory as described by Atkinson and Shiffrin (1968) allows retention of information for approximately five to nine seconds, unless a rehearsal strategy is used to extend the retention period (for example, subvocal repetition of a telephone number until it is dialled). It is capacity limited allowing the storage of seven, plus or minus two, items (Miller, 1956). On free recall tasks such as a word list, individuals remember more items at the beginning and end of the list. The recency effect (remembering the items presented last) may be a result of rehearsal in short-term memory. This articulatory rehearsal loop provides information storage for very little effort. The primacy effect (preferential recall of items occurring first) may be subserved by long-term memory. Baddeley and Hitch (1974) proposed that an executive system adopts strategies to form associations, rules and relations between items. The idea of an active, working memory was developed in an attempt to explain the systems and processes used by individuals in tasks like arithmetic, verbal reasoning, prose comprehension or free-recall learning.

Long-term memory storage can be usefully conceptualized under the headings procedural and declarative (episodic and semantic) (Tulving, 1983). Procedural memory can be thought of as the store of acquired patterns of behaviour unmediated by cognition. Procedural 'knowledge' is not available to introspection, information is accessed through the performance of the skill (e.g. riding a bicycle). Procedural memory has been inadequately researched and has, until recently, been thought to play a minor role in human memory. There is, however, increasing interest in investigating procedural memory. Lewicki and co-workers in a series of experiments (Lewicki, 1987, 1988) have examined the ability of individuals to acquire relatively complex procedural knowledge. Results demonstrate that non-consciously acquired knowledge can automatically be utilized to facilitate performance without conscious awareness. What is particularly interesting about the series of tasks reported by Lewicki and colleagues is their extreme complexity. Although the skill acquisition is likely to be via procedural learning, the tasks were far more complex than those normally thought to be subserved by this memory system. The process described by Lewicki and co-workers differs from the automatic processing of Shiffrin and Schneider (1977) which involves the utilization of knowledge which was once consciously controlled. Procedural learning allows subjects to make use of much more experience than can be mediated by cognitively controlled channels.

Declarative memory has its greatest development in man with extensive elaboration of medial temporal structures (Squire, 1986). Unlike procedural memory, information in this store is available to introspection. (It includes the majority of information learned in institutional education, e.g. scientific facts and historical dates). Declarative memory may be divided into semantic and episodic memory. Semantic memory is organized knowledge about the world, which is normally not tied to context (Tulving, 1972). In contrast, episodic memory stores information about temporally dated events, and the temporal-spatial relations between these events (Tulving, 1972). It refers to 'historical' information specific to the individual. Tulving maintains that the learning and retrieval of information (from the episodic or semantic memory systems) constitutes an episode. One implication of this theory is that the act of remembering is recorded in the episodic memory store thus changing its overall contents. The semantic memory store assists in the interpretation and storage of information about episodes. The episodic memory store is prone to interference and forgetting, whereas the semantic memory store is relatively stable. The permanent structure of concepts protects the stored information.

An alternative view deserving mention is the 'levels of processing' model of Craik and Lockhart (1972). These authors suggest that coding of information could vary in 'depth' from the higher sensory level to deeper semantic levels. They propose that retention of information is dependent on the 'depth of encoding' and that merely maintaining the information does not lead to long-term storage. Learning will only occur when the information is processed to a deeper level.

Types of memory dysfunction

Recent evidence suggests that information storage is far more complex, widespread and mediated at a more fundamental level than was thought hitherto (Black *et al.* 1988). Considerable progress is being made in understanding the neuroanatomical correlates of memory functioning. Specific neuroanatomical structures must be intact for memory processes to operate normally. Damage to the medial aspect of the temporal lobe and the midline of the diencephalon, including the hippocampus, corpus callosum, and mamillary bodies, obstructs the encoding of new memories and impairs the ability to retrieve some memories encoded prior to injury. Short-term memory is independent of the medial temporal and diencephalic regions but long-term memory depends on these structures functioning. Damage to the hippocampus results in rapid forgetting, suggesting that the hippocampus is involved in the encoding of material actually stored elsewhere in the cortex (Lynch and Baudry, 1984). The fact that repetition can result in 'semantic' learning, but that it is stripped of context, is one line of evidence among many suggesting that the hippocampus has a specific role in encoding contextual associations (O'Keefe and Nadel, 1978). Certain cells in the hippocampus have been shown to respond to single items preferentially during new learning of word lists or a series of unfamiliar faces. This evidence suggests that the hippocampus contributes specific information during the retrieval of recent memories (Heit *et al.*, 1988).

Damage to brain structures associated with memory function can occur as a result of trauma, infection, or vascular injury, and may produce profound impairments in the individual's ability to acquire information. Inability to maintain directed attention in the face of distractors (arising either internally or externally) may result from frontal impairment and significantly impair memory functioning. In addition, impaired drive and difficulty in planning and regulating complex dependant sequences of action may result in patients not completing the internal mental 'behaviours' they need to do in order to remember (see also discussion of 'nested sequences' and 'checking' below). Parkin (1984) has reviewed the literature on memory and concluded that even the extreme of memory disorder, amnesia, does not represent a unitary syndrome. Damage to a widely distributed array of brain structures can result in general or specific memory difficulties. Given the frequently diffuse nature of traumatic brain injury following trauma, it is not surprising that a particular individual's memory deficits are not perfectly predictable from the type of injury or location of brain damage.

Retrograde and anterograde amnesia

Retrograde amnesia describes the period of disturbed memory function affecting memories for events prior to the neurological insult. Retrograde amnesia has a temporal gradient with the severest memory loss immediately preceding the trauma. Levin *et al*. (1985) studied the influence of personal salience on remembering pre-injury events during and after post-traumatic amnesia (PTA: characterized by difficulty in establishing new memory traces). Two groups of patients, one during PTA and one shortly after the resolution of PTA, and a control group, were tested on the recall of episodic events which had no specific importance to them. The task required patients to select from four alternatives the title of a weekly evening television programme which had been broadcast on a major network for a single season. The individuals with brain injury did not perform as well as the controls and those in PTA performed worse than patients in whom PTA had resolved. The two brain-injured groups were also tested on the recall of autobiographical details with personal salience. The results were similar, but there was a clear trend in the PTA group for more remote events in the person's history to be recalled better than more recent events. The authors concluded that partial retrograde amnesia was demonstrated in both PTA and post-PTA patients, and the patients in PTA showed a temporal gradient in personal but not general episodic material (Levin *et al*., 1985).

Anterograde amnesia refers to disordered memory function for events occurring subsequent to the neurological event. Following the resolution of coma there is a period of memory disturbance referred to as post-traumatic amnesia. The duration of the memory disturbance is related to severity of injury.

Levin *et al*. (1988b) examined learning and forgetting during post-traumatic amnesia (PTA). The authors wanted to determine if PTA was primarily a problem of learning or forgetting. Learning time was manipulated so that retention of test material at ten minutes was the same for a group of brain-injured persons in PTA, a comparison group no longer in PTA and a control group. Due to the nature of the paradigm a number of potential participants (presumably those with the most profound memory impairments) were unable to reach criteria for initial learning. Provided that initial learning was controlled for, patients out of PTA demonstrated a rate of forgetting very similar to that of a control group. However, those still in PTA demonstrated an accelerated slope of forgetting even when patients were matched on indicators of severity of injury. Levin *et al*.'s (1988b) results suggest that training provided during PTA may have less robust effects than those provided after PTA has resolved, i.e. it is not only that patients have a more difficult time learning new material, they also have more difficulty retaining the material once it has been acquired.

Many individuals who continue to have memory disorders after the resolution of PTA can remember small amounts of information, such as a string of numbers, as well as those without a memory impairment. Patient's memory problems occur when attempting to remember large amounts of information which exceed short-term memory capacity, and in trying to retrieve information after a delay or following distractions.

Episodic memory is the most vulnerable to impairment. Deficits may be very mild – such that it takes an extensive assessment period to determine that they exist – or so severe that the individual is incapable of remembering any individual discrete event. Though deficits in acquiring new semantic information probably occur in tandem with episodic memory deficits, semantic memory stores may still be accessed (i.e. learning may take place) via frequent repetition of information. Procedural memory appears to be relatively preserved following most types of brain trauma. It is likely to be phylogenetically old and subserved by very diffuse brain structures (Giles and Fussey, 1988). Beatty *et al*. (1987) examined the proposition that an individual's procedural learning capability could be intact for psychomotor and cognitive tasks, even when the declarative memory system was impaired. Their results show that some but not all amnesic patients perform normally on tasks, which are thought to measure procedural learning. The much-studied patient, H.M., was able to learn and retain the skill of mirror writing, improve performance on a pursuit motor task and a visual maze without recollection of any previous experience of the tasks (Milner, 1962; Corkin, 1968; Milner *et al.*, 1968). Memory-impaired patients are capable of learning complex-domain specific knowledge. For example, they can acquire the knowledge needed for operating and interacting with a microcomputer (Glisky *et al.*, 1986). Patients could learn to manipulate information on the computer screen, to write, edit and execute simple computer programmes, and to perform disk storage and retrieval operations. The learning process was, however, slow relative to controls. It is not unreasonable to hypothesize that the slowed rate of learning was as a result of more heavy dependency, by the brain-injured, on the procedural memory system. An amnesic patient's performance can be influenced by recent exposure to material providing that conscious recall is not required for subsequent performance.

Mishkin and Petri (1984) account for the learning ability of amnesics by suggesting that there are at least two forms of retention, only one of which is impaired in amnesia. They suggest that experiences are stored in both a memory system (which is impaired in amnesia) and in a habit system (which is not). Each successful trail strengthens the habit. Mishkin and Petri (1984) suggest that habits subserve both semantic memory and procedural memory. Evidence from our intensive studies of patients J.B.R. (Giles and Morgan, 1989), M.F. (Giles and Shore, 1989b) and others, would suggest that they can learn procedures which may vary in specific content, and which may be available to introspection. The generation of habits is central to the work of the occupational therapist in rehabilitation of the severely memory-impaired patient.

Category specific knowledge

A number of workers have investigated the categorical organization of knowledge (Warrington and McCarthy, 1987). Warrington (1981) has demonstrated that individuals can have selective impairments of not only broad categories of semantic knowledge but also subsets of categories. Patients have been noted to have impairments in the recognition of inanimate objects but no impairment in the recognition of food or living things. One patient described by Warrington and Shallice and also seen by the current authors (J.B.R.), (Giles and Morgan, 1989; Giles and Clark-Wilson, 1988a) demonstrated relative preservation of the categories of mechanical and garden implements but was severely impaired in the recognition of fruits and vegetables. Within the class of objects, Warrington and McCarthy (1987) have demonstrated selective impairments of recognition of manipulatable objects as opposed to large man-made objects. Patients most frequently described with categorical knowledge impairments have suffered from encephalitis or cerebrovascular accidents but the traumatically brain injured may show similar deficits (Giles, 1989).

Confabulation

Confabulation is frequently associated with severe disorders of memory but does not occur in all cases of amnesia. Berlyne (1951) defined confabulation as 'a falsification of memory occurring in clear consciousness in association with an organically derived amnesia'. In mild cases, where insight is relatively preserved, an individual may realize that his view of reality is, on consideration, unlikely, but more often, confabulation is not accompanied by any insight. Kopelman (1987) delineates two types of confabulation. He calls the first type spontaneous confabulation, which could be a result of the combined deficits of frontal lobe dysfunction and amnesia (which may include PTA). Spontaneous confabulation is often grandiose, sustained and wide-ranging with the subject making obviously absurd claims about events which have never been part of his or her experience. The second type of confabulation described by Kopelman is provoked confabulation which is normally the result of questioning and may reflect a normal response to tasks beyond the subject's memory capacity, i.e. it is a normal process demonstrated to an abnormal degree as a result of reduced memory capacity. It may include the out-of-context representation of overlearned or exceedingly familiar material.

LANGUAGE

Language is central to a wide range of human functions and influenced greatly by other cognitive disorders such as attention, perception and memory. In some clients slowed speed of information processing or impaired attentional capacity may adversely affect an individual's language comprehension. Perceptual deficits or memory disorders can influence understanding of the contextual details required for comprehending or reading material.

Language deficits (communication)

Following brain injury, the complex processes which underly normal communication may be disrupted. Left hemisphere lesions, particularly in the parietal and left temperoparietal lobes, cause receptive and expressive communication disorders but damage is more likely to be diffuse and affect widely separated areas of brain tissue. This could lead to, at one extreme, severely disordered linguistic ability and at the other, sub-clinical linguistic disorders. Sarno (1984) reports that over one-third of all individuals with closed head injury significant enough to cause coma have hidden linguistic deficits. Once the patient emerges from coma therapists begin to assess the degree of the patient's understanding and their ability to communicate. Frequently, unrecognized language difficulties interfere with the patient's performance of functional skills.

The term 'receptive dysphasia' describes difficulties in understanding spoken or written language. Processing deficits and attentional disorders influence the amount of information understood in reading and conversations. Individuals can often only understand one or two-stage instructions and are confused by more information. Most patients retain basic phonologic, syntactic and semantic relationships in language (Hagen, 1972), however, some patients have difficulties in recognizing letters, understanding words and appreciating complex grammatical sentence constructions. Examples of the type of syntactical structure where these are apparent are conditionals. In conditional sentences, the order of performance does not always follow the order in the sentence construction, for example, 'place the blue square on the yellow square after placing the yellow square on the red circle'. The frequency of words, types of sentence construction and the hierarchy of concepts included will affect the individual's comprehension of spoken or written language. Patients may understand each word but be unable to comprehend the more abstract or complex meaning.

The term 'expressive dysphasia' describes difficulties in language expression. Non-fluent dysphasia is characterized by sparse, effortful and hesitant speech, word retrieval difficulties and the over-use of non-specific words to compensate, such as 'thing'. Content words (nouns and verbs) are lacking and articles, conjunctions and prepositions predominate. Material frequently violates syntactic rules and may contain paraphasias, where either words or syllables are substituted or neologisms (new words) are used. Compensatory strategies are frequently used to provide the listener with greater contextual cues, for example, associations, descriptions or gestures. The written productions of an individual with non-fluent dysphasia may contain an abundance of starters, fillers, circumlocutions, and substitutions. In written work misspelling words, grammatical errors and lack of punctuation are also often evident.

Fluent dysphasia is marked by rapid production of unsubstantive speech. The language deficits may be so severe that the speech or written work becomes completely incomprehensible (jargon aphasia). Some individuals perseverate their language production so that words or phrases are repeated, whilst others echo words from another person (echolalia). The content of the language may become distorted and disordered. Linguistically intact statements could be made that lack relevancy to the conversation, and expression could be circumlocutory, confabulated, tangential or lack a logical relationship to their previous thoughts or expressions. These types of language disorders markedly affect an individual's ability to communicate effectively and are usually related to other cognitive deficits.

Compensatory strategies can be used to ameliorate the functional impact of some of these deficits, and rehabilitation can help patients overcome deficits which impact vocational and interpersonal abilities. These communication deficits are discussed in Chapter 11.

The role of language in behavioural regulation

In addition to its role in communication, language assists in the regulation of behaviour and mediates internal cognitive processes such as memory and problem solving. There is considerable evidence to show that interference with a subject's subvocal language behaviour significantly impedes the acquisition of a novel motor task (Giles and Gent, 1988). There is growing evidence to show language helps individuals initiate and monitor complex behaviours, for instance, saying then doing for self-instruction; saying whilst doing for self-monitoring. Patients who have damage to the medial frontal lobes may retain the ability to understand and express themselves but be unable to use language (self-statements or instruction) to govern their behaviour. The verbal command may be remembered but loses its controlling influence on behaviour.

> Patient L.A. had a swallowing disorder three months following a left frontal aneurysm. It was explained to her at each meal that her swallowing disorder meant that she should eat slowly, swallowing all the food in her mouth before taking another bite. L.A. understood and remembered this information. She was however unable to use this information to govern her behaviour, requiring a staff member to sit with her to physically interrupt her stuffing food into her mouth.

Disruption of these very complex processes need not be associated with any distinct site of lesion, although in severe, diffuse brain injury some damage to the medial frontal areas may be presumed.

PROBLEM SOLVING AND PLANNING

Although early research suggested that the primary difficulties of patients with frontal lobe impairment was perseverative interference from previous modes of response (Milner, 1963), more recent evidence suggests that the picture is more complex with patients also having deficits in abstract thinking and planning. Freedman *et al.* (1987) examined the ability of closed head-injured patients to forward plan, using a relatively simple conditioning paradigm (a shuttlebox-analogue avoidance task). When compared to a group of patients after a cerebro-vascular accident, the closed head-injured patients demonstrated greater anticipatory behaviour deficits despite the fact that the two groups did not differ on escape behaviour, and that the closed head-injured group were equivalent or better on performance of individual tests of the Halstead-Reitan Battery and Wechsler scales. Neither clarification of the instruction, additional trials nor enhancement of the warning cue appeared to ameliorate the anticipatory behaviour deficit. The authors suggested that patients with anticipatory behaviour deficits would show deficits in situations where current behaviour should be regulated on the basis of expected future consequences.

After brain injury, individuals demonstrate greater difficulty in considering options, classifying or organizing ideas and prioritizing information. Vilkki (1988), using a task similar to the token test but with more ambiguity, found patients with frontal lobe deficits failed to identify the appropriate categories for sorting, thus exhibiting abstract thinking deficits. Cicerone *et al.* (1983) found that subjects with frontal lobe lesions failed to systematically explore a hypothesis (general concept formation) and failed to discard inappropriate hypotheses. The authors suggest that the deficit may be the result of disturbance of an attentional control mechanism which is involved in the ongoing monitoring of feedback from the environment and segregates relevant from irrelevant sources of information.

Many instances of 'problem solving' deficits are more likely to be difficulties in planning. Brain-injured individuals may not engage in the internal behaviours necessary for planning and subsequently executing complex dependant sequences of action. There is increasing evidence that this impairment in planning underlies some types of high-level cognitive disorders. The literature however primarily investigated performance of those with focal non-traumatic injuries so we are extrapolating from these studies to the traumatically injured. Shallice and Evans (1978) attempted to explicate some of these issues using a novel research protocol. They noticed that many of their patients with frontal-lobe impairment demonstrated a gross inability to produce adequate cognitive estimates. The authors asked the patients questions which tapped areas of knowledge which most people possess, but which required material to be accessed and manipulated in novel ways. Answering such questions adequately involved the selection of an appropriate plan to answer the question and check putative answers mentally for error. Examples of the questions posed by Shallace and Evans to the brain-injured and to the unimpaired control subjects inclued 'On average how many TV programmes are shown on one TV channel between 6.00 p.m. and 11.00 p.m.?' and 'What is the length of an average man's spine?' In the latter question, one must compare the spontaneous estimate of an average person's height with the percentage of an individual's height accounted for by his spine. The patients with anterior lesions performed considerably worse than either patients with posterior lesions or normal controls. The authors interpret this finding as a deficit in planning and checking answers against multiple types of data for bizarreness and inconsistency.

Shallice (1982) proposed a model to show non-routine tasks could be impaired independently from performance of routine tasks. Shallice used a task similar to the tower of Hanoi puzzle and found patients with left-anterior lesions had considerable difficulties. These patients were not more impaired than patients with lesions in other areas on other tasks such as the block design sub-test of the WAIS or on a measure of short-term memory. Shallice's model shows that in order to carry out complex behaviours, the initiation of various behaviours is required over time to develop a plan and initiate a check, act/wait cycle. In this cycle, the individual compares 'plan time' with real time in order to determine whether he needs to initiate a plan component or wait. Many patients, particularly those with marked frontal lobe impairment, appear unable to initiate this type of planning behaviour to develop the action plans required for the check/act cycles. Treatment for these types of frontally-mediated impairments is problematic. It is possible to teach patients to externalize and form a routine for these internally and frontally-mediated behaviours. Treatment approaches are discussed in Chapter 10.

SUMMARY

Chapter 4 has begun the discussion of some of the most important types of deficits found following brain trauma. It should be emphasized again that, although these deficits are discussed separately, real functional impairments are usually the result of a complex interaction of deficits. Disorders of attention are a common feature of the early stages of recovery and many patients simply get better. Disorders of attention, when they are severe and long-lasting, are profoundly handicapping. The types of attentional problems likely to persist are discussed in detail. Evidence was reviewed which suggests that attention-to-task is a prerequisite for learning. The more frequently encountered perceptual deficits are discussed and theoretical models for understanding visual and somatic neglect elaborated. It is noted that the testing procedures may have led to an underestimation of the frequency of right-sided neglect. Memory deficits are discussed in depth. Emphasis is placed on the differential impairment of memory systems because of the importance of this factor in the development of functional retraining programmes. A brief overview of language disorders is included. We also mention the important (but little understood) role of language in regulating behaviour. In the final section of this chapter we discuss problem solving and planning. These deficits are accounted for primarily in terms of a reduced level of internal mental 'behaviour'. Plans are not formed well and those formed are not reviewed or checked against relevant data. Later the authors argue that this failure to initiate certain types of mental behaviour is central to understanding the otherwise perplexing presentation of many of our patients. In Chapter 5 we review the psychiatric disturbances associated with brain injury.

5

Psychiatric changes following brain injury

INTRODUCTION

The term neuropsychiatric disorder is used here to refer to personality, psychiatric and some types of behavioural disturbance occurring as a result of brain injury. Since the work of Davison and Bagley (1969), brain injury has been recognized as a cause of serious psychiatric disorder. Patients with brain injury have a higher rate of psychiatric morbidity and are considerably more prone to suicide than the general population (Hillbom, 1951; Achte *et al.*, 1969; Lishman, 1978). Lezak has reported that 45% of a group of severely brain-injured adults treated by her exhibited behaviours usually associated with psychiatric disturbance (Lezak, 1987). Interest has centred on pharmacological and behavioural interventions for the treatment of these disorders (Eames and Wood, 1985a) and on psychotherapy (Prigatano *(Ed)*, 1986). In this chapter, neuropsychiatric conditions and possible pharmacological interventions are described. The treatment of behaviour disorders is considered in more depth in Chapter 10 and personality and sexual disorders following brain injury are discussed in Chapter 13.

Premorbid personality, pre-existing psychiatric disturbance and genetic predisposition undoubtedly play a part in psychiatric complications after brain injury but the contribution of the physical and neurochemical disruption to the brain is frequently underestimated. The range of psychiatric disturbances which may follow brain injury is extensive and embraces most of what can be found in psychiatric symptomatology (Lishman, 1972). Lishman's (1968) study of 670 soldiers with penetrating injury showed a direct relationship between severity of injury and the degree of psychiatric disorder. Follow-up one to five years after injury demonstrated that the relationship was maintained when variability due to intellectual impairment was controlled for. Psychiatric disorders closely tied to severity of injury were depression, apathy, euphoria, behaviour disorder, disinhibition, facile or childish behaviour and lack of judgement and consideration for others (Lishman, 1968). Other frequently encountered problems include obsessionality, paranoid ideas, aggressive behaviour, problems in initiating behaviour and changes in sexual behaviour. Patients' lack of insight into changes may be a further complicating factor (Lishman, 1978; Lezak, 1978). More recently, Bernstein *et al.* (1989) found that in a group of 125 patients with predominantly mild brain injury (unconsciousness of 20 minutes or less), neuropsychological disturbance was positively related to emotional disturbance. It is particularly interesting that in this group of mildly injured patients, duration of unconsciousness, post-traumatic amnesia, post-traumatic epilepsy and the presence or absence of skull fracture were not related to emotional adjustment. Normally personality and environmental factors play a role in outcome (McFarlane, 1989) but in this study group, differences in personality adjustment were only related to the degree of neuropsychological deficit. It is known that children who have traumatic brain injury have an increased likelihood of developing psychiatric disorder and that this likelihood is increased by poor home conditions (Shaffer *et al.*, 1975).

ASSESSMENT

Neurofunctional assessment assists in determining the relative contribution of factors leading to psychiatric dysfunction and is described in detail in Chapter 6. Psychiatric assessment of the brain-injured individual includes recording patient history incorporating information about childhood, home and social situation, and previous psychiatric impairment. Interview may be an important source of self-report and observational data. Considerable skill is required in observational assessment as psychiatric disturbances such as mood or anxiety disorders may be confused with cognitive deficits and learned behavioural problems. Observation in a range of settings is essential. Reports from the family about the individual's level of functioning, personality changes and socially interactive abilities all facilitate diagnosis and the implementation of appropriate treatment. The Katz Adjustment Scale (Katz and Lyerly, 1963) uses self-report in conjunction with a social reference (most usually a family member) to rate adjustment. Five scales attempt to address the following domains: clinical adjustment, freedom from symptoms of psychopathology, social functioning, personal adjustment and social behaviour. The patient completes measures on all these areas. The relative completes measures of these domains with the exception of personal adjustment. There is an attempt to capture the relative's level of satisfaction with the patient's social functioning by them rating both the patient's actual social functioning and performance of free-time activities and 'expected' levels of performance. Self-esteem (the development of which may be an appropriate goal of therapy) may also be assessed using self-report measures (Robson, 1989). A variety of other self-report scales assessing symptoms are available such as the Beck Depression Inventory (Beck *et al.*, 1979). The rating of behaviour disorders is discussed in Chapter 10.

BEHAVIOURAL DISORDERS

Wood and Eames (1981) characterize behavioural problems as positive or negative. Positive behavioural disorders, such as aggression, are spontaneously exhibited and may occur with high frequency. In contrast, negative behaviour disorders are characterized by apathy, lethargy, and aspontaneity. The individual is unable to generate sufficient effort to overcome obstacles to independent functioning, and often appears depressed and impassive, thus demonstrating a generalized poverty of behaviour. Although the distinction between positive and negative behaviour disorder is helpful, some patients are passive until placed under pressure and then demonstrate a positive disorder. Other patients can be very active in working to avoid activity. Conceptualizing patients on a continuum of active-avoidant-passive is therefore preferable.

Episodic dyscontrol, characterized by violent, usually short-lived, outbursts of aggression with no (or minor) provocation, has been reported frequently following severe brain injury. Outbursts of uncontrollable rage are not confined to the brain-injured and have been associated with epilepsy and other neurological abnormalities (Tunks and Dermer, 1977). Monroe (1970) proposed that episodic behaviour disorder represents a continuum of, at one end, neurologically mediated behaviour and at the other end, a learned pattern of deviant behaviour.

In a small percentage of patients, violence may be purely epileptiform in nature. In these patients the violence is usually non-directed though in rare cases it appears purposeful (Delgado-Escueta *et al.*, 1981). Fenwick (1989) described the differential diagnosis of seizure-related aggression as requiring a detailed exploration of the following factors. (1) Behaviour prior to the episode; when the patient's aggression is related to a seizure their behaviour prior to onset is quite normal and there will be no specific triggers for the outburst. The behaviour will occur if the patient is with others or alone. (2) Onset of seizure related aggression; in an aggressive episode due to a seizure, onset is always sudden, usually occurring in a matter of seconds. The behaviour is inappropriate to the setting and can occur anywhere. Witnesses often report that the patient suddenly stopped, started to stare and exhibited simple motor automatisms and seemed confused. (3) Nature of the aggressive episode; seizure-related aggression lasts from one to three minutes (post-ictal aggression may last longer) and usually includes the characteristics of complex partial seizures and automatisms, the behaviour makes no psychodynamic sense, is uncharacteristic of the patient and memory for the incident is not usually retained (Fenwick, 1989).

Although not clearly epileptiform in nature, many patients demonstrate abnormal electrical activity (often with a temporal lobe or limbic focus) in conjunction with aggressive behaviour. It is believed that limbic structures (the amygdala, the hippocampus and the hypothalamus) subserve intense feeling states. Damage to the temporal lobes and limbic system may produce increased intensity of feeling, irritability and paranoid misperception, all of which leave a patient more prone to aggressive behaviour (Lewis and Pincus, 1989). Cassidy (1990a, 1990b) has suggested a typology for considering organically-mediated aggression (for a discussion of a proposed neurochemical substrate for the types of aggression, the interested reader is referred to the original papers). Cassidy describes three types of aggressive behaviour: predatory aggression, affective aggression and non-directed aggression. Predatory aggression does not involve increased irritability or autonomic arousal, and is sudden and goal-directed. Individuals (or objects) entering the patient's visual field are at risk of attack (often with lunging or biting behaviours). Affective aggression is accompanied by autonomic arousal and characteristically escalates in relation to some form of provocation. Those who know the patient well can predict the occurrence of the aggressive outburst. Non-directed aggression may involve a brief period of autonomic arousal and the behaviour is generally short-lived.

Treatment centres around the use of carbamazepine (Elliot, 1977; Tunks and Dermer, 1977; Yudofsky, 1981) and to a lesser extent lithium and propranolol (Yudofsky, *et al.*, 1987), all of which have been used in combination with behaviour therapy. Recently, an animal model of episodic dyscontrol has been developed involving the phenomenon of limbic kindling. This model suggested that both the epileptiform disorder and environmental conditions are involved in the genesis of episodic dyscontrol (Post *et al.*, 1982).

A 19-year-old college student fell from the back of a pick-up truck and sustained a severe brain injury (coma duration three weeks). One year after injury, the patient was severely amnesic, tests of intelligence showed he was in the normal range and the results of an EEG were unremarkable. Some stereotyped behaviours were present (e.g. only walking on the white tiles on a patterned floor) but no fixed obsessions were present. Most handicapping were aggressive outbursts violent enough to keep him in a locked psychiatric facility. The outbursts occurred between one and six times per week and were precipitated by apparently minor frustration. Outbursts were unpredictable but staff reported that they could tell when he was at risk because he would become more sullen and childlike. Of particular note was that staff described the patient as weak and out of condition other than during episodes of dyscontrol when he was described as extremely strong, requiring up to six staff members to restrain him (sometimes continuing to struggle for three hours). Over the course of the year, the patient had developed some recognition of the existence of these episodes which he ascribed to his brain injury.

In some patients, brain injury appears to exacerbate a previously existing tendency to aggressive behaviour. As a result of the brain injury these individuals could enter the domain of medical rehabilitation services. Patients may meet the criteria for the category of organic personality syndrome (explosive type) in the Diagnostic and Statistical Manual of the American Psychiatric Association (DSM-III-R) (1987). In a recent review, Lewis and Pincus (1989) suggested that severe aggressive behaviour in some patients may be the result of a complex array of factors including cognitive impairment, brief episodic psychotic symptomatology (characterized by paranoid ideas and misperceptions) and a history of having been exposed to physical abuse or having watched such abuse in infancy. Many of these patients have a prior history of brain injury. The individual's ability to exercise behavioural control is further compromised by the trauma.

Brooks and co-workers (1983) showed that threats of violence and inappropriate behaviour were present in nearly a fifth of patients during the first year after severe brain trauma. Brooks *et al.* (1986) in a five-year follow-up found relatives reported no reduction in patients' emotional disturbances, but an increase in the descriptions of personality change. The relatives perceived a considerable increase in disturbed behaviour, including bizarre, violent and inappropriate social behaviour. A fifth of these relatives described the patient as having episodes of physical violence, sometimes involving an actual assault on the relatives. Reports that family members were afraid of the patient were not unusual. One-third of the patients were reported to have been in some trouble with the law since the accident, but more than a third also had some contact with the law premorbidly. Wood (1987) has stated that the brain-injured have a less stable pattern of behaviour, including a reduced tolerance of stress and a coarsening or blunting of social skills, with the result that the person may often behave inappropriately, without concern for the feelings of others.

Aggression may be the result of the individual's inabilities to tolerate frustrations or to control anger in situations where previously this would have been accomplished without difficulty. Frustrations may include being dependent on others, waiting for people to meet their needs or being unable to accomplish previously easy tasks.

M.S. was admitted to a rehabilitation centre due to aggressive outbursts. At admission, two years after injury, he had a severe memory disorder and obsessional characteristics (coma duration unknown). His behavioural outbursts were precipitated by frustration and characterized by screaming, and waving his fist in a threatening manner towards the person or object with which he was frustrated. These behaviours could be precipitated by people staring at him, jokes, requests to complete a task, or minor environmental stressors such as too much water in the washbasin.

For some patients aggressive behaviour is learned post-injury and an instrumental quality to the behaviour is apparent. The behaviour disorder often develops when the patient has moderate to severe cognitive deficits, and appears to assist the patient avoid non-preferred activities or control people in his environment. Some patients learn to use aggressive behaviour to gain attention or commodities and these aggressive attention-seeking behaviours can be frightening for care-givers. When threatened it can be easier for the family or staff to give the individuals what they want, rather than managing the behaviour in a way designed to reduce its frequency of recurrence (see Chapter 11). Unfortunately, meeting the patients' demands and allowing the patients to manipulate others inappropriately decreases their receptivity to new learning and thereby limits their rehabilitation options.

C.P. had a severe brain injury (coma duration 2 weeks) as a result of a motor cycle accident three years previously. C.P. had learned to manipulate her care-givers into giving her commodities. She would shout 'tea' repeatedly, while banging her hand onto the table. When she did not get her own way, C.P. screamed profanities and made lewd and suggestive gestures, and banged the table harder. When her tea arrived she would smile disarmingly, and say 'thank you' and kiss the hand of the person who provided the tea. At home and at previous treatment sites, she usually had the commodities given to her quickly to ensure she maintained her equanimity.

Following brain injury many individuals are disinhibited, reactive to their environment, extreme in their behaviours and unaware of the effect of their behaviour on others. Disinhibition may result in novel maladaptive behaviours or an exaggeration of previous characteristics. Patients may be unable to inhibit desires, and appear socially unskilled. They may make childish and fatuous comments, display exaggerated emotions inappropriate for the situation, make lewd and suggestive verbalizations, stand too close to others, or attempt to be the loud, centre of attention in social settings.

B.T. was seen in a rehabilitation unit 13 years after her brain injury sustained as a nine-year-old pedestrian in a road traffic accident (coma duration unknown). B.T. was quick to engage in interpersonal conflicts, confront every situation and never back down. B.T. became agitated when she did not get her own way, and shouted at others when upset. Even when she was relaxed, she would cry easily (at least once a day), stand too close to others, talk too loudly and was always attempting to be the centre of attention by directing conversations towards her own concerns.

Alterations in the patient's level of arousal and drive may also contribute to aggressive behaviour. Arousal is the tonic level of responsivity of an organism. Drive is the tendency for an organism to engage in behaviour directed towards a specific goal. Disorders of arousal and drive frequently follow brainstem, frontal or diffuse cortical injuries and result in the individual's being unable to carry out functional tasks, because of the amount of effort required to initiate and maintain activity. In extreme cases, the individual may be unable to exhibit any spontaneous movement, while in less severely affected patients the effort involved in activity results in rapid fatiguability and a tendency to be impersistent ('run out of steam') during an activity.

C.V. had a severe brain injury (coma 6 weeks) following a traffic accident, and sustained a severe brainstem injury and diffuse anoxic damage. He was severely overweight, had hypertonus on his left side, severe dysarthria, hemianopia, and displayed impulsive aggressive outbursts, usually when being helped in daily activities. After his admission to the rehabilitation setting, he spent six months in his bed or wheelchair, without spontaneously initiating any activity except when food was placed immediately in front of him. When food was placed any further than three feet away from him he made no attempt to reach it.

Aggressive behaviour may be associated with other psychiatric conditions occurring after brain injury, for example, psychotic states and mania. Management of these disorders is discussed under the relevant sections.

AFFECTIVE DISORDERS

Depression

Depression of one form or another is extremely common following brain injury of all levels of severity. Lishman (1968) divided the causes of psychiatric disturbance after brain damage between psychological repercussions, as the individual struggles to meet social demands for which he is no longer adequately equipped, and direct results of the neurological damage. This separation of psychiatric disturbance into psychological reaction and direct results of neurological and neurochemical disruption may be particularly appropriate for understanding mood disorder.

Tyerman and Humphrey (1984) examined changes in self-concept approximately seven months after the traumatic brain injury and found very marked psychological distress in terms of both anxiety and depression. On the Leeds anxiety and depression scale, 60% of patients studied had scores indicating clinical depression and 44% had scores indicating severe anxiety. On a measure relating to reaction to physical limitations, 28% felt that they were no longer whole people. Thirty-two percent thought they were a lot of trouble for other people. In social relationships, 40% thought others pitied them and 32% complained 'everyone stares at me'. Thirty-six percent of respondents thought they would be considered inferior by others, 48% thought they would be less able than they otherwise would have been but 88% stated that they wished to make their own way in the world. Newton and Johnson (1985) found that 72% of their sample of the severely brain injured reported high social anxiety and low self-esteem.

Robinson and co-workers (1988) have attempted to assess the

contribution of organic pathology to depression following brain trauma by examining mood in patients following circumscribed cerebrovascular damage. This group of workers found that left-frontal lobe and basal-ganglia disorder are strongly associated with major depression following stroke (Starkstein *et al.* 1989). Patients with right-sided lesions who are depressed are most likely to have lesions in the parietal cortex while undue cheerfulness was likely to be associated with lesions in the right-frontal area (Starkstein *et al.*, 1989).

Grafman *et al.*, (1986) studied Vietnam veterans with penetrating brain trauma. Injuries were categorized as orbitofrontal, dorsofrontal or non-frontal. The study indicated that patients with right orbitofrontal lesions were prone to abnormally increased edginess/anxiety and depression whereas patients with left dorsofrontal lesions were prone to abnormally increased anger and hostility.

The presentation of a severe depressive illness may be atypical after brain injury. In addition, the absence of a stable behavioural baseline and the range of other cognitive and behavioural consequences of brain trauma may make diagnosis problematic. None the less, the cardinal signs of depression (dysphoric mood, appetite disturbance and alterations in sleep patterns) are often present. Threats of suicide and actual suicide are not uncommon and may be carried out in up to 5% of patients. The complexity of the treatment issues makes consultation with a specialist in the psychiatric consequences of brain injury essential.

A 49-year-old woman who had undergone mitral valve replacement five years earlier was found by her husband on the floor of their home after cardiac arrest. Duration of the cardiac arrest was at least fifteen minutes. Eight months later the patient exhibited a severe agitated depression, complicated by an amnesic syndrome. She would pace the facility ceaselessly, and become extremely tearful and distraught at any mention of her current disabilities. Staff were unable to retrain her in specific activities because of her agitated behaviour. Treatment with very small doses of an antidepressant resulted in an almost immediate reduction in the patient's distress and allowed rehabilitation staff to train her to develop the behavioural control required by her family to allow them to care for her at home.

Mania

Brain injury may precipitate mania. Krauthammer and Klerman (1978) first suggested that mania should be regarded as a syndrome with multiple causes. Among the causes they listed were drug intoxication (steroids, stimulants and toxins), infection, neoplasms and epilepsy. Robinson and co-workers (1988) note that mania appears to be more frequently associated with damage to frontal areas of the right hemisphere in conjunction with the limbic system. They also note that mania was principally seen in patients where there was a family history of affective disorder, suggesting that hereditary factors may play an aetiological role in mania following traumatic injury. Robinson and co-workers have now demonstrated similar findings relating to location of lesion and secondary predisposing factors in a large series of stroke patients (Starkstein *et al.*, 1989) and in patients with lesions of diverse aetiology (Starkstein *et al.*, 1988). Shukla *et al.* (1987) described 20 patients who developed mania after closed brain trauma. Thirteen of the patients were classified (using Russell's criteria) as having had severe brain trauma, four had moderate trauma and three had mild trauma. Ten patients had seizure disorders (temporal or temporoparietal abnormalities were present in nine of these). Fourteen of the patients experienced recurrent mania without depression and the sample as a whole showed more manic than depressive episodes. A phenomenological breakdown of acute manic symptoms revealed a predominance of irritable (85%) rather than euphoric (15%) mood, and assaultive behaviour was frequent (70%). Psychotic symptoms were present in only 15% of the sample. Other typical manic symptoms, such as impaired judgement, grandiosity, pressured speech and flight of ideas, were seen in the majority of patients. Reports of treatment have primarily been limited to single cases (Cohn *et al.*, 1977; Sinanan, 1984) and have supported the effectiveness of lithium therapy in the treatment of mania following brain trauma.

PSYCHOSES

Schizophrenia-like disorders

Large population studies suggest that the incidence of schizo-phrenia-like illness is significantly higher in brain-injured sub-jects than in the general population (Shapiro, 1939; Davison and Bagley, 1969; Lishman, 1978). It is noteworthy that 15% of schizophrenic patients present with a history of brain injury preceding the first psychotic episode (Davison and Bagley, 1969). Thomsen (1984) reported that six out of 40 (15%) severely brain-injured patients followed up 10–15 years post-injury were hospitalized for psychotic states one year or longer post-injury. There is no evidence implicating a genetic predisposition in patients who develop schizophrenia after brain injury (Davison and Bagley, 1969), and whether the neurophysiological causes of the schizophrenic disorders are the same in patients with or without brain injury is unknown. It is also not determined if the social and environmental factors which may place indi-viduals with schizophrenic illness at increased risk for relapse, affect those with trauma-precipitated schizophreniform dis-order.

Nasrallah *et al.* (1981) describe a 22-year-old man with no family history of psychiatric illness who developed chronic schizophrenia subsequent to severe brain trauma (coma approximately 16 days). Thirteen months after injury the patient was hospitalized with a diagnosis of depression. He responded rapidly to medication and was discharged. Two months follow-ing this hospitalization there was an apparent change in his thinking. The patient expressed concern that others thought him homosexual and he felt he was part of an experiment which involved his accident. The patient's mother reported that he complained of voices on the radio accusing him of homo-sexuality within hours of emerging from coma. The patient continued to be followed up for a further five years during which time the patient had eight psychiatric hospitalizations. Symptoms included delusions of reference, influence, thought control and persecution. Treatment with neuroleptics produced symptomatic improvement but the patient stopped taking the medication after discharge and he relapsed on each occasion.

Paranoid disorder

Mild paranoid states are a very frequent consequence of brain trauma. Left temporal dysfunction may be associated with paranoia and there is often involvement of limbic system with the 'emotionalization of experience'. Meissner's work on the role of personality characteristics in the formation of paranoid thinking suggests that patients prone to paranoid thinking frequently reveal intense feelings of inferiority or inadequacy. They show a propensity for self-punishing or masochistic behaviour, especially directed at a once-loved object or person. The paranoid patient reports considerable depression and feelings of deprivation. Situational factors may play a significant role in the pathogenesis of the disorder (Meissner, 1978).

Delusions and paranoid ideas are well-known amongst other groups who have severe cognitive or perceptual deficits. Prigatano *et al.* (1988) described an increased occurrence of paranoia in patients who demonstrated severe cognitive impairment or who had poor pre-morbid psychiatric functioning. In contrast, examination of a series of 37 patients treated at a transitional living facility, suggested that those with paranoid features were more likely to have coma of a short duration and that focal lesions predominated (Giles, 1989 unpublished data). Clearly further study is indicated. Reducing the level of stress, supportive counselling and allowing patients to regularly describe recent experiences of their life may be helpful. Reviewing the day's events may help clarify misperceptions before they can become emotionally laden and delusional.

Delusional disorders

Delusions are false fixed beliefs about the self or others, which cannot be corrected by experience or reason. Family members or friends are unable to dispel or explain the patient's beliefs (Prigatano *et al.*, 1988). Delusions may occur following a large number of types of cerebral insults including metabolic disturbance, encephalitis and trauma (Cummings, 1985). Acute delusions are not associated with any specific site of injury (Levine and Grek, 1984) and may be distinguished from confabulation by being a continually re-occurring theme. These acute delusions are likely to be simple and may or may not incorporate aspects of the environment. Variants of these acute delusional disorders are probably extremely common following traumatic brain injury (see below, this section, and other clinical examples in Chapter 8). Enduring complex delusional systems are associated with specific sites of lesions (Toone; 1981: Trimble, 1981). As noted by Cummings (1985), central nervous system functions relevant to delusion formation include verbally mediated conceptual abilities of the left hemisphere and visuospatial, perceptual and affective functions mediated by the right hemisphere. Left-sided lesions are particularly associated with psychotic behaviour (Cummings, 1985; Hillbom, 1960; Davison and Bageley, 1969). Herpes simplex virus often affects the temporal lobes and limbic system with resultant paranoia and delusional states. In conjunction with the limbic system, frontal and temporal systems assess the emotional significance of ongoing experiences.

> Patient L.T. was a popular student and on the high school football team. L.T. was hyperventilating to get 'high' with his friends when he fell and hit his head on a rock. He was taken to the local community hospital. Seven hours later, following a rapidly deteriorating course, he was transferred to a major university hospital. A large bilateral subdural haematoma was surgically removed whereupon the course of medical recovery was uneventful. L.T. had a severe expressive aphasia and severe motor abnormalities. His recovery was marked throughout by bizarre ideation. He believed that the hair on his fingers 'meant' that he was dead – the real L.T. had died in the accident. During the early stages of his recovery he became convinced that he would only get better if he did not eat and he had to be hospitalized on two occasions for this reason. Two years following injury L.T. was being treated at a post-acute rehabilitation centre to develop personal, domestic and community living skills. His anti-convulsant was changed from phenytoin (epinutin/dilantin) to carbamazepine to reduce sedating side-effects. Two results of the change became apparent almost immediately. The first was that L.T. rapidly developed considerable insight into his circumstances. Rather than stating that he would be fully recovered in six months (a consistent theme for him since injury) he began to say that he accepted the idea of doing as much as

he could for himself within the limits of his current deficits. This viewpoint was maintained approximately 60% of the time. The second effect of the medication change was a marked exacerbation of relatively short-lived but intensely held overvalued ideas. For example L.T. would hold a mirror up to his mouth when talking, claiming that if he did this for three days his speech would return to normal. He became extremely distressed and belligerent when thwarted. As the time period he had set himself passed, he recognized what he had thought before was foolish. He apologized for his behaviour but would, within hours or days, produce another *idée fixe*. Due to L.T.'s language disorder it was difficult to assess whether he was having auditory hallucinations or was thought-disordered. A short course of a neuroleptic was administered. After three months the neuroleptic was discontinued and L.T. has not relapsed (one year later).

Weston and Whitlock (1971) describe a case of Capgras syndrome after severe brain injury. In Capgras syndrome the patient believes that friends or family members have been replaced by identical doubles, who are imposters. The patient was a 20-year-old male with no previous psychiatric history who developed Capgras syndrome after a severe brain injury (coma duration in excess of 1 week). After six months the patient's condition improved and the delusional belief was no longer present. The authors of the report ascribe the origin of the disorder to a hallucinatory experience early in the recovery process when the patient thought he saw his parents being murdered in the courtyard by Chinese communists. The recollection of hallucinatory episodes which occurred during a period of delirium is known to figure in some cases of delusional belief. The misinterpretation of an apparently ordinary experience was implicated in a case of Capgras syndrome following traumatic brain injury reported by Alexander *et al.* (1979). The patient insisted that he had two families of identical composition. The patient insisted that the two wives had the same given names, looked very similar, came from the same town and so on. He described positive feelings towards both wives. The patient's belief in the reduplication of his families apparently stemmed from a relatively trivial change in the routine of how his wife picked him up for a

home visit. Although reportedly distressed by the implaus-
ibility of his story he could not be shaken from it. Despite
the patient's continued recovery he could not reorient his
experience which surrounded the reduplication into reality.

Reduplications for place have also been reported following
brain injury. Paterson and Zangwill (1944) describe two
patients and Benson *et al.* (1976) three patients, all with acute
(and transient) paramnesia for places. In each case the patient
believed their hospital was located in an environment which
was more familiar to them (e.g. in part of their own house).
In each case as the patients developed an increased ability to
perform on reality-tests they became more and more uncer-
tain about their views until they were recognized as
erroneous.

NEUROSES

Anxiety disorders

Anxiety may be a marked symptom following brain injury
(Tyerman and Humphrey, 1984). In some individuals, this
anxiety may have an organic component and onset of the disorder parallels the clearing of consciousness. Anxiety is probably under-diagnosed and under-treated. We have seen a
number of patients in whom the primary cause of functional
deficits was marked anxiety. Phobic disorders may also occur.

A.F. sustained a severe brain injury (coma duration 4 weeks)
when the motor cycle on which he was a passenger was
struck by a bus. During the acute hospitalization he
developed fixed delusional beliefs of being physically abused
by care staff. On admission to the TLC he repeatedly sought
assurance that he was not going to be beaten even though
he no longer believed that he was being beaten. He attempted
to convince staff that he had been a boxer at college so (as
he said later) staff would be less likely to attack him. At the
same time he was constantly seeking reassurance from staff
and had a great deal of difficulty tolerating more than a few
minutes by himself. This was to such a degree that he wanted
male staff with him in the bathroom when he took a shower.
He was very frightened that his girlfriend would leave him.

A.F.'s attention and memory, self-care and community skills were profoundly disrupted by his level of anxiety. He asked questions constantly ('is my girlfriend really going to visit', 'are you going to beat me', 'please don't lock me in my room'). The staff's responses to these questions were forgotten immediately. Treatment involved the careful titration of a benzodiazepine and behavioural training directed at inappropriate statements, time alone, and asking questions (recording information).

L.R. a female factory worker without a previous history of psychiatric disturbance, suffered a severe brain injury at work when her head was caught in a machine press. She sustained unilateral damage to fifth and seventh cranial nerves affecting the right side of her face and lost vision in her right eye. She had mild cerebellar ataxia and moderate cognitive sequelae. L.R. was discharged from acute hospitalization after ten weeks and spent the following 18 months at home with her mother (who had a substance abuse disorder). While at home she had developed a serious depressive disorder and agoraphobia, resulting in her never going out on her own. She was treated by her psychiatrist with imipramine (Tofranil) and psychotherapy with some improvement. She was however requiring 12 hours of attendant care per day primarily as a result of her anxiety and 'illness behaviour'. At the TLC, treatment included systematic desensitization for her agoraphobia and gradually increasing degrees of responsibility and independence with training in appropriate systems to maximize functioning, given her cognitive deficits. She was subsequently able to move to her own apartment, live independently and attend local college.

OBSESSIVE–COMPULSIVE DISORDERS

Obsessive-compulsive disorders (OCD) are known to be associated with a variety of organic disorders including epilepsy, encephalitis and traumatic brain injury. OCD was well documented in patients following the epidemic of encephalitis lethargica following World War I. A number of patients with obsessive-compulsive disorders following herpes simplex encephalitis have been described (see Giles and Morgan, 1989). Incidence in post-traumatic brain injury patients has been estimated to be between 0.3% (Lishman, 1968) and 3% (Hillbom, 1960). McKeon *et al.* (1984) described obsessive-compulsive disorders following mild brain injury (three cases) and severe brain injury (one case). Premorbidly three of the patients were reported as having normal personalities and one as being mildly obsessional. Onset was very rapid in all four cases. These authors conclude that brain injury may be a contributory factor in the development of obsessive-compulsive disorders. Drummond (1988) has reported a case of OCD occurring six months following traumatic brain injury. Behavioural psychotherapy proved largely ineffective but the settlement of a relatively minor compensation claim led to a considerable reduction in symptomatology. Basing her discussion on the work of Gray (1982), Drummond suggests that OCD may occur if the septohippocampal system (a component of the limbic system) becomes overly sensitized to a stimulus. This might happen following a range of life events, trauma being one, and frequently occurs in conjunction with depressive symptoms. The septohippocampal system becomes overaroused and stimuli become emotionally charged as aversive (Drummond, 1988; Maloy, 1987). Elsewhere in this volume we have argued that many of the difficulties of brain-injured persons result from not manipulating available information mentally, e.g. planning, checking ongoing plans and monitoring available environmental information. OCD appears to be the opposite and involves compulsive planning, checking and monitoring rituals.

Hysteria

Hysterical phenomena have recently been defined by Miller (1987) as symptoms of a kind that would normally be associated with a disease process, for which no pathological process can be found and in which, in many cases, a pathological process appears unlikely. Hysterical phenomena can result from neurological insults and have been observed in patients with mild to severe brain injury. It is only usually with mildly injured patients that the differential diagnosis centres on hysteria. In Chapter 2 we have described a model of illness behaviour which can help clinicians avoid dichotomous thinking. Patients are seen who complain of memory deficits whose pattern of loss does not accord with known patterns of memory disorder, despite having sustained a severe injury. On the other hand, dissociative disorders (such as the Ganza syndrome) are known to occur in the severely brain-injured adult.

Denial

Denial is one of the most complex disorders encountered by rehabilitation professionals. Problems of denial and lack of insight frequently impair the ability to utilize standard rehabilitation interventions. The degree to which denial of deficit is a result of neurological damage is unclear. Individuals, who are not known to have suffered brain injury, are reported to deny deficits. For example, up to 20% of patients treated in a cardiac intensive care unit 'seriously doubt' whether they have had a cardiac arrest. For some, denial by patients can best be regarded as a disorder of self-image and like other 'agnosias' the individual has particular difficulty in learning information in this area. Some individuals become belligerent and refuse to listen to any information regarding their deficits. Others reluctantly admit their disabilities on confrontation but then forget this information very rapidly. Some people deny the deficit, for instance memory impairment, or alternatively deny the deficit's impact on their performance of daily living skills. Patients frequently attempt to undermine the relevance of any evidence disconfirming their ability, for example, 'I never have been able to do that', or 'I will be able to do that when I am at home'. In some cases, particularly immediately following injury, family members deny the severity of the individual's deficits, again suggesting that denial in the patient is not solely the result of neurological damage. It is possible to identify two different forms of denial: verbal and performance. To assess verbal denial, the interviewer may ask whether the individual has noted any changes in himself since his injury, whether he is aware of what other people have noticed or told him about his performance and from this, evaluate the individual's understanding of what these changes might mean to him. To assess performance, observations of denial can assess whether the patient attempts to perform activities he cannot accomplish.

One client injured in an automobile accident (coma duration

nine days) was sure that she could return to work immediately. When confronted with the very poor quality of her performance on a minor clerical task exclaimed 'I can't believe I can't do that' and burst into tears. She later backed away from that position and it took many such encounters before she could acknowledge the areas on which she needed to improve performance before returning to work.

Rehabilitation of denial involves the therapist talking about what the patient currently can and cannot do. While avoiding speaking in absolutes, the patient should be helped to achieve an understanding of his current deficits. The therapist should provide information in a clear, consistent and highly-repetitive manner related to the client's present performance. The client should not be deprived of all hope of improvement. Gentle and consistent confrontation around the individual's deficits can assist in the development of a stance (being in the world) which allows the client to see him or herself as a valid human being with deficits. It is essential, therefore, while the therapist is trying to undermine views which hamper rehabilitation in the client, to also build self-esteem and highlight what the individual can do. When the patients perform activities at which they fail, feedback given immediately can be effective. If repeated often enough, it can help the patient become aware of the reasons for failure and develop a positive approach to overcoming the problems. Since the patients' experience of themselves is similar to what it was before the accident, external feedback is essential to develop knowledge of difficulties. Additional treatment approaches are discussed in Chapters 7 and 13.

Prevarication

To lie, an individual must be conscious of the falsity of a statement and have an intent to deceive (Ford *et al.*, 1988). The phenomenon of lying, while to some degree ubiquitous in our society, can be seen as pathological when it becomes persistent and is destructive to the quality of an individual's life. Though distinct from confabulation, lying may be on a continuum with it and is often associated with frontal lobe impairment. Some patients appear to be seeking attention but for others the content of the lie may be a result of processes of ego maintenance as clients attempt to present themselves as being competent and important.

Hyperactivity

Hyperactivity may be associated with an arousal problem and presents as inability to inhibit motor activity. Paradoxically, in some patients the disorder may be exacerbated by sedatives.

Sleep disorders

Prigatano and co-workers (1982) studied sleep disorders occurring 6–59 months following brain injury. Patients showed less rapid eye movement (REM) sleep and more frequent awakening than age-matched controls. However, neither the time spent in REM sleep nor scores on the Wechsler Memory Scale were related to complaints of decreased or absent dreaming.

Benyakar and co-workers (1988), studying patients in the later stages of recovery, did not find an overall decrease in dreaming although they did report changed content of dreams, for instance, a decrease in dreams involving sexual content and an increase in dreams of a threatening nature. Narcolepsy, a disorder in which the sufferer is overtaken by irresistible attacks of sleep, is occasionally seen following brain trauma (Fernando Miranda, personal communication). As with individuals whose narcolepsy is of non-traumatic origin, treatment with Methylphenidate (Ritalin) has been recommended (Silverstone and Turner, 1988).

MEDICATION

Medication intended to address both psychiatric and/or medical conditions may exacerbate psychiatric disorders, further compromising the patient's ability to function. The therapist should be conversant with most common side-effects of medication and their impact on patient functioning. Pharmacological treatment may be directed towards four goals: potentiating the recovery process; remediating neuropsychological deficits; amelioration of specific neurological disorders such as headache, spasticity and epilepsy; remediating psychiatric symptoms (Gualtieri,

1988). Lack of research literature in drug therapies with this population necessitates extrapolation from evidence derived from other populations. Mechanisms of action, contra-indications and doses are the responsibility of medical personnel and are not included in this brief discussion. Many individuals with injured nervous systems may however be treated with drug doses lower than those customarily used with the general psychiatric population.

Therapists should have an understanding of the pharmacological agents used in the treatment of the individual with brain injury, especially those which could interfere with the retraining of functional skills. Observation of the individual's performance and behaviour in functional activities can be invaluable to the physicians in the diagnosis and prescription of medication. Pharmacological interventions should rarely be used in isolation from other interventions with the brain-injured population.

Psychostimulants

A number of workers have reported single-case studies of the use of psychostimulants with the post-acute, brain-injured individual. There is considerable evidence that these drugs have a positive effect in both children and adults with disorders of attention, hyperactivity, impulsivity and emotional lability (Wender *et al.*, 1985; Gualtieri, 1988). Evans and co-workers (Evans *et al.*, 1987b) administered the psychostimulants methylphenidate (MPH, Ritalin) and dextroamphetamine (DEA) to a young man with attention, memory and initiation difficulties two years after a severe traumatic brain injury. The medication trials were double-blind, placebo-controlled dose response studies. With the active drug condition, improvements were noted in memory and attention with a greater response to DEA than MPH. The patient reported considerable improvement in his daily life functioning. More recently Gualtieri and Evans (1988) reported a double-blind, placebo-controlled trial of MPH with 15 closed head injury patients who were post-acute and functioning at a high level. Results indicated 14 subjective responders and 10 with both subjective and objective evidence of a treatment effect. Group analysis did not indicate a robust treatment effect on many of those measured. A *post hoc* statistical analysis which separated objective responders from non-objective responders suggested more marked effects. Treatment effects did not appear to be sustained at the one-year period as placebo substitution in three patients did not result in deterioration. The authors tentatively suggest that this last phenomena may be the result of a permanent change of neuronal responsiveness as a result of MPH treatment. The authors conclude that their results support the notion that some symptomatic improvements may be the results of low dose stimulant treatment. They also conjectured that stimulant treatment may advance the course of recovery. Further research would be of particular interest to occupational therapists. Work should examine skill learning with or without medication and the transfer of skills from medicated to non-medicated conditions.

Recently there have been a number of reports of the use of anti-parkinsonian medications with the severely brain injured (Guidice *et al.*, 1986; Lal *et al.*, 1988). Methodological difficulties with these studies are profound but continuing trials are probably warranted. Patients following traumatic brain injury may demonstrate akinesia, bradykinesia, profound lethargy, mask-like expression, depression and mental slowing, all features of Parkinson's Disease. Some authors have suggested a therapeutic window, for instance, an effective time schedule of action for the use of these agents.

Anti-convulsants

Anti-convulsants are frequently prescribed routinely after brain injury. In the acute stage, phenytoin (epanutin/dilantin) is becoming increasingly regarded as the drug of choice, because of its effectiveness in protecting the brain from ischaemic damage. Treatment with anti-epileptic drugs may be maintained for considerable periods after the acute stage for reasons of prophylaxis, often needlessly. This is particularly unfortunate as many anti-convulsant medications have side-effects of sedation, depression, motor impairment and memory impairment. Frequently used anti-convulsants are phenytoin (epanutin/dilantin), carbamazepine (tegretol) and sodium valporate (VPA/epilim/depakene/depacoat). Carbamazepine is generally well-tolerated and it is used primarily for the treatment of generalized and complex partial seizure disorders. It appears to be useful in the treatment of aggressive patients with abnormal

EEGs, particularly those with temporal lobe epilepsy. It also appears to have an effect on a range of other disorders seen after brain-injury including mania, affective disorders (a mild antidepressant), emotional instability and aggressive disorders of non-epileptiform origin.

Lithium carbonate

Lithium carbonate is prescribed in the general psychiatric population for the prophylaxis of unipolar and bipolar affective disorders. Its effect on those with manic aggression is well-known and a number of single-case reports have appeared of successful treatment of juveniles with manic disorders apparently induced by brain trauma (Cohen *et al.*, 1977; Sinanna, 1984). It may also help patients who can be broadly described as cyclothymic and can be effective in some patients with recurrent rage outbursts. Recently, a number of studies have reported toxicity reactions in patients on combined carbamazepine-lithium therapy where both medications are at acceptable blood levels (Parmelee and O'Shanick, 1988; Shukla *et al.*, 1984).

Beta blockers

The beta blocker propranolol has been used in the treatment of aggression (Greendyke *et al.*, 1986). Possible side-effects may include dysphoria, hypotension and bradycardia. Propranolol has also been used in the treatment of anxiety disorders after brain trauma. Gualtieri (1988), after reviewing the literature, suggests that its effectiveness with anxiety disorders may be limited to those individuals who have a strong somatic component to anxiety-precipitating aggression.

Medications for affective disorders

The presentation of affective disorders after brain injury may be atypical. The tricyclic anti-depressants, while the drugs of choice, do appear to cause a raised incidence of seizures, and could affect memory and motor performance. This will be reduced by the selection of a tricyclic with a minimal anticholinergic effect. Tricyclics have also been used in the treatment of agitation (Jackson *et al.*, 1984).

Antipsychotic medication

Antipsychotics (phenothiazines and busipherones) may be used to treat the individual with psychotic episodes after brain injury. These medications are also sometimes used in the treatment of severe agitation and assaultiveness, particularly in the patient emerging from coma. Yudofsky *et al.* (1987) have noted that there is little evidence that antipsychotic medications are specifically effective in treating aggression. They advise against using them because of their sedating side effects, limited effectiveness, possible paradoxical effects and the risk of serious complications such as dyskinesias and a reduced seizure threshold. Gualtieri (1988) noted that the rare injury-induced Tourettes syndrome, may respond to neuroleptic medication.

Sedatives and hypnotics

Like antipsychotic medication, sedative and hypnotic medications, for example, the benzodiazepines and barbiturates, are sometimes used to treat acute aggressive episodes. Their use on a repeated basis is probably contraindicated due to a paradoxical releasing effect, chronic oversedation and interference with learning. Patients who are highly anxious may respond positively to a small dose of a benzodiazepine. Levine (1988) has suggested that buspirone, a new anxiolytic medication, may be effective in the treatment of agitation. Buspirone (Buspar) is unrelated to the benzodiazepines and does not appear to cause sedation.

Therapists should have sufficient knowledge of medication to help physicians evaluate the medication's effectiveness. Whyte (1988) has recently noted the difficulties involved in making an assessment of drug efficacy. Patient performance over time can be extremely erratic, and vary greatly with other stimuli. Staff tend to concentrate on problematic components of behaviour. The effects of the introduction of medication may not be so dramatic as to make it obvious that it is responsible for the change. Whyte advocates the use of standardized baseline recordings, individualized for each patient and compared blind to placebo. Selective videoing of patients in relevant real-world activities before, during and after the drug has been withdrawn with the staff viewing and rating the randomly ordered videos on pre-selected parameters, can be valuable for establishing the effectiveness of drug therapy.

SUMMARY

Chapter 5 has described the psychiatric consequences of brain injury. Almost any symptom complex which can occur in the general psychiatric population can occur following brain trauma. Disturbed patterns of behaviour may become apparent as the individual emerges from coma or onset could occur later, possibly as the individual attempts (and in many cases fails) to resume their past lifestyle and reintegrate into the community at large. For some the injury provokes an exaggeration of a previous tendency but for many the psychiatric difficulties represent a major behavioural change. As well as psychiatric disturbance in the early recovery period, brain injury also represents a risk factor for later psychiatric problems. Prolonged social isolation may be a factor increasing patient risk. Particularly striking is the increased risk of suicide among brain-injured survivors. In the next chapter we discuss the principles underlying assessment of the brain-injured adult.

6

Assessment of the brain-injured adult

INTRODUCTION

Several distinct frames of reference may be used in the assessment of the brain-injured adult. The approach adopted depends in part on the discipline performing the assessment. Perspectives could include the neurological, psychological, psychiatric, psychodynamic, educational, physical, functional, social and vocational. Functionally oriented therapists are principally concerned with social, functional and vocational independence. In order to assist brain-injured individuals re-establish independence, the therapist determines their retained abilities: home, social and work environments; and the limitations resulting from the brain injury itself. Furthermore, the therapist should understand the strategies that individuals use when attempting to overcome deficits and consider the methods which could facilitate their learning. Treatment focuses on areas which require the minimum amount of learning and lead to the maximum improvement in function.

Neurofunctional assessment considers the dynamic inter-relationship of the individual and the environment. The implicit and explicit demands of the environment are relevant in determining functional abilities. Cognitive, behavioural, physical and social abilities are examined in the environmental context in order to establish the brain-injured person's level of disability and handicap (see below). The demands of the environment need to be determined before drawing conclusions about the individual's functional abilities. Utilizing the natural context (or contexts) in the assessment process increases the ecological validity of the data. For example, a person's ability in a wheelchair in their community will be different according to the type of community in which they live. Standardized tests requiring inference about function (and functional scales from which composite disability or independence scores are derived) provide useful adjunctive data but should not be used in preference to naturalistic observation and description.

This chapter is not intended to supply the reader with an exhaustive list of assessment tools but discusses the fundamental principles of the assessment process. Specific assessment methods are discussed in the relevant chapters.

The aims of a neurofunctional assessment are:

1. to identify retained functional skills;
2. to identify deficits limiting independent functioning;
3. to identify environmental factors which support independent functioning;
4. to identify the demands placed on the individual by the environment;
5. to identify the strategies used to overcome functional deficits;
6. to identify methods to assist the relearning of functional skills;
7. to identify the changes required to enable the individual to function in his or her environmental context.

Functional data can be used to determine current status, optimal retraining methods, appropriate provision of follow-up or for litigation or research purposes. Functional assessment establishes a baseline of functional ability to monitor progress and forms a basis on which to establish goals or target behaviours required for the rehabilitation team's integrated treatment plan. Retained abilities may be used in the process of remediating or compensating for deficits (Cohen and Anthony, 1984; Ylvisaker, 1985). Functional assessment can be applied to personal, domestic and community activities of daily living, social and interpersonal skills and vocational status (Crewe and Turner, 1984). Assessment is not a static event but a cyclical process where the patient's response to therapy is considered on a continuing basis.

THE NEUROFUNCTIONAL ASSESSMENT MODEL

The neurofunctional model of assessment presented in this chapter incorporates aspects of the medical, psychosocial and educational models which are outlined below and is cognizant of the model of illness behaviour discussed in Chapter 2.

a) Medical

The medical model is concerned with disease and is discussed in general terms in Chapter 2. Current medical views of dysfunction include a three-point classification scheme of impairment, disability and handicap (World Health Organization, 1980). Impairment refers to loss or abnormality of psychological, physiological or anatomical structure or function (Wood, 1980). Disability refers to the functional consequences of impairments defined in terms of cognitive, emotional and physical performance (Nagi, 1976). Not every impairment results in disability and similar patterns of disability can result from different impairments. For example, two brain-injured individuals may be dependent on community mobility, one as a result of motor impairment, the other because of a memory disorder. Handicap refers to an individual's disadvantage in a society because of an inability to fulfil socially approved roles. For example, inability to work is a handicap when it was the major role prior to the injury and the patient suffers deprivation as a result (Wade, 1987). Impairment can be measured and interpreted in comparison with a fixed norm, whereas disability and handicap requires comparison with an evaluative norm. Although the nomenclature varies between authors there is increasing consensus on a number of points: recognition of the imperfect relationship between an impairment of a diagnosed condition and the extent of functional limitation; a distinction between discrete human capabilities (e.g. hearing) and broad human adjustment phenomena (e.g. vocational success); and understanding that not only functional limitations but also environmental factors affect adaptation in major social roles such as work (Sigelman *et al.*, 1979). Beyond the level of analysis represented here by handicap one can consider life outcomes.

Vreede (1988) has criticized what he calls the negative triad of impairment, disability and handicap and has suggested replacing this with an elaboration of the positive term ADL. Vreede's suggested tripartite definition would distinguish between the physical or mental operations needed for daily living activities (ODLs), the functional activities themselves (ADLs proper) and the individual's daily pursuits or human endeavours (IDLs) or ideas of daily living. Vreede's proposed system is hierarchical in that an ADL can only be performed if the prerequisite ODLs are available. However even when the ODLs are present an ADL may not be performed if it is not part of an IDL (Vreede, 1988).

b) Psychosocial

The psychosocial model concerns handicap and the individual's inability to overcome impairments and disabilities in order to return to established or desired roles. The person is approached in relation to their environment and ability to interact with it in a constructive way. Psychosocial assessment is concerned with adustment, self-esteem and related concepts which may be central to determining life outcome.

c) Educational

The educational model is concerned with the process involved in assisting clients to live with their disabilities in their environment (Trieschmann, 1980). The functional assessment aims to enlarge the person's opportunities to pursue a wide array of activities consistent with their personal goals, and is concerned with how the individual actually functions in normal environments. The model is essentially that of 'learning' in the recovery of behavioural competencies.

Functional assessment is used by the therapist to understand all aspects of the brain-injured individual's impairments, disabilities and handicaps. Data concerning the individual's goals and motivation towards recovery assist the rehabilitation process.

1. IDENTIFYING RETAINED FUNCTIONAL SKILLS

Information regarding degree of independence and personality prior to brain injury assists in determining changes in function. Level of independent functioning will depend on a wide range of factors including motivation, cognitive impairment, ability to communicate needs and physical disabilities. The therapist is concerned with competence and is not solely pathology-oriented. Functional assessment should consider both the patient's best performance and what the patient habitually does, as performance after brain injury is often highly variable. Consideration of the individual's general skills over a period of time establishes whether the behaviours observed are normal and customary for the patient, and ascertains a realistic 'tonic' level of ability. The fact that the person can carry out an activity once, such as preparing lunch in an occupational therapy department, does not mean that they are able to carry out the same task on a regular basis against a background of the other competing demands of their specific natural environment.

2. IDENTIFYING DEFICITS LIMITING INDEPENDENT FUNCTIONING

Assessments performed by all professional disciplines provides considerable information of use to the functionally oriented therapist. Assessments which may be available to the therapist include medical and neurological evaluations, neuropsychological test data, occupational therapy, physical therapy, speech and language evaluation, and educational and behavioural assessments. The majority of these assessments – which may overlap in content – employ standardized test procedures or interviews. These reports, in combination with the functional assessment, help the interdisciplinary team understand how the individual's brain injury impacts overall functioning. It also allows all aspects of assessment to be co-ordinated into a coherent and rational rehabilitation plan.

Knowledge of the assessment procedures of other professionals (and their frames of reference) assists therapists to understand the reports of other disciplines. Here we briefly review the information available from some of these reports.

i) **Medical assessments** describe the individual's medical condition by taking a medical history, and by investigation of neurological, medical and orthopaedic signs and symptoms. The examination is usually divided into a mental state and physical examination. Specific medical disciplines conduct special diagnostic investigations, such as CAT scans, pathology tests or nerve conduction studies. Diagnoses are made and medical treatment determined.

ii) **Neuropsychiatric assessment** determines the psychiatric sequelae after brain injury through assessment by a semi-structured interview and observation (psychiatric sequelae after brain injury are discussed in Chapter 5). Specific nomenclature may be used such as the terminology of the DSM III (Revised) of the American Psychiatric Association (1987). The neuropsychiatrist relies on accurate observation and assessment by staff of the person's behaviour under varying conditions in order to determine what, if any, psychoactive medications are warranted.

iii) **Neuropsychological assessment** evaluates the areas of intellectual functioning: attention, concentration and alertness; problem solving and judgement; flexibility of the thought process; academic functioning, such as reading, writing and arithmetic; sensory and perceptual functioning; language comprehension and expression; memory and learning; rate of information processing; effects of feedback upon performance; temporal and spatial conceptual abilities; fatigue and motor functioning; mood state and vocational interest (Baxter *et al.*, 1985; Lezak, 1987). Anastasi's *Psychological Testing* (1988) provides an excellent introduction to psychometric theory as well as providing useful descriptions of the most common tests of intellectual functioning. Lezak's *Neuropsychological Assessment* (1987) provides an excellent introduction to the subject. In addition, some psychologists use projective techniques to assess personality and areas of personal concern.

iv) **Physical therapy assessment** provides an evaluation of an individual's motor and sensory system. Investigation includes analysis of dynamic disorders of movement caused by spasticity, flaccidity and ataxia, tremor, rigidity, apraxia, and alteration of sensation, for example, tactile, proprioceptive and kinaesthetic senses; and static disorders of movement caused by contractures and other orthopaedic conditions. The need for assistive devices, for example, ankle foot orthosis (AFO) and equipment to aid mobility will also be evaluated. The assessment also frequently determines the individual's ability to carry out basic physical activities such as rolling in bed, coming to sitting from lying and ability to ambulate for specified distances with or without assistive devices. Various assessments measures and scales may be used.

v) **Occupational therapists' assessments** of motor and sensory abilities, cognition and social functioning in personal, domestic and community activities of daily living. In addition, occupational therapists may perform pre-vocational and vocational assessment. Both clinical and standardized assessments may be used but clinical assessment methods usually predominate.

vi) **Speech and language assessment** involves standardized and non-standardized procedures designed to identify the factors responsible for the disruption of speech and language functions (Beukelman *et al.*, 1984). Speech and language function is assessed in order to retrain the individual to communicate more effectively. More recently speech and language pathologists have begun to consider 'pragmatics', a term used to describe how an individual uses language in social discourse.

vii) **Education assessment** aims to identify academic ability and the capacity to integrate academic skills and perform complex cognitive tasks (Baxter *et al.*, 1985). Education skills include reading, writing, and arithmetic in practical situations. In adult patients, the educator works closely with the speech and language therapist and occupational therapist on activities such as bus timetables, writing application forms or handling money (Edney, 1988).

viii) **Behavioural assessment** procedures may be used by any member of the treatment team. Behaviour assessment helps to pinpoint maladaptive behaviours and determine the environmental contingencies which maintain unwanted behaviours (Giles and Fussey, 1988). Assessment in this area assists the rehabilitation team establish behavioural programmes in order to reduce abnormal behaviours and re-teach the brain-injured appropriate functional and social skills (see below and Chapters 11 and 12).

ix) **Social and emotional assessment** establishes the psychological needs of the individual and family via a social history, and by establishing home, family and work situations. This enables appropriate counselling and interventions to help the brain-injured individual and family adjust to their sense of loss and the (frequently) rapidly changing circumstances of life after injury. Family assessment is designed to help assess the family's dynamics and the family's response to their brain-injured 'loved one'.

Therapists will find that assessments performed by other professional disciplines assist in the understanding of functional skills deficits. On many occasions a conjoint analysis by an occupational therapist and a psychologist, speech therapist or physical therapist is required to determine the cause of a specific functional deficit. A standardized test performed by a member of another discipline cannot replace a true functional assessment. While there is a place for some types of psychometric testing by therapists the most important type of assessment to be done by therapists is clinical as the therapist wishes to investigate performance. This investigation is more like an experimental study of an individual (ideographic) than an attempt to relate the performance of the individual to a tested population (nomothetic). Psychometric evaluations generally are designed to measure the probability that an individual will succeed or fail at a task. The place of the functional assessment is made more central by the fact that psychometric testing and other standardized tests are not powerfully predictive of everyday function. Heaton and Pendelton (1981) reviewed attempts to relate neuropsychological tests to patient's everyday functioning. They found that some tests predicted broad functional outcome within certain population groups, but stated that clinical assessment was superior to neuropsychological prediction. There is no accepted rationale for making inferences about a person's functional skills based on measures of symptomatology. This failure of signs or symptoms taken in isolation to predict outcome is not limited to neuropsychological testing. Measures of psychiatric symptoms have been shown not to predict vocational rehabilitation outcome (Green *et al.*, 1968) or to correlate with vocational skills (Ellsworth *et al.*, 1968). In comparison, measures of work adjustment skills, i.e. inferences from a subset of real behaviours, predict vocational rehabilitation outcome (Green *et al.*, 1968).

Assessment should attempt to account for inabilities to perform functional activities. Functional skills deficits may be the result of physical, behavioural, cognitive or emotional/psychiatric difficulties and are most usually the result of their complex interrelation. Assessing in functional situations through observation and graded degrees of assistance, establishes the deficits which are hampering the individual's performance (see below). By attempting to establish the patterns of deficits underlying performance, greater understanding of the individual's level of functioning is possible. In addition the nature of the neurological deficit underlying functional skills deficits may have implications for recovery of function. Analysis of tasks facilitates an understanding of the skills required to perform functional activities and knowledge of a normal activity sequence is often required for retraining purposes (Giles and Shore, 1989a). More complex functional tasks incorporate more numerous basic skills – the more complex the skill the more likely it is to be disrupted.

3. IDENTIFYING THE ENVIRONMENTAL FACTORS WHICH SUPPORT INDEPENDENT FUNCTIONING

Functional assessments include evaluations of the future home, work or social environments. The context in which an assessment is conducted affects the number of available environmental cues influencing performance. A brain-injured person in hospital with unfamiliar procedures to follow is likely to have more difficulty than in more familiar home, work or social settings.

Under the heading 'environmental factors' are included all the resources individuals have to assist them. These resources could be the patient's family and friends who are prepared to provide care or the institutional support services available to play a role in determining the patient's likely level of independence. Examples of services include sheltered housing, sheltered workshops and transportation (Bowe, 1979). Some charitable societies, such as Headway or the Carers Association can also provide very significant support for families of the brain-injured and patients.

Social and cultural factors are able to help or hinder a patient's ability to function, for instance some extended families are able to care for a severely impaired individual better than a typical nuclear family. Financial resources also play a role, as money, allowances and grants open alternative opportunities for greater independence and satisfaction, for example, buying labour saving devices or paying for extra time and help from a carer.

The physical environment and social contacts should be assessed both on a macro (urban/rural) and micro level. Differences range from the amount of support which could be available from neighbours to physically help the patient, to the distance it is necessary to travel to get to the grocery store or bank. Robinete and Vondran (1988) demonstrated systematic variation in kerb heights and the amount of time that street-crossing signals allowed for crossing streets. Large population centres have higher kerbs and allow less street-crossing time than small towns.

In some instances the patient is best advised to relocate to an environment where the relevant services and amenities are available. The environment may need altering to enable the individual to gain more independence or make it easier for the family to care for the patient. Adaptations, such as house extensions or hand rails, could be considered for the physically-disabled individual but only when a realistic view of further recovery potential is predictable. Overly rapid alterations of the environment could increase the individual's dependency on physical equipment or cues, thereby impeding their ability to function without adaptations. Conversely excessive delay in the introduction of adaptations prevents the individual from learning to use the adaptations and results in a lower level of independence so that the person requires more supervision on discharge to the community. It is, for example, inappropriate to introduce an electric wheelchair to a client one week before discharge from an acute rehabilitation setting.

Environmental factors should be considered in designing retraining programmes. For example, McClain and Todd (1990) in their discussion of food store accessibility point out that large grocery stores tend to be more accessible than local stores (this may be due to the architectural demands of the use of shopping trolleys). These factors should be considered in training individuals where to shop.

4. IDENTIFYING THE DEMANDS PLACED ON THE INDIVIDUAL BY THE ENVIRONMENT

To understand the demands placed upon the brain-injured individual it is necessary to assess his roles, routine and culture. The therapist should develop an understanding of the person's own functional goals and appreciate the social pressures on him and his family. Role and status within the family, work and community influence perceptions of the person's degree of loss after brain injury and expectations for recovery. People occupy multiple roles, which vary with age, gender, social class and personal history. Family roles are 'repetitive patterns of behaviour by which family members fulfil and carry out regular functions' (Bishop *et al.*, 1984). People engage in activities which are meaningful to them and the family unit. Actual roles differ from any typical or normative roles because of the way the person perceives and defines his or her own situation. Social and community roles are perceived within the context of their environment but these are defined expectations of behaviour in social settings. After brain injury, the individual may be unable to perform tasks and fulfil roles that had symbolic significance for his family or which served to maintain social status. The patient becomes more dependent, 'forcing' certain aspects of his pre-morbid roles onto others, usually relatives who may resent or feel ill-equipped to perform them (Williams, 1984, 1987). The psychological impact of these changes may affect all aspects of community integration.

Functional assessment and the rehabilitation process should respond to the demands and expectations placed on the individual by himself, his family, and the social and work community. This requires developing an understanding of the person's typical daily routine, the number and type of tasks actually completed during the day, the degree of help given to him, and how he could incorporate new skills into his day. Assessment defines family members' roles and considers methods for achieving community reintegration. When staff have not understood the 'meaning' of the patient's deficits either for the patient himself, or his family, it becomes difficult to set realistic goals or to adequately address interpersonal issues. An assessment of the staff or family's expectations of the brain-injured person's recovery and discussion of potential rehabilitation approaches to improve level of functioning, will improve communication and reduce misinterpretations and distress.

5. IDENTIFYING THE STRATEGIES USED TO OVERCOME FUNCTIONAL DEFICITS

There are many different ways to perform functional activities. Assessment should establish the approaches previously used by the individual and the methods attempted since the injury, so alternative strategies can be constructed to aid overall performance. In some cases, the strategies spontaneously employed by the brain-injured individual may be helpful and can be supported and developed by the occupational therapist (Giles and Morgan, 1989). In other cases, the patient may have developed self-defeating and inappropriate compensatory behaviours such as manipulating others to gain help, or not performing the task at all (Giles and Clark-Wilson, 1988b). Some individuals are unable to develop strategies and attempt to perform the task in novel ways on every occasion. Teaching specific adaptive strategies, which can be practised until mastery is achieved, is central to the rehabilitation process.

The health and daily living form (Moos *et al.*, 1988) may be used to assist in the assessment of coping methods in mildly impaired individuals. Of particular interest are the scales relating to methods of coping, which include active cognitive coping, active behavioural coping and avoidance coping. In addition there are scales relating to the focus of coping which include logical analysis, information seeking, problem solving, affective regulation and emotional discharge. Hinkeldey and Corrigan (1990) investigated the symptoms and psychological functioning of 55 severely head injured patients. These authors found that the patients they studied were significantly more likely to use avoidance coping than were a community sample in dealing with a major life event. The head-injured people were, for example, more likely to report that they 'took it out' on others than the community comparison group. Under focus of coping the head-injured people were found to make lessened use of logical analysis or of information-seeking in their attempts to cope.

6. IDENTIFYING METHODS TO ASSIST THE RELEARNING OF FUNCTIONAL SKILLS

As discussed in Chapter 7, even the most severely impaired brain-injured adult has the ability to learn (change behaviour in response to systematic changes in the environment). While the basic set of techniques available to therapists for retraining functional skills are limited they should be adapted to meet the patient's needs. This portion of the assessment is initially an educated process of trial and error. It is important to determine if patients are able to use auditory, written, pictographic or modelling cues so the relevant details can be incorporated in programme designs. Careful analysis of the activity, graded interventions and evaluation of functional ability should help the therapist provide the minimum number of cues required for performance. Whilst assessing or teaching functional skills, excessive variability in executing an activity impedes learning, therefore a sufficient number of cues should be given to ensure similar behaviour each time the activity is practised.

The functional tasks can be analysed (see Chapter 7) to identify the steps involved in the process. One assessment method which emphasizes functional activity and retraining procedures is Portage (Wilson, 1985). This approach can be adapted for use with individuals with acquired neurological injury. Family members are taught specific (behavioural) interventions which are carried out by them in their home environment. By using a home-based programme, problems with generalization can potentially be avoided. In addition it is hoped that a functional focus could be maintained, and carers would be more equipped to cope with future functional problems.

7. IDENTIFYING THE CHANGES REQUIRED TO ENABLE THE INDIVIDUAL TO FUNCTION IN AN ENVIRONMENTAL CONTEXT

A functional assessment requires an understanding of the actual difference between current performance and that required for independent functioning. Neurofunctional assessment is out-

come-oriented. 'Recovery' is a relative term and is not an appropriate goal of treatment after the acute stage of recovery. The
therapist should focus on outcome and placement. Most of
the factors considered above are relevant for determining the
minimum criteria to be achieved to allow the client to function
in his environment. For example, a severely impaired patient,
M.F., could be cared for at home by his parents but only if he
was able to perform basic independence skills like transfers and
washing and dressing himself. Once these goals were achieved,
he was discharged from an in-patient unit, and other goals to
increase his independent social functioning were addressed on
an out-patient basis (Giles and Shore, 1989a). The question the
therapist should ask is 'what are the minimum changes required
by the client to allow him or her to live in their environment?'

TIMING OF ASSESSMENTS

The therapist needs to observe, identify improvements and
institute retraining procedures at the appropriate time. In the
early period of recovery, a brief assessment determines the
patient's level of responsiveness, ability to communicate, orientation to time, place and person, physical abilities and some
aspects of cognitive functioning. Attention is directed towards
the patient's physical state to ensure that contractures are prevented. It is not helpful to spend long periods assessing functions which are changing rapidly. Brief assessment procedures
such as use of passive range of motion (PROM) recordings and
the GOAT (Chapter 8) are recommended (Levin *et al.*, 1979).
In-depth assessment at this early stage is likely to result in an
overestimation of deficits, because levels of arousal and attention are insufficient to allow a clear appraisal of higher cognitive
functions. A patient that is constantly distracted by aspects of
his environment will show poor performances in tests of diverse
functions. In the acute stage, rehabilitation is often 'deficit
driven', leading the therapist to focus on remediation of impairments. As the patient progresses, assessment becomes more
functionally driven: the therapist attempts to help the patient
develop skills specifically needed to function in his environment.

Performing an activity once does not guarantee that the
patient is independent in the task. Performing the activity on a
regular basis in natural settings is a more robust indicator.

Assessment should be of sufficient duration to ensure a representative sample of the person's characteristic behaviour, and should be performed at regular intervals to show the individual's rate of recovery. By the time the post-acute stage is reached, standardized and descriptive assessments can be focused on the individual's level of ability, as a baseline from which changes can be evaluated. In practice the therapist will make judgements about which skills to assess in the light of the extent of impairment. For example, if a patient cannot perform basic self-care skills due to amnesia, an evaluation of work skills may not be thought appropriate (though this position has been challenged by some, see Chapter 14).

METHODS OF FUNCTIONAL ASSESSMENT

Specific assessment goals should be established as these influence the content, method and focus of the assessment. Data may be obtained from documentary information, interviews, questionnaires, observations and standardized testing.

Documentary information

Hospital case notes and medical records may include family and social history, pre-morbid functioning and history of the present illness. Relevant medical data includes diagnosis, history of substance abuse, psychiatric illness, concurrent medical conditions, allergies and treatment contra indications, time and cause of injury, type of brain injury, Glasgow Coma Scale score, length of PTA, residual neurological deficits, medical and nursing procedures, and other specialist reports. It should be remembered that errors may be included in the patient's record and it is advisable to check important features of the patient's history.

Interviews

The purpose of an initial interview is for the participants to give and receive information and establish rapport. A variety of interviewing methods could be used depending on the requirements of the assessment. A formal interview elicits information by using a structured schedule of questions. An informal interview is more conversational in style and may allow more detailed examination of problem areas (Moore, 1977). The unstructured interactional aspect of the interview may provide a significant amount of data. The brain-injured individual may be unable to give accurate information because of memory deficits, behavioural problems or denial. An experienced interviewer can compare the person's answers, and with the observational data derived from the interview, gain valuable information. In interviews, the therapist needs to be careful not to encourage answers he or she expects to hear and keep in mind that an individual's statements about the reason for his or her behaviour may have little connection with the actual cause of the behaviour. For example, a patient with problems in initiating activity reported that he did not want to perform the task, because he had other work to do, was expecting visitors and so on. In reality the patient had a generalized inability to initiate behaviour as a result of frontal lobe damage.

When interviewing and observing individuals after brain injury, the discussion could follow many themes and styles of approach. The main aim is to keep an open questioning mind. Table 6.1 provides some ideas for interview observation.

Questionnaires

Many different questionnaires can be administered to brain-injured persons, their families or care staff. Questionnaires can address aspects of biography, social settings, abilities in the home and rehabilitation setting, or alternatively attempt to assess a range of hypothetical constructs, such as 'self-esteem'. Severely impaired brain-injured people are frequently unable to complete lengthy questionnaires because of confusion, attentional deficit, restlessness and agitation or language deficits. Priddy *et al.* (1988) have shown the unreliability of the Minnesota Multiphasic Personality Inventory (MMPI) with patients in PTA and the decreased reliability of the MMPI in patients following PTA, when compared with normal controls. Individuals with behavioural deficits may underestimate their behavioural problems (McKinley and Brooks, 1984). Assessment by questionnaire is best directed towards the patient's family or friends (though they have their own biases) (McKinley and Brooks, 1984) and toward the brain-injured adult with mild to moderate impairments. Comparisons between the patient's and the

Table 6.1 Interview observation

Appearance
Dress and grooming. Does the client maintain eye contact?

Motor Activity
Body posture and activity level, gait, eye movements. Is there an appearance of paresis? Does the client move one side more than another? Is tremor present?

Speech
Is the verbal output of the client informative? Is it understandable (dysarthric), circumlocutary, concrete, too loud, too quiet, pressured or does the client show evidence of thought disorder?

Mood
Mood includes anxiety, depression, euphoria (excessive self-confidence, boastfulness). Does the client appear to have insight into his deficits? Does the patient's mood fluctuate (lability)? Does the client laugh or cry uncontrollably or inappropriately?

Alertness, attention and concentration
Is the client drowsy or immobile? Does the client maintain contact and attention throughout the interview? Does the client appear distracted and lose the theme of conversation?

Cognitive functioning
Does the client remember previous points in the conversation? Does the client perseverate on themes? Does the client appear concrete in his thought processes?

Perceptual functioning
Is the client perceiving the environment adequately? Is the client experiencing auditory or visual hallucinations?

The client's attitude during the examination
Is the situation or questions during the interview misperceived? Is the client anxious, paranoid, belligerent, co-operative or overly friendly?

---

family's reports can be revealing (Sunderland *et al.*, 1984) and some assessment devices, such as the Katz Adjustment Scale, have deliberately incorporated a self-report and relative-report measure (Katz and Lyerly, 1963). One example of a question-naire intended for the mildly brain-injured population is the Subjective Memory Questionnaire of Bennett-Levy and Powell

(1980) which samples everyday memory skills. The questions are directed to frequently occurring situations which involve memory and the subjects rate themselves on various aspects of memory functioning (Bennett-Levy and Powell, 1980).

Observation

Functional assessments should be conducted under conditions that closely approximate those the person will experience following rehabilitation. Functional assessment therefore differs from other types of testing which demand highly standardized conditions. The rigorous control of variables necessary for the pursuit of science is sacrificed in favour of ecological validity. There are many variables which influence performance in real world situations, for example the presence of setting events, cues or environmental conditions. Willems (1972) studied variations in patient behaviour relative to a hospital environment. He found that patients spend most of their time on the ward, particularly around the nurses' station or in hallways, with considerable time also spent in physical therapy, occupational therapy, the cafeteria and recreational therapy. He also found that the areas in which patients displayed the greatest amount of independence behaviour was the cafeteria and hallways. The ward environment essentially allowed very limited independence.

In addition to the environmental context, the presence of an observer may influence behaviour. Gold (1958) differentiated four types of observation, by the degree of participation of the observer. In Gold's type I observation, both the observer and the fact that observation is taking place are concealed from the subjects. In type II, the observer is completely removed from the activity of the subjects, his role is unknown to them but the observer is not physically hidden. In type III the role of the observer is known to the subjects but the observer is a non-participant. In the type IV interaction, the observer is closely involved and identified with the activity. Type III and type IV observations are most likely to occur in therapeutic situations. Therapists are likely to influence the brain-injured individual's behaviour during observation. For example, one patient was able to cross the street safely when accompanied by the therapist, but the patient's performance deteriorated when the therapist observed from the other side of the street.

The ability to make accurate observations is a skill acquired with training and experience. Most therapists do not emphasize observation or appreciate the importance of establishing a picture of what the client does unconstrained by external cues or demands. The person being observed needs to be put at ease, and the clinician should be able to state the purpose of the observation in a value-free fashion. One should not stare at the person being examined or interviewed in a cold and calculating way or maintain a critical aloofness while examining their every move (Aiken, 1987).

Recording observational data

Written descriptions of the individual's behaviour can be completed during the assessment, notes being made as events occur. It is impossible to record everything but crucial aspects of behaviour can be recorded. Recall tends to involve a selective reorganization in the light of subsequent events. Observation of the brain-injured individual can yield a pattern of deficits which may not be apparent in standardized testing or identified in an interview or by questionnaire. Where many people are involved in an observational protocol (such as when there is an attempt to determine the total number of times a behaviour is exhibited in a given period), a highly structured observational schedule must be used (see under methods of behavioural recordings). The development of a consensus as to what does and does not constitute an instance of the behaviour is a prerequisite.

Methods of behavioural recording

Frequency recordings measure the number of times a specified behaviour occurs in a set time period. This is simple to use because the observer only has to count the occurrences of the behaviour. A frequency measure is used when the target behaviour is discrete, brief and has a clear beginning and end (Kazdin, 1978). Interval recording is based on units of time rather than the frequency of behavioural responses. A period of time, for example a day, is divided into smaller units of time, for example half hours, and the number of periods in which the individual is engaged in the behaviour is recorded. Rather than a single observation once per day, clients can be observed at various times during the day and in different settings. Duration recording actually measures the time spent in particular behaviours. This type of recording is simple, involving starting and stopping a stopwatch, but may be inaccurate when the boundaries of a behaviour are ill-defined. Some computer tasks have this duration recording feature built into the system.

Audiovisual techniques provide an observational record of the individual's performance, but have practical and ethical limitations. The information is highly selective and may be biased by the presence of the equipment.

Standardized assessments

Many standardized procedures are available which assist in comparing level of function with the performance of a normative group. A standardized assessment is a specific test designed to explicitly define and measure a construct, such as hand function. The construct may be composed of a number of related concepts which can be operationalized. The standard assessment consists of specific instructions for the application of the test and indicators to measure the person's performance. These scores can be compared with group norms, for instance, expected standards of performance available for a specific age or occupation group. By using the same indicators, the same test and the same administrative rules for subjects and by scoring the results in a standard way, a reliable measure of an individual's ability on the test can be determined. Therapists may use standardized tests for a variety of assessment purposes. Some of these are discussed in the chapters of this book which refer to the particular domains of functioning.

Check-list and rating scales

Check-lists fulfil the useful function of ensuring that the therapist has not omitted a significant area of function from the examination. Check-list data is nominal and a useful way of presenting an individual's basic abilities in functional activities. Rating scales may be used for a variety of purposes and for some scales inter-rater reliability may be known or could be established. Some of these structured observations may be relevant to particular stages of recovery from injury (e.g. the Disability Rating Scale of Rappaport *et al.*, 1982). Most check-lists and rating scales can be completed by many staff on the treatment team.

Scales of measurement and recording

Individuals' functional abilities may be conceptualized as occurring in a hierarchy from small, goal-directed movements to highly complex, orchestrated sequences of actions often performed intermittently over an extended period. Where one chooses to enter this hierarchy depends on the type of information that is required. A wide variety of scales are used to rate activities of daily living. Screening scales used for placement decisions may treat a domain of behaviour, for example washing and dressing, as all-or-none, or, in other words, independent/dependent. Other scales analyse activities into component parts and those scales which examine functional behaviour in detail are more valuable for retraining purposes (Klein and Bell, 1982). A number of scales describe the degree of assistance required to perform tasks (for example, complete independence to total assistance).

The types of scales used in ADL assessments have distinct properties which affect how they should be interpreted. Scales may be one of the following: Nominal scales, where recordings are placed into either two or more categories, for example sex: male or female. Ordinal scales which have properties of nominal scale, but are ordered along a continuum in terms of a given criterion, for example A is bigger than B but the distance between the items is not known or is unequal. Interval scales which have characteristics of ordinal scales but with a specified distance between each point on the scale, for example temperature recordings. Ratio scales which have very similar properties to interval scales, but have a fixed zero, for example age. ADL scales vary widely on scoring systems. Bruett and Overs (1968) reviewed 12 scales; one was an interval scale, eight were ordinal scales, and three were nominal scales.

Reliability and validity

Reliability is a relatively straightforward concept. Reliability refers to the consistency of results of a test when administered by different people or at different times. Validity is a more complex concept but relates to whether a test actually measures what it purports to measure. Adequate reliability is a prerequisite for most types of validity (Anastasi, 1988). In addition to reliability and validity, an adequate rating scale must be brief enough for clinical application, complete enough to address relevant functional domains and sensitive enough to capture changes of functional relevance.

The use of the rating scales and other objective measures to assist therapists construct individual treatment plans has been emphasized. In addition to this, functional scales are increasingly being used to manage cases, compare intervention strategies and evaluate programme effectiveness. There is considerable risk associated with 'objective tests' or functional evaluations being put to these uses. The presumption of unidimensionality (that only one thing is being tested) is usually erroneous. For example, summed functional assessment measurements should not alone be used to measure the hypothetical construct 'independence' or compare clients. Multifaceted functional assessments are unlikely to reliably predict in individual cases either 'independence' or 'level of care' (see Wright and Linacre, 1989 and related correspondence for a discussion). For example, when comparing patients with brain injury and impaired social/interpersonal skills with a patient with a low spinal cord injury, the former are likely to be erroneously rated as more independent than the latter. The fact that unidimensionality is necessary for generalization results in any comprehensive ADL scale having limited generalizability. Scales can provide measures of progress of individuals but even here the distance between points on the scale (where the measure is independence, impairment or burden of care) should never be presumed to be equivalent. This problem is exacerbated by the fact that many of the scales used currently were not developed specifically for use with the brain-impaired and are based on a conceptual framework not appropriate for this population.

SUMMARY

The therapist can obtain documentary information, interview, observe and test the brain-injured individual in many situations and settings. The therapist can determine the individual's functional, social, behavioural, cognitive and physical abilities and how he attempts to compensate for deficits. Interviews and observations of the family's interactions with the patient helps therapists develop an understanding of the patient in his family context. As the patient's strengths and deficits become evident in functional situations, priorities are discussed with him, his family and the rehabilitation team. Where natural recovery is unlikely, rehabilitation programming is focused on areas where improvement will significantly impact future independence. Assessment of learning ability indicates the most effective types of retraining for each patient. The priorities of retraining should be re-evaluated at regular intervals. Assessment is cyclical with a constant process of goal setting and therapy. Neurofunctional assessment systematically determines what the client can or cannot do (or does and does not do), defines areas which require intervention and demonstrates the progress the individual has achieved to reduce his disability and handicap.

This chapter has presented a neurofunctional approach to brain injury assessment, involving seven factors. We have argued for a truly functional approach to assessment, stressing observational data in natural environments. The importance of standardized tests is recognized but they are not central to the functional approach. Check-lists and behavioural recording methods are discussed and are regarded as valuable methods of structuring observation.

7

Learning approaches following brain injury

'Skill does not develop from practising the skill per se, but rather from practising consistent components of the skill'.

Schnieder *et al.*, 1984

INTRODUCTION

Miller (1980) has argued that retraining in independent living skills is central to rehabilitation after brain injury. The extent and location of brain injury places constraints on human learning but the ability to acquire new behaviours is retained in all but the most severely injured (i.e. those in a persistent vegetative state). Miller found that the severely brain-injured patients he studied improved rapidly with practice on a novel psychomotor task (Miller, 1980). The ability of the severely impaired to learn functional skills following specialized retraining has been demonstrated (Giles and Clark-Wilson, 1988a; Giles and Morgan, 1989; Giles and Shore, 1989a).

Learning can be defined as a relatively permanent change in behaviour resulting from practice or experience. A complex interaction of many types of learning processes are probably utilized in the acquisition of functional skills. Assessment ascertains the skills to be learned and methods to assist learning. Debate continues as to the contribution of various types of learning in recovery from brain injury. Behavioural or associative learning has been distinguished from cognitive learning. People have different learning strategies (Pask and Scott, 1973) and these may be taken into account when designing interventions. The more cognitively impaired the patient, the greater the need for the therapist to organize the patient's environment to facilitate learning.

ASSOCIATIVE LEARNING

Both classical (Pavlov, 1927) and operant (Skinner, 1938) conditioning concern associations between environmental events and behaviour. Oakley (Oakley, 1983; Goldstein and Oakley, 1985) has related a number of studies with experimentally brain-damaged animals to rehabilitation with traumatically brain-injured persons. Goldstein has used these studies to illustrate that certain types of associative learning (those dependent on subcortical brain structures) may remain relatively unimpaired after brain injury. Goldstein and Oakley (1985) have suggested that application of association learning techniques (behavioural therapy) to those with behavioural disturbance may lead to the development of adequate behavioural control thus allowing cognitive therapies to be effective.

Reinforcement and skill building

A reinforcing event is one which increases the likelihood of the behaviour which immediately precedes it being repeated. Reinforcers may be primary (social attention, praise and tangible reinforcers) and intrinsically desirable or secondary, such as points and tokens which can be traded for primary reinforcers. Reinforcement principles are discussed more extensively in Chapter 11.

There is some evidence that reinforcement aids learning (Dolan and Norton, 1977; Lashley and Drabman, 1974). The importance of tangible reinforcement, in addition to social praise, is less clear and results have been inconsistent. Dolan (1979) has suggested that the inconsistency may result from the level of motivation towards the activity that needs to be learned. Where there is high motivation, tangible reinforcement is likely to be irrelevant. Knowledge of result and knowledge of performance (discussed further in Chapter 9) may act as reinforcers where individuals are motivated towards learning the task. The reason that reinforcement increases learning is unknown but could be related to the ability of reinforcement to help direct attention toward the central aspects of the task to be learned.

Reinforcement has a number of major functions in addition to directing attention in skill building programmes. Some of these might be regarded as irrelevant by a learning theorist, but the authors have found them to be clinically useful. Reinforcement can help patients retain a positive attitude towards developing skills, especially when some activities may be extremely effortful and intrinsically unrewarding. A suitable reinforcement schedule can assist the patient in his participation and practise of a skill when co-operation with the programme is problematic. Reinforcement schedules help staff remain oriented to the task at hand and retain a positive attitude to treatment, even when the behaviours which are the target of treatment are aggravating. For higher-level clients, rewards provide recognition for the amount of effort they are devoting to relearning and may be used to introduce the concept of self-reinforcement. Table 7.1 lists factors to be considered when developing learning programmes.

Table 7.1 Behavioural facilitations to learning

a) Consistency of approach
b) Organization of material
c) Reinforcement – social/tangible – knowledge of performance/results
d) Achievement-orientated
e) Goal-directed
f) Practice

D.P. was amnesic following severe brain injury (coma in excess of 3 months). He was unable to perform basic hygiene activities independently due to profound memory impairment, and an inability to sequence his behaviour in the absence of external prompts. A computer programme was designed to help him internalize an appropriate sequence. Reinforcement schedules were constructed to give him tangible reinforcers for correct performance on the task, and graded according to his scores. For example, he earned a piece of chocolate for completing the programme, a cigarette for achieving 60% of correct answers and five cigarettes for errorless performance. Within six weeks, he learned the computer programme and this improvement was demonstrated when transferred to his morning hygiene programme (Clark-Wilson, 1988).

Task analysis

Task analysis involves a process of dividing tasks into component parts that can be taught as units and chained together
into a functional whole. The analysis provides a method of
organizing behaviours to make them easier to learn. The components of a task analysis may be converted to verbal or visual
prompts and the learner's attention is directed to each step of
the activity sequentially. These can be built into subgroups
of contiguous core skills or identified as functional clusters of
behaviour. These clusters can be taught as a single instructional
step to learners who are more competent. A functional cluster
is defined as a sequence of 2–4 component contiguous 'core
skills' that have a meaningful relationship and constitute an
identifiable and potentially teachable segment of a whole task.
An example of a core skill could be establishing an appropriate
sitting posture, whereas an example of a functional cluster could
be all the steps to enable transfer into a wheelchair.

When using a task analysis to develop a set of verbal cues, the
number of cues depends on the patient's ability. For example, in
developing a washing and dressing programme some patients
require only a few prompts such as 'wash your face' to produce
complex behavioural chains. Other patients require several
prompts, for example 'pick up the wash cloth, put soap on the
wash cloth, wash your face, rinse the wash cloth.' One patient
reported elsewhere (Giles and Clark-Wilson, 1988a) had a washing and dressing programme, which initially consisted of 70
prompts. After six weeks this was reduced to 34, then again
after three months to 17 and finally to four. The final prompts
were to get her clothes out, wash, clean her teeth and brush
her hair. O'Reilly and Cuvo used an interesting variant of this
procedure in attempting to train self-treatment of cold symptoms to an anoxic brain-injured adult. Three levels of cueing
were used: generic prompts (non-specific subject headings),
specific prompts (based on a specific step by step task analysis)
and individualized prompts where specific prompt sequences
were provided only where the client failed to provide the appropriate behaviour to the generic prompt.

Where clients are able to respond to verbal or visual prompts
to carry out procedures, the authors have found it most effective
to use a whole task system in which prompts are provided for

each step until the task is completed. An exception to this general rule applies to clients who are so slow that attempting to train the whole task is too demanding. Where this is the case, specific functional clusters may be selected. Where patients are unable to make use of visual or verbal prompts, forward or backward chaining may be used. Backward chaining maximizes the contextual cues available to the learner.

B.N. had suffered a very severe brain injury (coma duration unknown) two years prior to admission. The injury had been penetrating and since that time he had suffered multiple brain abscesses. B.N. had profound attention and memory deficits and an inability to initiate behaviour. Initially he had great difficulty putting his trousers on the right way round and in putting his shoes on the correct feet. He needed specific and repeated prompting to engage in extremely simple activities, for example 'Pick up your T-shirt'. He frequently responded with sterotyped phrases 'I will do if I can do' or 'I bloody will'. Initially, because of B.N.'s profound deficits, treatment staff were pessimistic about being able to help him become independent in washing and dressing. A programme was constructed which was as simple as possible and involved a series of 12 activities. Backward chaining for each functional cluster was used and B.N. was required to perform the 12th activity then the 11th and the 12th and so on. As the activity was reliably performed he received less and less assistance. After 4 months' treatment, B.N. had progressed from requiring 50 prompts and considerable physical guidance to independently completing the activities involved in bathing, washing his hair and getting dressed. In a sense we had been rather too successful as B.N. spontaneously engaged in the washing activity a number of times per day. Since B.N. was safe this was regarded as acceptable, but shows one of the possible consequences of increasing the probability of a behaviour in a profoundly impaired amnesic individual.

Prompts

Events which facilitate the production of a behaviour are called prompts (or cues). A prompt assists an individual produce the target behaviour which may then be reinforced. In many instances prompts are available in the environment but they are no longer sufficient to guide behaviour or they have lost their meaning entirely (for example, arriving at a busy junction no longer cues safe routines when crossing the street). The therapist adds additional prompts to those already available in the environment. Therapists can facilitate the learning of skills with a range of differing types of prompts: visual (pictures), written lists, physical touch or guidance, modelling and verbal instructions. Once the skill is reliably carried out, the prompt can be faded until performance occurs without the additional aid to initiation. O'Reilly and Cuvo (1989) used picture prompts teaching self-treatment of cold symptoms to the anoxic brain-injured adult. The authors did not demonstrate any transfer of training to real-life settings but the study is of interest because of the use of pictures, repeated practice and feedback.

Shaping

Shaping refers to the reinforcement of closer and closer approximations to the desired behaviour. Tasks are graded in difficulty so they are achievable. As competency is demonstrated the task's requirements are increased. For example, one patient seen by the authors would pace the corridors of the treatment facility when not engaged in an activity by staff. The goal of intervention was to enable the patient to sit with others and engage in appropriate conversation. Initially he was reinforced (with attention and food) if he remained in the unit day room. Later he was only reinforced if he was sitting down, and finally only if engaged in appropriate conversation.

Control of a behaviour by antecedents

For many therapists, applied behavioural analysis when applied to brain-injured persons has been synonymous with operant conditioning. Antecedents, the 'A' in the ABC chain, may be altered in an attempt to change behaviour. This is a method of setting the environmental conditions – the stimulus events – to increase the possibility that the patient will emit the desired behaviour. Elsewhere we have reported the use of posters containing specific information in an attempt to 'prime' the individual in certain activities (Giles and Clark-Wilson, 1988b). The control of specific antecedents may be of particular usefulness in working with patients with profound memory impairment. Discussion of attempts to control behaviour disorder by antecedents are reserved for Chapter 11.

Zencius *et al.*, (1989) systematically studied the effect of altering antecedents. The effects of altering antecedents were compared with the effect of varying consequences in three patients with marked memory disorder following severe brain-injury. In the first patient reported, Zencius and co-workers (1989) found that posting a sign regarding breaktimes at the work station drastically reduced the number of unauthorized breaks. In another client, the most effective way to increase her use of a cane, a goal of the rehabilitation team, was to provide her with a cane to use during her morning activities of daily living. This technique was found to be more effective than social praise, a contract for money or someone to escort her to get her cane when she was found without it. In a third patient, the authors found that a map and a written daily schedule was more powerful than a contract for money in increasing therapy attendance. The alteration in the antecedence produced behavioural improvements, whereas previous attempts to alter behaviour by consequences had proved to be, at best, only marginally successful.

Behavioural momentum (Mace *et al.*, 1988) may be considered a special subclass of antecedent behavioural methods. It refers to the tendency for low probability behaviours to be more readily performed to request when embedded in a series of high probability behaviours. The greater the rate of reinforcement available the greater the momentum. Interventions based on this notion can address non-compliance or delayed compliance. But preceding a low probability request (i.e. an activity which the subject does not normally perform) with high probability means the likelihood of compliance is considerably increased. The research of Mace and co-workers (1988) with a mentally handicapped population demonstrated that these effects are independent of experimenter attention, but the behavioural momentum was only effective when the high-probability commands occurred immediately prior to the low probability commands (Mace *et al.*, 1988). Wahler and Fox (1981) have advocated a shift in focus from molecular units of behaviour to an analysis of setting events. A setting event is a stimulus which facilitates or inhibits the response to follow it. Conceptually there is no reason to discount the ability of an event occurring hours earlier to influence later behavioural events (see Chapter 15 for a further discussion of setting events).

Overlearning

Overlearning (in this context) refers to the practice of a skill well beyond the point where mastery has been attained. Overlearning increases the chances that a skill is consolidated – becomes automatic – in the individual's repertoire of skills and reduces the amount of effort required for performance. When a skill becomes automatic, it becomes the easiest behaviour to initiate from an array of possible behaviours. The goal of rehabilitation can often best be met by ensuring a degree of overlearning. For example, a street crossing programme should not be terminated on achieving the functional criteria, but on meeting the criteria with extra practice sessions designed to make the behaviour automatic. The number of additional sessions required to develop automaticity is unclear but depends on how difficult it was for the patient to initially learn the behaviour. Automaticity is assessed by ongoing monitoring on the patient's behaviour in conjunction with distractors.

Fading

When learning a task, patients could depend on a range of environmental cues. Some of these are deliberate objects of manipulation by the therapist and other cues occur without the conscious control of the therapist. Verbal cues can be faded by forming clusters of prompts from the task analysis, after the individual has learnt to complete the behaviour in response to the original prompts. Another method of fading is to increase the time between completion of the previous behaviour and the provision of the subsequent prompt. This delay procedure should only be used however when the patient has already developed the skill to the point where they can be 80–90% correct, as otherwise they are likely to 'practise' the propagation of incorrect responses – a situation to be avoided. Questions like 'What's next?' or instructions telling the individual to 'go ahead' can help the individual initiate the activity and decreases dependence on prompts. Verbal cues are faded more easily than visual cues, but it is possible to gradually reduce the amount of information available even in pictograms.

Not all of the cues used by the patient to guide behaviour may be immediately apparent to the therapist. For example, when teaching a patient to be assertive the personal character-istics of the therapist may cue assertive behaviour. Consider-ation of the cues present during teaching of the skill by the therapist need to be reduced gradually so the individual becomes able to perform the task without either subtle or obvi-ous cues. For example, physical presence in a washing and dressing programme or the therapist's physical proximity during a road safety programme, can be altered to a system of intermittently 'checking' with reinforcement for appropriate activity in the former case, and distant observation in the latter case.

C.H. (seven years post injury; coma duration unknown) was taught to control his movements in a structured washing and dressing routine. During the fading of the programme, he was checked regularly on the physical activities in the task. The staff checked six times during his programme, to see if he was positioned in the way he had been taught to stabilize his movements. Each time he was observed to be performing the activity correctly he was given a token which he exchanged later for a previously agreed upon reward of his choice.

Encore procedure

When an individual demonstrates an infrequently displayed skill without prompting, he or she can be prompted to produce several more correct responses. For example, C.P. (whose demanding ways were discussed in Chapter 5) was learning to attract peoples' attention appropriately before asking questions or making requests in social skills groups. On any occasion when she asked correctly, by saying the person's name, or 'excuse me' and then asking a question, she was given social and occasionally tangible reinforcement. She was then asked to repeat the sequence of behaviours again whereupon she was reinforced again.

Rehearsal strategy

Rehearsal strategies can facilitate retention of new material. J.B. had a severe amnesic disorder following herpes simplex encephalitis, and used verbal rehearsal strategies to remember the information he needed. For example, he looked at the programme in his room, checked his watch and rehearsed statements about what he was going to do, for instance going to work. If J.B. wished to consolidate a new fact he would simply state it over and over to himself for hours, a technique which allowed him to memorize a considerable amount of information. Bjork and Allen (1970) demonstrated that the spacing of repetitions of an item has large and clear effects on measures of performance. Teaching the patient to repeat statements containing information of use to them, may have an effect on behaviour. There are however both theoretical and practical reasons for training verbal behaviour and physical behaviour in tandem.

Highlighting

Many individuals after brain injury have problems in distinguishing the central aspects of a task. Highlighting refers to a strategy that promotes the discrimination of the crucial elements of an activity, by exaggerating the perceptual salience of some stimulus features. Prompts are progressively faded once the patient is consistently making correct discriminations. Highlighting might be achieved by emphasizing phrases, pointing, touching or by providing specific reinforcement.

Even profoundly brain-injured individuals can be trained to perform basic functional skills. The patient is often unable to introspectively determine the nature of their difficulties and treatment centres around modifying their previous automatic responses and replacing them with new and more adaptive ones. The individual may not even know that he has learned anything despite markedly improved performance. Many more complex behaviours, no matter how overlearned they become, continue to be effortful. These behaviours are usually available to introspection and often involve conscious initiation. They involve a combination of control and automatic processing. An example of a controlled and automatic process combination is the use of a diary. With practice a patient may automatically check in the diary. Practice in how to make entries and what information to enter reduces the difficulty of these tasks but these procedures remain partially effortful. Purely automatic behaviours can be developed in individuals who do not have insight, by practice and appropriate reinforcement contingencies. This is not possible when effortful control processes make up a significant proportion of the activity. Where effortful control processes are required (on an ongoing basis), it is almost impossible for the patients to learn and utilize procedures without their active co-operation and understanding.

COGNITIVE LEARNING

Cognitive learning involves the formation of rules about regularities in the environment (Goldstein and Oakley, 1985). These rules often involve linguistic representations in man and depend on the neocortex and hippocampus (see Chapter 4). Cognitive learning requires the use of attention (Goldstein and Oakley, 1985), memory, language, perception and problem solving. Many deficits influence the ability to engage in and make use of cognitive learning. Both perceptual and attentional deficits can hamper the understanding of environmental events, and memory deficits limit the use of information. Continual loss of information results in personal data not being updated on a regular basis so the individual's view of themselves and of the world may increasingly deviate from reality. With these impaired memory stores, new information becomes harder to place in context. Damage to the frontal lobes results in difficulties in generating and executing plans and in the use of language-based programmes to control behaviour. Not all learning deficits seen after brain injury are a result of trauma. As noted in Chapter one, developmental disorders are very common in individuals who later have a traumatic brain injury.

The individual's psychiatric status affects his attitude towards learning and others' reactions to the patient will influence his co-operation towards rehabilitation. The production of a positive mental attitude must have a primary place in all re-education (Franz, 1923). A negative response to brain injury may lead to compensatory reactions which, if somewhat successful, may inhibit or preclude the course of true recovery from the damage.

STRATEGY FORMATION/EXPERIENTIAL LEARNING

During the acute stage of recovery, patients are not called upon to organize their day-to-day activities, which are structured by hospital routine. As recovery progresses they should be expected to resume their normal daily activities and take over the responsibilities and organization of their lives. Following brain injury, the individual may find previously overlearned ways of performing tasks no longer effective due to physical or cognitive changes or changed life circumstances. Flexibility of thought and problem solving may also be significantly impaired.

It is often the combination of physical and cognitive disorders which prove most problematic. For example, an individual with severe physical deficits after brain injury may be unable to work out how to move around his environment in an electric wheelchair. He would potentially have managed had he remained ambulatory. The practical problems of community mobility and other complex functional tasks are very different for someone using an electric wheelchair than they are for someone who can walk.

The therapist's role is to supervise the patient in setting his own goals, and developing his own strategies to perform functional tasks. For example, a patient who has been working on improving his community mobility might set himself the task of finding the way to a specific novel location. The patient would then have to develop for himself, with the assistance of the therapist, a knowledge of the parameters involved in the task, such as available means of transportation, time requirements, cost, finding the way and so forth. Initially limited time periods should be set aside for the individual to learn to 'self schedule' as he could find the activity stressful, become inactive without continuous support, be side-tracked, or demonstrate behavioural deterioration. As the patient demonstrates increasing competencies, longer periods of time and more complex tasks can be set for him. Eventually long periods of the treatment day should be devoted to the patient pursuing his own goals, periodically checking in with the therapist who can ensure that he remains critically self-aware. The therapist's goal is to set tasks and direct the patient's attention on how his current experience can be incorporated into strategies to improve his future functioning. Tasks could include enrolling in evening classes, college programmes, or finding social activities.

After a severe brain injury and a prolonged period of hospitalization, patients are likely to have difficulty in maintaining the tonic level of activity required for community living. Gradually increasing the individual's responsibility for his own day-to-day activities can assist him in achieving the considerable degree of activity necessary for independent functioning. This may take a long time. Occasionally patients need to be prevented from overestimating their own abilities and attempting to do too much. Ultimately the goal of strategy formation and the use of experiential learning should be under the control of the brain-injured individual. They need to learn to evaluate functional strategies and incorporate these into their own behavioural repertoire. Each new experience should be designed to produce a useful and effective strategy.

INTERACTIONS WITH BRAIN-INJURED INDIVIDUALS DESIGNED TO FACILITATE LEARNING

Goal statements

The incorporation of goal statements in each session has a number of advantages in helping brain-injured individuals learn. It can increase participation, help them attend to the to-be-learned aspect of their activities (this discriminatory aspect may need to be repeated throughout the session) and it communicates respect from therapist to patient. For patients with a lack of insight, it orients them to their deficits and cues them as to how the therapeutic activity to be undertaken will help them achieve their own goals (usually to get out of the treatment facility). The use of goal statements may cause some therapists to be anxious, for fear of causing an aggressive or confronting response from the patient. They may wish to present the session as a scientific endeavour, in which either the therapist or the patient is allowed to have incorrect notions, but in which an empirical question is examined. Alternatively the therapist could present the activity against the background of a shared goal, for example, independence. With some patients, however, active agreement with the therapeutic intervention is not attainable, and the therapist seeking agreement will only side-track the patients and derail the therapeutic endeavour. Therapists are not advised to abandon the goal of developing functional skills by waiting until the patient knows that he has deficits. Goal-directing statements, for example for five minutes at the beginning of each session and interspersed throughout, orienting patients to these issues, is frequently indicated. For example, 'as you know, as a result of your severe brain injury you have needed some help in washing and dressing yourself – we are working with you every morning so that you can develop a system to be independent – you can now perform all but three of the activities of washing and dressing completely independently'.

Debriefing

Regular debriefing about performance (knowledge of results) is indicated in producing positive behavioural change. Telling the patient they have done well is encouraging, but non-specific and damaging if untrue. Feedback about results should be concrete and accurate. Written materials the patient can refer to, such as graphs or logs, should be used where possible (particularly when the patient has a memory deficit). Feedback of performance, for example the areas completed well or those that could have been better, should be given to the patient with the reasons why the therapist makes those judgements. For example, feedback given to a client who was asked to carry out a complex collating task for an assessment of office vocational skills was as follows: 'Although you started slowly you worked accurately and with minimal supervision. Your previous employment has led me to believe that you would have performed more rapidly prior to your injury (I think it took you about twice as long as it would have before). Also, organizing the photocopying task was difficult for you: it took you 10 minutes and eight copies to get it correct. The areas of speed and the new photocopying task were problems but you kept going, were methodical and got the task accomplished. That is a lot of what an employer looks for and is a positive achievement. I will be asking you to work on a similar task tomorrow to see if you can improve your performance'. Not only was the patient encouraged, she was also told why she was asked to perform the task; what the therapist learned from her performance of the task; what the next step was going to be; and that the ultimate goal of the activity was return to vocational work.

For many individuals who have difficulties in learning about their deficits, performance debriefing may be of assistance. A patient, known to one of the authors, was evaluated for his local topographical orientation and safety in crossing roads (he was told before going out that these skills were going to be observed). He got lost on a simple, local route and made impulsive errors like stepping into the street without looking. On one occasion, he was attempting to light a cigarette as he walked, stepped into the road and had to be restrained to prevent him from being hit by a car.

Patient:	So am I approved to go out on my own?
Therapist:	I think that with some work you will be able to be safe in crossing the street: but you demonstrated in the last hour that when you are not paying attention you can be unsafe (patient interjects).
Patient:	What was unsafe?
Therapist:	On four occasions out of six you stepped into the street without looking. On one occasion you did not seem to be aware of a car coming from the right and I held you back. You became confused about the route back, even though you have walked it with me twice before and once with another staff member. [Rather than talking in generalities the therapist fed back concrete examples]. Right now I am less concerned about your getting lost than about being in another accident because you are not paying attention when you cross the street. I know that you work very hard and I am confident that you can be safe after some more practice. I know that you want to get these independent skills back as fast as possible [positive re-frame].

Patient: When can we go out again?
Therapist: I am going to write down exactly what I want
             you to practise. If you can fulfil these require-
             ments for ten trips out I think that you will
             be able to be independent in our local area.

It is the patient who really trains the patient; the therapist is
only the guide. Friends and family can be trained to give verbal
reminders to facilitate correct performance, to keep track of
progress on goal attainment sheets, and to provide moral support for the work carried out in residential rehabilitation settings.

CASE REPORT

M.F. a 20-year-old right-handed male, sustained a closed head
injury from an automobile accident on 7 May, 1986. A CT scan
at that time revealed a right frontal contusion and some mass
effect. The patient required mechanical ventilation and underwent a tracheostomy on 1 June, 1986. Duration of coma was
approximately four weeks and the patient remained in a stuporous state for the following five weeks. Acute hospital care was
followed by five months of rehabilitation services, provided
within an acute rehabilitation unit. Following the acute rehabilitation phase and on admission to the Transitional Living Centre
(where the programme described here was conducted), the
patient was mobile indoors in a wheelchair. The patient's
memory was severely impaired. Attention span was within
normal limits (digit span 5.3), but immediate recall of the 'Logical Memory' subtest of the Wechsler Memory Scale (1945), was
negligible with delayed recall non-existent. The patient had a
severe left-sided hemiparesis, more pronounced in the lower
extremity, and right elbow extension was limited by 10 degrees
due to heterotopic ossification. When first admitted to the unit
at the beginning of December 1987, M.F. was eight months'
post-injury and dependent in activities of daily living. Scores
on the relevant Adaptive Behaviour Rating Scale (1974) were
dressing, 2 and undressing, 3.

Procedure

The patient was observed on three consecutive mornings by the occupational therapist and the methods used spontaneously by the patient to wash and dress were noted. It was observed that the patient was assisted by one attendant (the patient's wife) who provided between 25 and 30 instructions to the patient as well as physical assistance on between three to seven separate occasions each morning. The patient's wife stated that the patient had been performing at this level for the previous three months (confirmed by chart review). Two central problems were noted. Firstly, the patient was attempting to dress in a way in which he could not be physically independent. He attempted most of his dressing activities by arching his back whilst lying on the bed and did not wash at all (he did clean his teeth and comb his hair). Secondly, his attempts to dress were erratic in order and content, changing from day to day, disrupting any practice effect which could have helped him to learn.

The occupational therapist (who had determined a series of steps used to order washing and dressing from informal questioning of his wife) developed a programme for M.F., incorporating M.F.'s own reports as to his pre-injury washing and dressing habits. In this way, it was hoped that the new programme would require the smallest amount of new learning to aid the patient in becoming independent. During the initial observations the precise nature of the behaviour which could be expected as a consequence of cueing was assessed. For example, it was determined that M.F. could produce an adequate washing sequence to 'wash your face' only if the words 'wash, rinse and dry' were added. The most difficult behaviours for M.F. to acquire were the new behaviours used to overcome physical handicaps. These involved moving from lying to sitting on the bed; transferring to the wheelchair; manoeuvering himself in his wheelchair and to a stable sitting position in front of the wash-basin; grasping the sides of the wash-basin and using this to assist him in standing, utilizing methods that would inhibit spasticity. Standing occurred twice in the programme, once to undress preparatory to washing and once to dress. The new physical routines often required multiple cues (for example, sitting on the side of the bed and standing using the sink required multiple cues) whereas pre-injury over-learned routines such as brushing teeth never required more than a single cue.

The new physical routines were practised in separate sessions as well as during the programme itself. Even so, up to treatment day six, verbal cues were insufficient and M.F. required physical positioning by the attendant in addition to verbal cueing.

Table 7.2 M.F.'s morning programme

---
1. Push back the covers.
2. Sit on the side of the bed.
3. Get into wheelchair.
4. Go to the sink (M.F. should sit directly facing the sink).
5. Take off shirt.
6. Clean teeth.
7. Fill sink.
8. Wash face (wash, rinse and dry).
9. Wash under arms (wash, rinse and dry).
10. Push wheelchair back from sink – grasp sides of sink with both hands – good hip bend – stand up – push down trousers and underwear and sit down.
11. Wash groin.
12. Dress top half.
13. Put on socks – underwear and trousers over feet.
14. Push wheelchair back from sink – grasp sides of sink with both hands – good hip bend – stand up – pull up underwear and trousers and sit down.
15. Put on shoes.
16. Comb hair.

Remember to give praise for good performance!

The analysis performed of the patient's behaviour resulted in all activities involved in washing and dressing being conceptualized as 16 steps and used as cues (Table 7.2). At each step cueing was provided if (1) behaviour compatible with the next step in the programme was not evident within approximately 5 seconds of the previous step being completed or (2) behaviour incompatible with production of the next step in the behavioural chain was demonstrated. When M.F. proceeded directly to the next appropriate behaviour after the completion of the previous behaviour he was congratulated and no cue was given. M.F.'s wife was trained in the procedure by observing the occupational therapist on the second day of treatment and carrying out treatment under the supervision of the occupational therapist on the third day. Subsequently days of treatment were divided approximately evenly between the therapist and his wife but co-treatments occurred every 4 days to ensure consistency. Ratings of independence, number of cues provided and the physical assistance required were recorded. In addition to the above, at least three times a day, a staff member questioned the patient about the sequence of behaviours involved in washing and dressing, stating that he had done well when he gave the correct response and telling him 'No! that was incorrect' when he made an error. The programme ran for 12 days, interrupted by weekends and a four-day vacation (see Figure 7.1). The patient's wife did not provide home treatment as the physical facilities were inadequate, although later alterations to the home allowed the patient to be independent at home.

Results

Figure 7.1 shows M. F.'s response to the morning washing and dressing programme. By day nine, M.F. was independently dressing himself but making some errors in the sequence of washing. By day 12 he was independently performing all procedures and was as a result not receiving any verbal cues. Relevant adaptive behaviour scale scores in a suitably adapted environment were, dressing 5 and undressing 5 (maximum scores). The occupational therapist continued to be present when M.F. washed and dressed for a further four days but no cues were required. Over the next two weeks, washing and dressing behaviour was monitored by periodic checking. After two weeks, this checking was discontinued and M.F. continued to dress himself in a timely way and was not malodorous. At a three-month follow-up the patient was observed and was found to be using the same techniques as he had been taught, despite the fact that he had changed rooms in the facility. No further treatment of washing and dressing behaviour has been required, six months since the programme ended, when M.F. was using the same techniques at home when attending the treatment facility as an out-patient with advanced treatment goals.

Discussion of case report

Central to the success of the programme was the evaluation of the patient's physical abilities and the design of a programme in which M.F. was immediately capable of partial success. Frequent repetition of a sequence of actions helped M.F. learn a method of washing and dressing despite a severe memory impairment. It should be noted that the introduction of the new system immediately resulted in a reduction of both the amount of physical assistance and cueing required (though a transitory increase in the amount of cueing is not unusual). By the end of the programme the time saved for staff and family were considerable and, more importantly, the patient achieved success.

A distinction can be made between the behaviours most difficult to learn and those most difficult to carry out in the correct sequence. The hardest behaviours to learn were the novel movement patterns required (physical assistance required to day 6). The most difficult activities for M.F. to sequence correctly were washing behaviours. M.F. learned the order of dressing before the washing activities. This may be due to the situational cues involved in dressing being more salient than those involved in washing. So for example, an individual can see the light is out, smell that breakfast is being prepared, notice he has his trousers half on and realize that he is dressing. He is less likely to remember whether he has cleaned his teeth, washed his face or combed his hair. The therapist, when teaching the cognitive overlearning element of the programme, concentrated on those short sequences, in which situational cues were at a minimum, but were central to the success of the programme. For example, while it is obvious that after pushing back the covers, the patient needs to transfer into his wheelchair, it is less obvious at which point he cleans his teeth. Learning a specific point in the programme at which the patient needs to clean his teeth is essential, if the patient is to do so each morning and not forget whether he has actually performed the task.

Both procedural memory and semanatic memory appear to be involved in the learning process described (Squire, 1986). The neuropsychological testing performed with M.F. revealed extremely limited declarative (episodic/semantic) memory, but an unimpaired procedural memory. It is reasonable to infer that

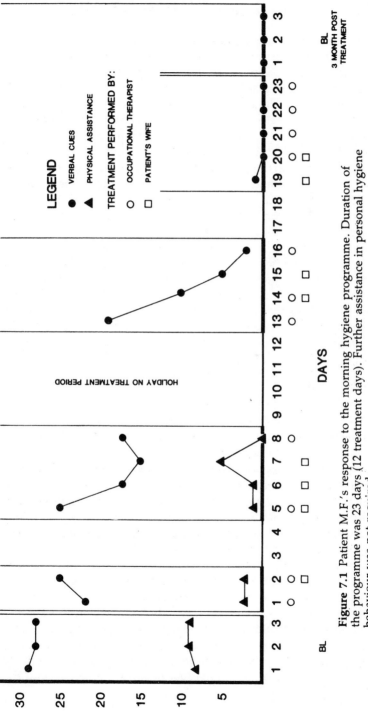

Figure 7.1 Patient M.F.'s response to the morning hygiene programme. Duration of the programme was 23 days (12 treatment days). Further assistance in personal hygiene behaviour was not required.

procedural memory could account for most (but not all) of the changes in behaviour. During the cognitive overlearning element of the programme, when the patient was questioned, he demonstrated clear learning of the prompt sequences (with the multiple repetitions and cues required initially). Yet it was not until two weeks after the completion of the programme that M.F. realized that he was able to wash and dress, a fact that gave him considerable satisfaction. This single case report demonstrates that a training approach to ADL may be successful where other methods have failed. Central to the programme is a highly structured repetitive approach using verbal cues when necessary and emphasizing the patient's achievement. This approach differs from most customary ADL methods which are instructional or stimulating rather than a specific training approach. M.F.'s response to the programme was rapid and resulted in independence in washing and dressing. As a result the patient became considerably easier to care for and presented with a much lower level of demand. Where an individual is not demonstrating rapid spontaneous recovery in the acute rehabilitation setting, it is recommended that a functional retraining approach be used.

SUMMARY

Only recently have the learning characteristics of the severely brain injured become a matter of more than academic interest. Researchers have begun to investigate the training of patients in functional tasks (Goldstein *et al*, 1985; Glisky *et al.*, 1986). The current authors have reported the day-to-day retraining of patients using practical techniques in self-care tasks, and demonstrated that even those who are many years post injury can improve performance to the point of independence in personal activities of daily living (Giles and Clark-Wilson, 1988a). The individual's psychiatric, behavioural and cognitive deficits may result in impaired learning ability (see Chapters 4 and 5). Assessment of the patient's abilities, deficits and their means of attempting functional tasks, environmental resources and the skills needed to function independently are reviewed in Chapter 6. From the process of assessment, functional priorities can be determined, and methods of retraining identified. The methods adopted depend on the individual's learning strategies and the techniques should be 'economical' in the sense of the amount of effort required by the individual to achieve each skill, and the overall rehabilitation programme. For example, learning to use a daily diary can assist a patient with multiple tasks. It is sounder rehabilitation practice to teach this skill, than spend a comparable amount of time and energy on learning an internal mnemonic strategy to aid recall of a shopping list. It is the therapist's task to determine a system which results in the maximum functional gain for the least amount of new learning. For example, when teaching an individual to wash and dress, incorporating pre-morbid habits can reduce the amount of new learning the patient has to do.

Fitts (1964) and Fitts and Posner (1967) describe the process of skill acquisition as one in which the individual initially uses cognitive control, which requires active attention, and in which subjects tend to verbalize each step of the task. The associative stage which follows is the practice stage where the skill is consolidated and the final autonomous stage, where a considerable level of skill has developed and the task places only limited attentional demands on the subject. Typically in the autonomous stage the subject loses the ability to verbalize the task (Fitts, 1964). Central to Fitts' notion is the idea that most complex tasks are learned as a number of simple procedures which are fitted together (and sometimes overlaid on one another). Learning is demonstrated not only by increased competency but also by a reduction in the attentional demands of the task. A programme of skill development should contain the components listed in Table 7.1. Methods used to teach a skill should be used consistently as inconsistency confuses patients who have learning deficits. The individuals' cognitive problems impair their ability to acquire information, remember the methods to be used, or retrieve the information when required. The patient's default response may be to return to previously used habits or spontaneously developed compensatory strategies. These may be both ineffective and detrimental to the patient's overall rehabilitation. For example, the individual with severe spasticity could use methods of transferring which increase the spastic pattern of movement. Specific programmes should be rigidly adhered to, if the patient is to learn, and practice and reinforcement schedules need to be determined.

Learning is demonstrated when the functional skill is used automatically in the relevant circumstances.

Glisky *et al.* (1986) demonstrated that individuals with severe brain injury could learn to use a computer, but were unable to adapt the skills to analogous (but different) circumstances. In a follow-up paper Glisky and Schacter (1988) reported that simple computer skills could be retained by amnesic patients for a considerable period (at least nine months). The difficulties in acquiring skills, and the problems experienced in transferring learned skills into novel contexts, mean it is important to determine and prioritize the skills that need to be learned. Goldstein and co-workers (1985) taught three amnesic patients a variety of useful behaviours, for example, walking to the institution's cafeteria, but the behaviour did not generalize to novel tasks. This underlines the importance of choosing behaviours with real functional significance which may also have implications for the patient's feelings of self-worth.

8

Management of the brain-injured patient in the acute stage of recovery

INTRODUCTION

This chapter provides an overview of the aims of treatment in the acute care setting, thus emphasizing the role of the therapist at the early stages of the patient's recovery. Models of recovery are discussed in Chapter two. The involvement of therapists in the acute medical setting depends on local practice, especially their 'role' in the intensive care unit (ICU). Therapists have an important role to play in the very early stages of recovery of function and their work assumes major importance in patients whose coma duration is protracted.

As noted in Chapter one, early accurate prediction of functional outcome is not possible. It is therefore reasonable for a treatment protocol to establish early and energetic management of possible complications. Bricolo and co-workers (1980) examined the evolution of level of consciousness in 135 individuals who sustained traumatic brain injury and were in coma in excess of two weeks. By one year post-trauma, 30% of the patients had died, 8% survived in persistent vegetative state, 31% survived with severe disability and 31% were rated as having made a satisfactory recovery. Within these groups the early clinical picture was not predictive of outcome. The restoration of wakefulness without awareness occurred in most patients between two to four weeks after the traumatic event. However not all patients appeared to go through this phase and individuals continued to emerge from the condition of wakefulness without awareness for up to one year. Recovery is less frequent after three months and unusual after six months. Risk of mortality increases with age and youth is associated with better outcome. The prognosis of patients with marked ischaemic or hypoxic damage is bleak. Nonetheless, failure to provide appropriate physical management during this stage could impede or prevent later improvement due to permanent damage to the musculoskeletal system. The fact that patients continue to emerge from PVS for at least a year warrants continuation of prophylactic care for a considerable period.

In the acute care setting it is essential to chart the patient's condition with special references to neurological changes. Decreasing responsiveness in a brain-injured individual suggests an active destructive process or space-occupying lesion and requires immediate management. Level of responsiveness is most frequently assessed by use of the Glasgow Coma Scale developed by Teasdale and Jennett (1974).

ASSESSMENT OF RESPONSIVENESS IN THE ACUTE STAGE OF RECOVERY OF FUNCTION

Assessment of coma (determining responsiveness)

A severely brain-injured patient in the intensive care unit (ICU) is likely to be ventilator dependent and to have intracranial pressure monitoring. Arterial and venous lines may be in place and the patient is likely to be catheterized. The patient in ICU may therefore present a terrifying prospect to the novice therapist. Guidance from an experienced therapist or nurse about the purpose of nursing procedures will reduce the new therapist's anxiety. Therapy evaluation of the brain-injured patient begins with a review of the patient's medical records. The therapist is interested in the mode of injury, results of investigative procedures (for example, CT scans), type and severity of injury, surgical and other medical treatment and associated injuries. The therapist should know the patient's spinal status and any other contra-indications for therapy intervention. The therapist should ascertain the types of medication the patient is receiving as this may affect responsiveness.

Assessment of responsiveness begins with the therapist loudly stating the patient's name, stating their own name and why they are there (i.e. auditory stimulation). The therapist notes whether the patient orients to the sound and whether they maintain eye contact with the therapist. The therapist notes the patient's resting eye position to assess cranial nerve function. Visual tracking may be assessed by noting if the patient can visually follow a moving brightly coloured object. An assessment of oculomotor function may be made by seeing if the patient tracks the object in all planes of movement. Some patients will demonstrate an orienting response but then be unable to track. If the therapist is able to gain the patient's attention then assessment may progress to determining the patient's ability to understand and communicate. If the therapist cannot gain the patient's attention by the use of auditory stimuli, then non-painful tactile stimulus is used. When the patient is not responsive to auditory and non-noxious tactile stimulation, the therapist could then elicit motor responses via more intense tactile stimulation (Boughton and Ciesla, 1986). Each extremity may be tested to determine the patient's ability to localize noxious stimuli. The type of reaction elicited should be noted for each extremity including quality and symmetry of movement. Noxious stimuli could include supraorbital pressure, pressure to the nailbed (administered with the eraser end of a pencil), sternal rub or pin prick. The therapist may then progress to a standard motor evaluation including range of motion, muscle tone, and reflexes. In addition the therapist should evaluate for musculoskeletal injury.

Many patients will be unable to speak (due to intubation, for example). Patients can be asked to follow one-step commands such as 'blink once' or 'move a finger'. It should be remembered, however, that abnormalities of tone, apraxia and slowed processing may disrupt the patient's responses. Once ability to respond has been established the therapist may evaluate orientation to time, place and person.

The Glasgow Coma Scale (GCS) of Teasdale and Jennett (1974) is a standardized assessment procedure for use with the patient in coma. The GCS uses three independently measured aspects of behaviour: motor responsiveness, verbal performance and eye opening. Patients are rated on their best response. The GCS can be applied rapidly and consistently by many members of the treatment team. Normally recording of GCS scores is completed on admission to the emergency room or neurological

Table 8.1 Glasgow Coma Scale* with explanations of terms

		Motor Responses
Obeys Commands:	6	Patient follows simple commands; care must be taken to avoid interpreting a grasp reflex or a postural adjustment as a response to command.
Localized pain response:	5	A stimulus applied at more than one site causes movement in an attempt to escape it.
Withdrawal:	4	A normal flexor response; patient withdraws from painful stimulus applied to nail bed with abduction of the shoulders
Abnormal flexion response:	3	Patient withdraws from painful stimulus applied to nail bed with stereotyped mass flexor pattern (including adduction at the shoulder)
Abnormal extensor response:	2	Patient withdraws from painful stimulus applied to nail bed with stereotyped mass extension pattern (including adduction and internal rotation at the shoulder and pronation of the forearm).
No response:	1	Usually associated with hypotonia (ensure adequate stimuli and absence of spinal cord injury).
		Verbal response
Oriented:	5	Patient oriented to time, place and person.
Confused conversation:	4	Patient can converse but the content indicates disorientation and confusion.
Inappropriate speech:	3	Patient utters comprehensible words but only in a random way (e.g. purposeless shouting and swearing)
Incomprehensible speech:	2	Patient utters grunts and groans only (no recognizable words)
No speech:	1	Self explanatory.

Table 8.1 *continued*

		Eye opening
Spontaneous eye opening:	4	Does not imply awareness (includes sleep/wake cycles)
In response to speech:	3	Patient opens eyes in response to some speech (includes shouting) but does not imply that the patient opens eyes to command.
In response to pain:	2	Patient opens eyes in response to painful stimuli applied to the chest or limbs.
Eyes do not open:	1	Self explanatory.

Glasgow Coma Scale score = sum of motor, verbal and eye opening score (3–15)
*After Teasdale, G. and Jennett, B. (1974) The Glasgow Coma Scale. *Lancet*, ii: 81–84.

trauma unit. A severe injury may be defined as a GCS of 8 or less (the lowest obtained score is three); a score of 9 – 12 indicates a moderate brain injury and of 13 – 15 a mild brain injury (Rimel *et al.*, 1981). Therapists may be trained to administer the GCS by nursing staff. However, when other staff are administering the GCS duplication is unnecessary.

Assessment in the early post-coma recovery period

After the stage of coma it remains important to be able to track progress and a number of more general scales are available and widely used for this purpose. An overall categorization of purposive behaviour is provided by the Rancho Los Amigos Scale (see Table 8.2).

An alternative to the Rancho Los Amigos Scale is the Disability Rating Scale (DRS) of Rappaport and co-workers (1982) which charts the progress of the recovery of the severely brain-injured patient particularly from the middle stages of recovery (for instance, the level of recovery seen in acute rehabilitation settings: early arousal from coma and early sentient functioning). The DRS consists of four categories. The first category measures arousal, awareness and responsivity and is adapted from the Glasgow Coma Scale. Unfortunately the scoring is reversed so the higher the number the greater the degree of impairment. This reversal may lead to some confusion for those

Table 8.2 Rancho Los Amigos Levels of Cognitive Functioning* with explanation of terms.
Not all patients go through all stages nor do all patients progress at the same rate

1. No response	Patient exhibits complete absence of observable response when presented with any stimuli.
2. Generalized response	Patient exhibits generalized responses to painful stimuli; may respond to repeated auditory stimuli with increased or decreased activity; responses are the same irrespective of the type or location of stimuli.
3. Localized response	Patient demonstrates withdrawal or vocalization to painful stimuli; may turn towards or away from auditory stimuli; responds to discomfort by pulling tubes or restraints.
4. Confused/agitated	Severely impaired processing of environmental information; patient responds primarily to internal state; attention span very limited; profound difficulty in encoding new information; behavior may be bizarre or aggressive; dependent in all aspects of care.
5. Confused/inappropriate Non-agitated	Patient is unable to respond to simple commands fairly consistently; patient is able to attend to some aspects of the environment but attention span remains limited; patient requires assistance or close supervision for functional tasks; performance deteriorates when structure decreases or complexity increases.
6. Confused/appropriate	Patient follows simple directions consistently; patient inconsistently oriented to time and place; completes overlearned tasks with supervision.
7. Automatic/appropriate	Orientated consistently; may retain significant memory dysfunction; initiates and carries out basic routines completely independently; displays some insight into disability but may be unable to realistically plan for own future.

Table 8.2 *continued*

8. Purposeful/appropriate	Patient is alert and oriented consistently; demonstrates more responsibility for self and may be able to plan realistically for own future; able to learn new tasks and can apply learned skills independently in new situations; may be able to work or be a candidate for vocational rehabilitation; may continue to show reduced ability relative to pre-morbid functioning.

*After Hagen, C., Malkmus, D. and Durham, P. (1972) *Levels of Cognitive Functioning*, Rancho Los Amigos Hospital.

used to the alternative method. The second category grades cognitive ability for self-care activities (feeding, toileting and grooming) and relates to the patient's knowledge of how and when to perform such tasks. Ability is rated as complete/partial/ or minimal. Rating is dependent on stating or demonstrating the requirements of how and when to perform, but not on their actual performance. Patients therefore can be rated as independent, but nonetheless fail to perform in real-world settings. The third category is level of functioning and is modified from that of Scranton *et al.* (1970). The patient is rated as completely independent, independent in a special (modified) environment and mildly, moderately, markedly and totally dependent. The fourth category is degree of independent employability the individual is likely to have in the job market. In the original study, inter-rater reliability were 0.97 to 0.98 and no patient was rated at discharge as being without disability. The scale can be learned easily and be applied rapidly (usually taking no more than 5 – 15 minutes).

GOAT

The Galveston Orientation and Amnesia Test (GOAT) (Levin *et al.*, 1979) is a test designed to chart changes in cognition and orientation during the subacute stages of recovery from brain injury. Longitudinal investigation of groups of patients with closed brain-injury has confirmed the prognostic significance of duration of post-traumatic alteration in memory functioning, and while retrospective assessment is possible (Russell, 1971) it is likely to be either as complete or reliable as prospective assessment. The GOAT provides a practical and reliable scale designed to evaluate the major spheres of orientation, for instance, time, place and person and may be used by various health-care workers. The GOAT also allows for estimation of the period following injury for which the patient is unable to recall events (Post Traumatic Amnesia: PTA) and for the period pre-dating the injury for which recall is absent (retrograde amnesia). All items are presented orally and include asking the patient to identify the town they are in and to identify the building as a hospital. The GOAT can be used at the patient's bedside or in the therapy department. Presenting a calendar may help overcome difficulties in assessing patients with aphasia or tracheostomy. Daily administration of the GOAT is recommended. The recording form and detailed scoring instructions are provided in the original report (Levin *et al.*, 1979). In a validity study of 52 closed brain-injury patients, the duration of impaired GOAT scores was strongly related to the acute neurosurgery ratings of eye opening, motor responsiveness and verbal responding on the Glasgow Coma Scale. Prolonged confusion as demonstrated by the GOAT is characteristic of patients with diffuse brain injury and those who have evidence on computerized tomography of cerebral swelling (for example, compressed ventricles). The patient's performance on the GOAT was related to severity of outcome. Prolonged disability resulted primarily from injury that produced confusion and amnesia which lasted in excess of two weeks following resolution of coma. Recently Davidoff and co-workers (1988) demonstrated that use of the GOAT aids clinicians in recognizing those spinal cord injured patients who have also suffered brain trauma. In their prospective study of 34 patients, nine would have been misclassified as being without brain injury had the GOAT not been used (Davidoff *et al.*, 1988).

Jackson *et al.* (1989) have described the orientation group monitoring system (OGMS). The OGMS provides a simple and reliable behavioural monitoring system for use in group setting. It allows for the tracking of orientation and the identification of deterioration (it is described further in Chapter 10). A comparison of the GOAT and the OGMS is instructive regarding the applicability of both (Mysiw *et al.*, 1990). Both are reliable and construct validity has been supported. A comparison of results of the GOAT and the OGMS on the same series of patients showed 71% agreement over the course of the study on whether the patient was or was not in PTA. The most common discrepancy was for patients to have results indicating recovery from PTA on the GOAT but not on the OGMS. In 10% of cases the GOAT showed PTA as having cleared while the OGMS never did. A disagreement in the reverse direction (i.e. the OGMS showing recovery and the GOAT indicating continuing PTA) did not occur. A number of factors may account for these differences. The OGMS attempts to assess memory function via events of the previous day. The events may be difficult to substantiate but this method has the advantage (snared by other portions of this test) of having limited practice effects. The OGMS appears less prone to false negatives than the GOAT. However the GOAT has the advantage of being an instrument designed for rapid bedside administration and which does not require a continuing group programme.

The BRISC

The Barry Inpatient Screening of Cognition (BRISC) (Barry, *et al.*, 1989) is a cognitive screening device which can be administered to subjects in the early stages of recovery from brain injury in about 30 minutes. It can be administered to a subject who is in bed, and provides a broad sample of cognitive functioning. The BRISC is most appropriate for subjects in the middle range of recovery; it has a low ceiling and is not a substitute for the more extensive neuropsychological tests required as the subject improves. The BRISC is divided into eight categories. The reading category asks the patient to read single words or short phrases printed in large bold type. The design copy category asks subjects to copy five simple shapes. The third category, verbal concepts, asks subjects to state in which ways common objects are similar and different. Category four assesses orientation. Category five is a test of mental imagery where the subject is asked to recite the alphabet and list all of the letters with curves in them. Category six, mental control, includes digits forward and backwards and a sequential alternation task (a verbal task analogous to trail making two). Category seven asks subjects to generate lists of items purchased in a grocery store or items of clothing. Category eight tests delayed recall of graphic and verbal items included earlier in the test. Inter-rater reliability was 0.94 and above and test–retest reliability after one week was also at the 0.90 level. The test appears to be valid with significant correlations with five frequently used measures of cognitive functioning (Barry *et al.*, 1989). For a general discussion of the timing and content of assessment in the acute stage of recovery see Chapter six.

Following the patient's emergence from post-traumatic amnesia the duration of PTA may be used to infer severity of injury (Russell and Smith's 1961 criteria are provided in Table 8.3). Prior to emergence from coma these criteria are not available.

Table 8.3 Russell and Smith's* criteria for brain injury severity

Mild	PTA under one hour
Moderate	PTA one—twenty-four hours
Severe	PTA one—seven days
Very severe	PTA over seven days
(Focal complications introduce qualifying factor)	

*After Russell, W. R. and Smith, A. (1961) Post traumatic amnesias in closed head injuries. *Archives of Neurology*, 5, 16–29.

MEDICAL PROBLEMS OF THE PATIENT IN THE INITIAL STAGES OF RECOVERY

During the initial period of recovery the purpose of intervention is to provide medical treatment, monitor physiological functioning, prevent complications associated with immobility and provide family members with information and support. Therapists should be aware of the medical conditions and nursing procedures which may complicate their treatment approaches. Endotracheal intubation is initially indicated for maintaining an airway and ventilation, the removal of secretions, and to provide hyperventilation which may be undertaken in an attempt to reduce cerebral oedema. Tracheostomy/intubation is usually performed if the coma is expected to be of extended duration. Complications of both endotracheal intubation and tracheostomy are common and could be life-threatening. Therapists should be aware that excessive tube movement during turning or during range of motion is contra-indicated. Due to the patient's decreased level of awareness and oral–bulbar status, intravenous fluids, nasogastric tube feeding or a gastrostomy procedure may be required to ensure that the patient receives adequate nutrition. In addition, tubes may be used to facilitate the administration of medications (such as anti-convulsants). Therapists should take cognizance of these in providing range of motion exercises and splinting, as well as recognizing that they are major irritants to confused patients.

Raised intracranial pressure is a major risk for patients in coma and many trauma centres now have ongoing intracranial pressure monitoring. Whether or not this monitoring is available, the therapist should be aware of the risks of raised intracranial pressure in some patients following range of motion exercises or other forms of excessive stimulation.

Medical problems do not cease on the patient's transfer to the acute rehabilitation setting. Kalisky and co-workers (1985) studied a consecutive series of 180 patients with severe brain injury admitted to a rehabilitation unit. Patients had a coma duration of greater than six hours or cerebral trauma confirmable on CT scan. The mean coma duration of the group of 144 males and 36 females was 55 days. Medical problems frequently originated in the acute hospital but were not always identified there. Of the entire series, 56% ($N=100$) had neurological problems which required further investigation. Ventricular dilatation was the most frequently encountered neurological disorder: 37% ($N=67$). Seven patients received shunts, four in the acute hospital and three in the rehabilitation unit. Post-traumatic seizures accounted for 13% ($N=23$) of the neurological problems, eight patients had their first seizure in the acute facility and the remainder developed the disorder in the rehabilitation unit. Four of these patients had an episode of status epilepticus. Other problems encountered in the rehabilitation phase included delayed subdural haematomas or hygromas requiring evacuation (three patients), meningitis (one patient) and subdural empyema (one patient).

Fifty percent of the population studied developed gastrointestinal problems (GI) ($N=90$) and impaired liver function occurred most frequently: 43% ($N=77$). Eleven patients had symptoms consistent with oesophagitis, gastritis or ulcer disease and this was confirmed in nine patients. In five patients, these problems originated in the acute hospital, while in six they first occurred in the rehabilitation unit. Upper GI bleeding occurred in five patients while on the rehabilitation unit. Of the total sample, 81 patients (45%) developed genito-urinary disorders with urinary tract infections (UTI) accounting for most of these 38% ($N=68$). Of the patients with UTI, 63% had indwelling Foley catheters. Bladder dysfunction was seen in 8% of patients ($N=15$) while urethral strictures occurred in two (1%).

Respiratory problems occurred in 34% of the total sample ($N=61$). Of this group, 26% ($N=47$) had a tracheostomy. All of those with a tracheostomy developed bacterial colonization of the site. Thirty-two patients developed pneumonia. Six patients had pulmonary embolism, two in the acute hospital and four at the rehabilitation site.

Fifty-eight subjects (32%) had cardiovascular abnormalities. Hypertension was seen in 19 patients (11%), ten were diagnosed acutely and one at the rehabilitation setting. Eight patients (4%) developed thrombophlebitis and one, endocarditis. Thirty-seven patients (21%) had skin problems while hospitalized and of the nine patients who developed decubitus ulcers, seven did so at the acute hospital site and two during rehabilitation. Thirty-four patients (19%) developed heterotopic ossification and osteomyelitis occurred in four patients. Eight patients (4%) had endocrine disorders. The frequency with which medical problems occur in the rehabilitation setting makes it important for therapists to be alert to medical complications which may occur in their patients.

Grosswasser and co-workers (1988) described the incidence and characteristics of patients with communicative hydrocephalus (CH), a deficit of reabsorption of cerebrospinal fluid. Almost 3.9% of the group of 335 severely brain-injured patients studied developed the disorder. Patients were suspected of developing CH whenever coma persisted, recovery was delayed, or there was an arrest in clinical improvement following initial recovery. Treatment involved ventricular–peritoneal shunts in 10 of the 13 patients (77%). Three patients were not provided with shunts despite progressive ventricular enlargement, due to additional frontal and temporal lesions. Seven of the patients were operated on whilst still in coma and the remaining three were operated on following an arrest of progress or deterioration following an initial period of progress. Duration of coma was longer in the CH patients, they had a higher incidence of behaviour disorder and poorer motor, ADL and occupational outcome than non-CH patients (Grosswasser *et al*, 1988).

Klingbell (1988) described problems of maintaining airways in patients with traumatic brain injury. Of 44 patients studied, four did not tolerate decannulation and were discharged intubated. Two patients required multiple surgical interventions due to complications arising from the tracheostomy.

Cosgrove, Vargo and Reidy (1989) performed the first prospective study of the relationship between traumatic brain injury and peripheral nerve lesions. The authors studied 132 patients admitted to a specialized brain injury unit. Patients fulfilling the research criteria of flaccidity, areflexia and abnormal motor patterns underwent neurodiagnostic evaluation. Fifteen electromyograph studies were performed leading to positive findings in 13 patients. There were 16 lesions, one patient sustained three injuries and another patient two. Thirteen of the lesions occurred at the time of injury and three pressure palsies occurred during hospitalization. There were eight brachial plexus injuries, three radial nerve injuries, two lumbosacral plexus injuries, two peroneal nerve injuries and one femoral nerve injury. At time of discharge three injuries had recovered fully, eight patients had minor deficits and five had major impairment or no recovery. Treatment during their hospital stay included the provision of orthoses. Two patients with radial nerve palsies were given extension wrist-hand orthoses and both had stopped using these by the time of discharge. Four patients were given ankle-foot orthoses and all were continuing to use them at three month follow-up. The patient with a femoral nerve injury had a concomitant left hemiparesis and was provided with a knee-ankle-foot orthosis which was also in use at the time of discharge.

THERAPY IN THE ACUTE STAGES OF RECOVERY OF FUNCTION

The therapist has the responsibility of developing close working relationships with the ICU staff. When nursing staff are fully appraised of the contribution which can be made by therapy professionals, they can facilitate appropriate referrals from the physician for evaluation and treatment. Therapy staff should attend the daily ICU staff meetings to allow for a comprehensive exchange of information on each client. Central to the role of the therapists in the acute stage of recovery from brain injury are work with the family, coma stimulation and the management of orthopaedic and neuromuscular conditions. The way in which the therapist interacts with the patient not only helps the patient manage his or her own behaviour, but also acts as a model for appropriate stimulation and interaction with the patient by others on the treatment team.

Working with the family

The families of brain injured people have to cope with many crises during the acute stage of recovery. Family members have usually had to change their entire routine to be at the hospital, causing disruption of domestic and work routines such as the care and support of children, or taking time off work. Meeting with medical professionals who know nothing of the person before the trauma, and whose focus is on the injury and not on the person known to the family, is also stressful. The reluctance of medical professionals to give concrete predictions regarding their loved one's future functioning could give the family the impression that they are not getting straight answers.

There are various stages of emotional reactions that relatives are likely to experience on learning of the traumatic incident. Therapists should keep in mind the possible stages of reaction to injury of denial, anger, mourning or depression, and finally adaptation. Initially family members are shocked and overwhelmed. Some appear very organized, presenting as 'coping relatives' in the initial stages, only reacting to the traumatic event later. Others are incapable of dealing with the situation and need guidance and support to develop a plan of action. Many relatives stay for long periods of time in the hospital environment and find it difficult to leave their injured relative and attend to their other responsibilities. During the slow (and often long) rehabilitation process, relatives may deny the existence of the individual's deficits, take over the caring role, become critical about the patient's physical care, display anger to the staff about certain aspects of the rehabilitation programme or the communication about their relative from one shift to another.

Family members contribute significantly throughout the recovery phase. Alliance with the family is enhanced by information sharing and empathetic recognition of concerns. Therapists play an important role in educating family members about the patient's motor, cognitive, behavioural, functional and vocational recovery. As part of the rehabilitation team each therapy professional provides a role model and an instructor in behaviour management.

The purpose of therapy at this stage in rehabilitation of the brain-injured patient should be explained. Family members may be encouraged to assist in positioning. They could also be encouraged to bring posters, photographs and the patient's favourite objects into the ICU. Whatever effect this has on the patient (and it undoubtedly has an effect after the resolution of coma) it helps the family feel more comfortable. It also enables the staff involved in the patient's rehabilitation gain knowledge and understanding of the persons they are working with. Many hospitals, national and local organizations, produce explanatory publications about brain injury for family members. One of these relevant booklets can be selected by the staff and given to family members. It is important for the therapist concerned to follow up with family members who have been given reading materials, to answer questions. Meeting other people to talk to, who have been through the experience of coping with brain injury in a loved one, can be beneficial. The local organization of Headway (UK) or the National Head Injury Foundation (USA) may provide this service. In our experience, family support groups are most useful after the patient has become medically stable. Family support groups are discussed in Chapter 13.

Coma stimulation

The therapeutic interventions known as coma stimulation were developed in an attempt to reduce those factors thought to impede the recovery of patients in coma. Analogies between a developing nervous system and a recovering nervous system led some to believe that the sensory depriving nature of hospital environments could be damaging to the individual recovering from brain trauma. Both human developmental models and animal models were used to justify this view (Ylvisaker, 1985). While it is recognized that an intensive care unit may be 'stimulating', this stimulation is random and unorganized (Le Winn,

1980). The aim of the originators of systematic stimulation of the comatose patient were (1) to augment the limited sensory stimulation present in the ordinary hospital environment; (2) to make the patient independent of mechanical life-support systems; (3) to hasten the patient's return to consciousness and hence reduce medical complications; (4) to enable the patient's family assume responsibility for intervention and (5) to achieve the earliest possible discharge from hospital.

Stimulation is applied to the five senses and includes loud noises, pain and strong olfactory stimulation provided by aromatic spirits of ammonia or lemon juice. Le Winn and Dimancescu (1978) advocated six hours of coma treatment per day and claimed remarkable results including a considerably reduced rate of mortality in comparison with those not provided with coma stimulation. These findings have not been replicated by other workers. Rader *et al.* (1989) reported a study designed to assess change in the responsiveness in comatose patients as a result of sensory stimulation. The patients were in a specialized programme for the treatment of minimally responsive patients and no significant differences in general responsiveness were found. Similarly no relationship was found between amount of treatment per day, frequency of family visits, pre-morbid education, age, time since injury or neurological status between patients who improved and those who did not. Many health facilities, particularly in the USA, offer sensory stimulation programmes to comatose brain-injured individuals (NHIF, 1989). As noted by Rader and co-workers (1989) Western culture does not easily allow medical personnel to take a passive role. Active interventions are welcomed by all those involved in the rehabilitation process. Structured stimulations, not contra-indicated by raised intracranial pressure, may assist in determining the patient's level of responsiveness. The aims of treatment for the minimally responsive (not comatose) patient are to increase level of response and overall awareness. Stimulation should be structured and broken down into simple steps and enough time must be allowed for a response, since the patient's response may be considerably slowed during this phase of recovery. However the more optimistic claims of the early proponents of coma stimulation are probably unfounded.

Positioning and handling

The avoidance of raised intracranial pressure is a central consideration in positioning and should initially be supervised by medical personnel. As noted by Palmer and Wyness (1988) the most consistent research finding regarding the effects of positioning and handling on ICP suggests the importance of maintaining the patient's head in the anatomically neutral position to allow unimpeded venous outflow. Maintenance of the head in the midline is also central in the avoidance of abnormal tonic reflex activity. Although acutely ill, brain-injured patients are predominantly maintained in supine; many patients could benefit from alternated periods of side-lying (see an introductory occupational therapy, physiotherapy or nursing text or a description of basic positioning and handling procedures).

The patient may display stereotyped posturing as a result of release of lower (sub-cortical) centres from the modulating influence of higher cortical structures. Proper handling and bed positioning limit abnormal posturing and its long-term consequences. Abnormal posturing is increased by excessive tactile stimulation, sudden movement, noxious stimuli, loud noise, cold or pull of a limb against restraint (Palmer and Wyness, 1988). A programme of therapeutic movement can be started for many patients in the ICU. It is recommended that this is accomplished as a combined treatment session with a physical and occupational therapist. Medical approval should be obtained and ICP, blood pressure, pulse, respiration, amount of perspiration and the patient's colour should be monitored to ensure that the patient can tolerate the change of position. When sitting on the side of the bed, with a therapist in front and another behind, a midline head position should be maintained, with the patient's hips and knees positioned at 90 degrees and feet placed on the floor (or a solid object if they do not reach the floor). Initially sitting may only be tolerated for five minutes or less. Some patients appear to become more alert when sitting, and a sitting programme gives the therapist the opportunity to provide range of motion through functional activity. Longer periods of time and reduction in the amount of support provided increase the challenge of the programme as the patient progresses.

When the patient is in prolonged coma or persistent vegetative state (PVS), a programme of wheelchair positioning must be considered. It minimizes the adverse effets of prolonged bed rest and decreases the risk of decubiti. Correct seating helps inhibit the production of abnormal reflex movements and aids in the prevention of joint contractures. An appropriate physical regime will help maintain hip and knee flexion, ankle dorsiflexion and spinal alignment. Adequate wheelchair positioning may require the use of positioning devices and standard guidelines for wheelchair positioning should be followed. For patients in PVS a Putney Alternative Position (PAP) chair or reclining wheelchair, with a custom fabricated 'U' shaped head rest and head band is recommended. Maintaining hip and knee flexion at 90 degrees or more inhibits abnormal reflex movement during transfers and positioning. If lifted into a reclining wheelchair a firm seat board should be in place to discourage internal rotation and adduction at the hip. Trunk positioning devices will be required and a lap tray for arm positioning. In the presence of hypertonicity, limbs should be supported in opposition to the position of contraction, i.e. the paralysed shoulder is positioned in abduction, the elbow, wrist, and fingers in extension, the hip extended and abducted and internally rotated. Uninterrupted periods of sitting in bed or chair, or continuous side-lying with the hips and knees flexed, can result in hip and knee flexion contractures. Such contractures predispose to decubiti, since bony prominences are more exposed to pressure and result in a considerable reduction in positioning options.

Fractures

Fractures should be stabilized as early as possible unless this is prevented by neurological or other systemic contra-indications. Orthopaedic management is always more complex in an agitated patient or in a patient who is minimally protective in response to pain. Failure to diagnose musculoskeletal injuries in the acutely brain injured patient is common (Garland and Baily, 1981). The therapist should be alert to the possibility of an overlooked injury; this is particularly likely with the shoulder girdle. Given the patient's inability to protect the fracture site, internal fixation is often warranted as external fixation could lead to further injury in the agitated patient. Traction may be required for patients who are medically unstable. Anaesthesia is contra-indicated where there is risk of increased intracranial pressure. Poor skin condition could also preclude operative intervention.

The most common injuries to the upper extremity occur at the shoulder girdle, scapula, clavicle and acromio-clavicular joint but because of lack of obvious deformity associated with these injuries they are regularly overlooked. Elbow injuries are associated with the highest incidence of heterotopic ossification in the upper extremity. As heterotopic ossification develops, the elbow becomes painful, warm and swollen and loses motion. Treatment of upper extremity fractures by stable internal fixation allows continued mobilization. Neuropathies frequently complicate elbow injuries.

Brachial plexus injuries are common after motor cycle accidents. The combination of upper and lower motor neurone damage may be particularly difficult to diagnose but lower motor neurone lesions usually lead to hypertonicity. Nerve conduction studies may be helpful in diagnosis but positive findings may not be evident until some time after injury.

Pelvic fractures are serious when they occur with a traumatic brain injury and are a common cause of hypovolemic shock. Pelvic injury occurs in 50% of pedestrians struck by fast moving motor vehicles (Garland *et al.*, 1979). Bladder and urethral damage are common complications of pelvic injury. Stable fractures heal rapidly, unstable fractures require fixation as slings and traction are contra-indicated in the agitated brain injured patient. Fractures involving the acetabulum carry with them an increased risk of heterotopic ossification. Femoral fractures are the most common lower extremity injury and reduction must be stable to prevent angulation as a result of hypertonicity with cast bracing advised for some difficult cases. Acute reconstructive surgery for knee ligamentous injuries are not advised. Tibial fractures pose no special difficulties and are treated with plaster cast immobilization. Botte and Moore (1987) state that fracture bracing is not used because patients tend to remove the brace. In open fractures external fixation is less than optimal because (1) the pins and bar are hazardous to the agitated patient and (2) ankle positioning is difficult to maintain in the non-agitated patient and far more difficult when the patient is agitated. Percutaneous pins and plaster offer considerable advantages and since the occupational or physical therapist will have to maintain ankle positioning in a patient with external fixation it is important to educate the orthopod to the preferred method of fixation from the therapy perspective.

Casting and splinting

Following brain injury many patients develop soft tissue contractures as a result of poor posture associated with hypertonicity. Range of motion exercises, positioning, stretching and the appropriate application of resting splints may prevent soft tissue contractures from prolonged immobility but may be insufficient to counteract the development of contractures where there is severe prolonged spastic posturing.

A contracture is the loss of range of motion (ROM) due to alteration in muscle and connective tissue surrounding a joint. Shortening of tendon, muscle, joint capsule, skin or bony changes may all contribute to the development of contractures. ROM limitations may also result from heterotopic ossification, fractures or ligamentous injuries. Serial casting would be contemplated if the patient has ROM limitations in conjunction with significant hypertonicity. Contra-indications to casting include marked oedema, open sores, skin grafts, vascular disorders, the limb being used for vital sign assessment or drug administration (Conine et al, 1990). Casting may also be contraindicated when there are fractures in the same extremity due to the risk of compartment syndrome (uncontrolled swelling in a fascia compartment leading to – if untreated – muscular necrosis) (Moore et al., 1989). Although an increased risk of compartment syndrome in patients with fractures in the same extremity treated with serial casting is thought to exist, its incidence is unknown.

Both casting and splinting may be used in an attempt to maintain ROM. Plaster is strong, weighty and inexpensive and can be repaired when necessary and bivalved. Disadvantages include time-consuming and messy applications and extreme caution is necessary to prevent pressure injuries. Weight may also limit the functional use of the extremity. Although research is limited there is some evidence indicating the superiority of non-bivalved casts over bivalved casts (Imle et al., 1986). The advantages of customized adjustable orthoses include the closeness of fit because adjustments may be carried out while the limb is in the orthoses. Removal of the device permits regular cleaning and skin inspection. The lightweight construction of orthoses allows functional activities to be performed with the splint in place. Disadvantages are the much higher initial cost and the high level of skill required for fabrication. The extra expense and difficulty is probably justified where abnormal tone prevents function, the patient's condition is stable, and the patient is cognitively able to perform activities they were not physically able to perform because of positioning.

When serial casting is used, the duration of each individual cast application is approximately 5–7 days. The affected joint should be put through the full range of motion available at each application, with 3–4 positioning casts used in a course of treatment. The final cast may be bi-valved and used as a day or night resting splint. See Sullivan *et al.* (1988) for a detailed description of application procedures and Leahy (1988) for a method of assessing appropriate patients for serial casting in the acute stage of recovery. The upper extremity problems most responsive to serial casting are elbow and wrist flexion and in the lower extremity, knee flexion and ankle equinus deformity (the most common contracture following brain injury) may respond well to this procedure. A variant of the serial cast is the drop-out cast which allows movement in the desired direction but restricts movement in the other direction. Knee casts may be articulated with a locking device to allow sitting during therapy sessions. Conine and co-workers (1990) have demonstrated the existence of clinically and statistically significant differences between patients before and after a serial casting procedure used to reduce equinus deformity in the acute recovery period.

The beneficial effects of serial casting with patients in the acute stage of neurological recovery may result from the prevention of muscle shortening. There is no evidence that serial casting is an active component in reducing abnormal tone as neurological recovery often leads to the progressive reduction in hypertonia. Whatever the cause of the poor posture, soft tissue changes will occur and minimizing contracture formation while the patient is recovering and tone reducing facilitates neuromuscular re-education when this is appropriate. Surgical release of contractures should not be considered until 18 months after injury – and not until after energetic conservative means have proved ineffective. Surgery should not be considered for purely cosmetic reasons and, where there is some retained function in the limb, possible gain should be weighed against the risk of decreased function.

Heterotopic ossification

Heterotopic ossification (HO) is the ectopic appearance of bone in soft tissue. The pathophysiology of heterotopic ossification in neurological disorders remains unclear but it most frequently occurs around large joints in spastic extremities of patients with severe brain injury and prolonged unconsciousness. Early signs and symptoms of HO include warmth, swelling, pain responses, and an elevated sedimentation rate. Therapists should alert a physician when the patient suffers progressive loss of motion. Treatment of HO aims to minimize the ultimate loss of range of motion and may involve surgery. Therapists should attempt to maintain range of motion to prevent ankylosis since the traditional belief that range of motion increases HO is unfounded. If ankylosis does occur there should be an attempt to ensure that this occurs in an optimal position. Surgery for HO is usually performed one to two years following an injury. Gennarelli (1988) has advocated a programme of HO prophylaxis involving the following.

1. An aggressive programme of ROM to prevent joint immobilization. Care should be taken to avoid limb trauma which may act as a focus for HO.
2. Diminish or reduce abnormalities of tone by available pharmacological intervention.
3. The early use of an agent specifically for HO prevention, for example etidronate disodium.

INTERACTING WITH THE PATIENT RETURNING FROM COMA

Confusion/agitation

On emerging from coma many individuals go through a period of marked agitation. Agitation may be defined as including one or more of the following: repetitive, stereotyped, or purposeless movement of the trunk (rocking) or extremities (thrashing);

attempting to hit, bite or pinch others; attempting to remove naso-gastric or intravenous tubes or catheters; shouting or attempting to get out of bed or chair. The patient may be given a Craig bed, which is a large mattress placed on the floor and surrounded by a low padded wall. The Craig bed is designed to allow the patient to move without restraint but prevents injury.

There is dispute regarding whether agitation is a stage all those with brain injury experience or if it is restricted to a sub-group of the brain-injured and whether it has prognostic significance. In the series reported by Rao and co-workers (1985), 25 of the 26 patients studied, all of whom were comatose for 24 hours or more, experienced agitation and in 11 cases the agitation was severe enough to be treated with medication. Levin and Grossman (1978) noted that 30% of their patients exhibited a significant period of agitation. Corrigan and Mysiw (1988) examined the relationship between agitation and confusion in the early post-traumatic period. These authors found that agitation was significantly correlated with measures of cognitive function and as cognition improved, agitation diminished. Marked agitation was associated with severe cognitive impairment. The degree of behaviour disorder in the acute stage may also be linked to cognitive impairment (Dr. James Wilson, personal communication).

Those patients who recover rapidly may not go through a period of agitation requiring intervention. For other patients agitation may be marked and the period of agitation may be extensive. Many patients may be managed by reducing enviromental stimulation and by the provision of a Craig bed. Some patients, particularly those whose care is complicated by fractures or other medical conditions, may require pharmacological or physical restraint. Major tranquillizers used to reduce agitation may slow recovery. Physical restraints have their own dangers. (Dube and Mitchell, 1986) Berrol (1988) describes the case of a young man recovering from a severe brain injury, who was strangled in a posy vest and suffered severe anoxic damage as a result. The tendency of staff to loosen the restraint to decrease patient discomfort could paradoxically increase this risk.

Other psychiatric/behaviourial disturbances which could occur in the acute stage include the development of *ideé fixe*.

One patient became convinced that he had to contact his brother Michael in Miami. This theme was with him for some weeks (and was remembered later in his recovery) even though, by this time, he knew he did not have a brother and knew no one in Miami. Another patient was convinced that the driver of the car which hit him was his Methodist minister. Other patients have produced bizarre ideas. One individual (previous occupation plumber) would talk at length about his job transporting circus animals and when asked how he received his brain injury stated he had been chasing monkeys down the freeway. On other occasions he recounted stories about being a soldier of fortune in the Philippines, which were, according to his family, not part of his personal history.

Interacting with the comatose patient

We recommend the following approach to patients who are in a coma or minimally responsive. These approaches may be followed during all contact with the patient, while performing range of motion, splinting, plaster casting, and assessment procedures.

1. Introduce yourself to the patient whether it is your first visit or one of many.
2. Say who you are, what your job is, and why you are there.
3. Tell the patient in short, clear statements what you are about to do or what is about to happen. Also tell him or her immediately before it happens (if the patient can understand they will nonetheless forget very rapidly).
4. Speak slowly and calmly.
5. Always assume that the patient understands what is said in their vicinity and do not discuss the patient's prognosis in front of them or other patients.
6. When you are with a patient devote your attention to him; do not talk to other staff while working with a patient other than when giving instructions to colleagues with whom you are performing a procedure.
7. Encourage family members to talk to the patient in the same way as outlined above. Topics should include non-stressful events in the life of the family or items of previous interest

to the patient. Interaction should be kept brief however so as not to be overwhelming.

Adopting the style of interaction described here is justifiable on multiple grounds. It is felt by some that interpersonal interaction is a form of stimulation which may aid in recovery. It is respectful and will not offend family members who may be present. It encourages slow and deliberate movement which will be less likely to lead to over-arousal and models appropriate handling of the patient by other staff.

Interacting with and treating the acutely confused patient

The aim of interaction with the confused or stuporous patient is to carry out medical care while not increasing agitation or confusion, and to engage the patient in therapeutic activities up to the level that the patient can tolerate. At this stage the individual remains 'stimulus bound' and stereotyped responses are produced to discomfort or over-stimulation as he or she cannot tolerate physical discomfort. If the patient becomes agitated during an activity, terminate the activity, wait until the patient is calm and then either reintroduce the activity, or if this leads to repeated agitation, proceed to something else. If the patient's agitation begins to escalate remove him from the environment. Attempting to calm him in an already over stimulating environment increases his level of stimulation and could exacerbate the situation.

Information should be presented slowly, calmly and softly, in as reassuring a manner as possible. The patient is likely to have profound memory and attentional difficulties, and preventing overstimulation can be attained by reducing ambient stimulation to a minimum. When speaking to the patient present information as concisely as possible.

Assessment at this stage in recovery can be problematic; it is often difficult to determine if the patient can give reliable 'Yes' or 'No' answers. The patient may be unable to speak, highly distractible, apraxic and/or have other difficulties impeding motor control. As the patient's level of consciousness improves he/she will be more able to follow (intermittently at first) simple one-step instructions.

The patient's environment should be arranged to provide

him/her with as much control as possible within the limits of safety. The aim of environment manipulation is to allow the patient to communicate and carry out simple activities as effectively as possible. Therapists should be calm, move slowly and not engage in activities which will distract the patient from the task in hand, for example, talking to others. Give one simple instruction at a time and wait for the patient to complete one task before giving another. Ensure the patient is paying attention and demonstrate tasks to help him understand the requirements. The more events can be associated with normal environmental activities (for example, lunch) and at regular times of day, the better. The patient should be told each time an activity/event occurs, the time of occurrence and relate it to other events. Placing activities in the context of other activities is especially helpful, for example 'You have been in occupational therapy for the half-hour (10.00–10.30) where you have been working on sitting upright and dressing yourself. You are now going to physical therapy where you are learning to walk'.

Automatic overlearned behaviours are the easiest for the patient to display, but activities should be performed in the same way each time to provide a practice effect. Initially the major focus of therapy should be communication, motor control, feeding, toileting and personal hygiene behaviours. Physical skills can be developed within the context of functional activities, for example, trunk stability and dynamic sitting balance when putting on a T-shirt. Some patients show marked motor weakness and use an external aid, such as an overhead arm support. This can, for example, allow a patient to write his name, blow his nose or eat independently. Often the patient will be unable to complete a task, either due to the physical demands or because of the conceptual requirements (generating a complex dependent series of actions). Continued prompting and redirection towards the next step in a task is often required. At this stage, patients are still likely to be unsafe and could engage in a range of bizarre activities, for example, attempting to clean their teeth with shaving foam. This type of behaviour probably occurs as a result of accessing the wrong behaviour sequence through mis-associations with contextual information.

The next step in treatment is to allow patients to carry out routine daily activities with reduced levels of supervision. Patients at this stage are beginning to perform activities which have adequate contextual cues. The therapist has to be especially wary of the potential for unsafe behaviours, for example, falls in the motorically impaired are common at this stage of recovery. The patient is still cognitively disorganized and requires a highly structured environment in order to function. More use could now be made of environmental cues: written checklists, a calendar, a schedule posted in the patient's room and a wall clock. Orientation activities can begin and end all other scheduled activities (see discussion of orientation training in Chapter 10).

Persistent vegetative state (PVS)

After severe brain injury from traumatic or medical causes, individuals could have a condition described as 'vegetative state'. Prognosis varies depending on the cause but implies a very severe injury. It has been estimated that there are between 5200 and 7800 PVS survivors in the United States (Berrol, 1986a); comparable figures are not available for the United Kingdom. After severe traumatic brain injury between 1–5% remain in PVS at 6 months (Jennett et al, 1977).

Clinically the patient presents with spontaneous eye opening, sleep-wake cycles, the absence of discrete localizing motor responses, no comprehensible speech, inability to follow instructions and the absence of sustained visual pursuit movements (Berrol, 1986b). The pathological substrate is severe diffuse damage to the cortex with relative preservation of the brainstem. The condition may manifest itself early (as early as one day after trauma). Roving eye movements are often present as well as blinking (spontaneously and in response to stimuli). This pattern of arousal may occur in conjunction with complete destruction of both cerebral hemispheres. Patients may progress though a vegetative phase and the condition should not be described as persistent until the patient has not demonstrated an improved level of responsiveness for one year. Progress from PVS to a higher level of functioning has been reported 3½ years post-injury (Arts *et al.*, 1985). Appropriate management of the patient in PVS decreases the incidence of complications and allows for precise evaluation. Even when improvement is no longer expected, appropriate management will maintain the patient in a condition which eases nursing management and is humane for both the family and the care staff.

SUMMARY

In the intensive care unit medical rescue of the patient is the primary concern. The work of therapists of all disciplines is adjunctive to that of the team of trauma physicians and nursing staff. In patients whose coma duration is protracted, physical and occupational therapy has an important role in preventing complications. Some therapists are convinced of the importance of coma stimulation in promoting patient recovery. Therapists also have an important role in assisting family members learn about and cope with what has happened to their loved one. The emotional distress associated with the injury of a loved one and the disruption of normal life often results in strong family reactions directed towards treatment staff. It is particularly important that lines of communication remain open. Careful assessment of the patient at this early stage allows the course of recovery to be charted. Therapists may be the first to notice a change in the patient's responsiveness, ability to sustain attention or endurance which may accompany one of the many medical complications which may occur in this early phase. Therapists are the acknowledged experts in positioning and handling of the head-injured. Although the increased tone and abnormal posturing of the severely injured is extremely difficult to manage on its own, this is made far more complicated by the presence of any associated fractures. Prolonged hypertonic posturing will cause contractures unless a way can be found to maintain the joint in an appropriate position. Ways of maintaining improved joint position are discussed. Heterotopic ossification is a potentially damaging complication of severe brain injury which needs to be treated early and aggressively. As the patient emerges from coma the therapist's role is to manage the environment and to interact with the patient so that the patient is stimulated to perform at his or her maximum level. The following chapters, beginning with Chapter 9 on motor skills, describe methods used to assess and maximize function in the middle and later stages of recovery.

9

Retraining physical skills in functional settings

'If a functional and usable activity is not achieved before therapy is discontinued, it is of no value to begin [the] . . . training program, because the activity will not be used at the end of the therapeutic program and will be forgotten.'

Kottke *et al.* (1978)

Assessment of brain-injured persons' physical functioning includes evaluation of sensory impairment, orthopaedic conditions (e.g. contractures), strength and disorders of motor control (e.g. altered tone, abnormal patterns of movement, lack of initiation of movement, and motor planning deficits). In addition, cognitive and behavioural deficits, the person's living environment and the expectations of the individual and his or her family about recovery should be evaluated. The patient's deficits in these various domains should not be viewed in isolation. It is the task of the skilled therapist to evaluate how the patient's physical and cognitive deficits combine and affect the whole person's real-world functioning (Hooper-Row, 1988). Thorough assessment is vital to evaluate the individual's functioning and to highlight problem areas which can be addressed as treatment priorities.

Balancing the patient's need to reintegrate into the community with the need for intensive motor skills training necessitates a realistic understanding of the individual's likely level of future functioning. The individual should never be asked to put their life 'on hold' to receive therapy. Developing the individual's use of compensatory strategies or environmental adaptation can facilitate the performance of functional tasks, but could impede long-term motor recovery. Motor retraining should emphasize normal movement in the performance of practical activities. In cases where normal movement is not emphasized, the individual may develop abnormal motor patterns potentially limiting recovery. Close interdisciplinary co-operation is required if motor skills learned in therapy sessions are to transfer to functional situations.

MOTOR LEARNING

Motor learning may be defined as a relatively permanent change in movement patterns brought about by practice (Magill, 1985; Sage, 1984). Models of motor learning have been developed, which place emphasis on diverse aspects of the learning process. Motor learning theory offers some valuable ideas for the facilitation of motor recovery following neurological trauma. The major theories concerning the acquisition and control of movement will be reviewed before discussing their implications for the treatment of the brain-injured individual.

Open and closed-loop theory

The open and closed-loop model of motor control (Adams, 1971, 1976) has been used to explain the acquisition and regulation of different types of skilled movement. Open-loop motor programmes include all the temporal and qualitative elements necessary for production of the desired motor response. Once initiated, an open-loop programme cannot be adjusted. Sensory inputs set the external parameters of the movement but are not used to regulate the movement during execution. Rapid ballistic movement and certain types of overlearned movements are in this category. Feedback or error regulation can only occur inter (not intra) trial. Unlike the open-loop system the closed-loop system makes use of continuous sensory feedback to control movements. Slow, precision movements and movements in the early stages of being learned are in this category. The closed-loop system compensates for deviations from the internal representation of the 'ideal' movement through feedback, error detection and correction. Two separate memory constructs are thought by Adams (1971) to be involved in closed-loop learning.

The memory trace is responsible for the initiation of movement while the perceptual trace is responsible for guiding the limb to the target position. The memory trace must be cued to start a movement (motor recall) and error correction during the movement is the responsibility of the perceptual trace. The strength of the memory trace grows as a function of practice, and the perceptual trace as a function of ongoing feedback. The perceptual trace influences the choice of direction and amplitude of movement and uses information about error in the last movement, and feedback regarding the moment-by-moment position of the responding limb.

According to this model, skilled movement develops as a function of trials and reinforcement. When a motor response occurs, if feedback matches the motor plan, the individual knows that a satisfactory action has been performed. When the stimuli fail to match the individual's model, an orientating reflex occurs. As a response to this 'error signal' the individual may momentarily consciously control the movement. This orientating reflex is common during the acquisition stage of learning and is extinguished during the course of normal motor learning (Anokhin, 1969; Sokolov, 1969).

Schema theory

Schema theory (Schmitt, 1975, 1980, 1982) suggests that a motor programme is a movement plan in which parameters are preset according to specific task demands, e.g. force and direction. A schema is an abstract memory construct that represents a rule or generalization about an event, perception or motor action. A schema is an abstract relation formed from experience about a particular class of movements. Four critical features establish the abstract rules which govern a movement (i.e. a schema). These are the conditions preceding the movement; the parameters or motor commands which were assigned to the generalized motor programme; the consequences of the movement (extrinsic feedback); and the intrinsic feedback from the response. Two types of schema are derived from these features: the recall schema responsible for movement production (the abstract rule that defines the relation between response parameters specified and actual movement produced), and the recognition schema (the abstract rule which defines the relation between the sensory consequences and actual movement produced).

Action theory

An individual intending to change his position in space or to perform a certain action, can never make the action take place simply by means of a single set of efferent, motor impulses to a moving extremity. The locomotor apparatus, with all its moveable joints, provides a very large choice of movements. Articulatory changes are involved in every movement and every stage of the sequence alters the muscle tone requirements. For movement to take place there must be constant correction of the initiated movement by afferent impulses providing information about the position of the moving limb in space and the change in tone of the muscles, so that necessary corrections in its course can occur (Bernstein, 1967).

Movement is dictated by the intentions of the individual and is usually purposeful and goal-directed (Luria, 1966). Motor tasks reflect the demands of the outside world and movement loses all its meaning if it is considered apart from action in the world. At the level of instinctive behaviour, with its elementary structure, these motor tasks are dictated by inborn programmes, but at the level of complex action these intentions are formed with the participation of speech and language which help to label movements and regulate human behaviour. According to action theory, every action consists of a chain of consecutive movements, each element of which must be completed to allow the next element to take place. In the initial stages of forming this motor behaviour, the chain of motor elements need developing as motor skills until they can be reduced into automatic complex movements and performed as a single 'kinetic melody' (Luria, 1966) or 'inner mental actions' (Vigotskii, 1962). Action theorists see movement as occurring as the result of an action plan. At its highest level this is not a representation of a series of movements but a function. This approach recognizes that many different methods can be used to achieve the same ends (Gibson, 1969; Reed, 1982). For example it is possible to sign one's name while sitting at a table, lying on the floor, or at arm's length on a blackboard, and the signature remains the same.

FACILITATIONS FOR MOTOR RELEARNING

Each model of motor learning discussed above suggests that certain performance and feedback variables are involved in the acquisition of normal movement. For the brain-injured individual with severe motor control deficits, motor retraining should incorporate techniques which aid the individual in learning to inhibit abnormal patterns of movements. Facilitations to motor learning include the following.

Functional goals

The brain-injured patient should be aware of the functional goals of treatment to help him maintain motivation and attention to task. It is hardly surprising that patients are often much more enthusiastic about working on walking (where the goal is easily recognized and practical) than they are about stacking cones (an apparently pointless task).

Task analysis

Task analysis (breaking the movement into subcomponents) is essential for training severely impaired patients' functional (motoric) skills. It is described at length elsewhere in this text. Following task analysis, retraining programmes can focus on the subcomponents of the activity with each subcomponent verbally labelled, so they may then be used as prompts. These small steps are sequenced together to teach the motor skills involved in fuctional independence (see case studies in this chapter).

The role of language in the acquisition of skilled movement

People instruct themselves as a kind of covert guidance during motor learning (James, 1890; Ho and Shea, 1978; Magill and Lee, 1987). Motor sequences are under conscious attention and under verbal control initially but this diminishes as learning of the motor skill proceeds. Appropriately formulated instructions increase the rate of motor skill learning and verbalizations help to form a basic understanding of the task. Language can be used to help the initiation and termination of activity, and the regulation of movement.

Feedback

The acquisition of a motor skill requires knowledge of perform-ance (KP) or knowledge of results (KR) either singly or in combi-nation. KR and KP are obtained through auditory, visual and proprioceptive feedback. The activity of a normal motor system can be regarded as a type of servo-system in which feedback from a response enters a comparator where it is tested against the image of an ideal response. This process results in detection and correction of movement errors. Normally people do not repeat unsuccessful movements, but attempt to correct their errors (Elwell and Grindley, 1938). Schema theory postulates that errors and variability of response (when accompanied by KR and KP) promote rule development by facilitating under-standing of the task requirements. The person attempts a move-ment, receives feedback about performance (KR and/or KP) and uses this knowledge to alter (improve) the next response. This process is the development of a new schema. The individual can only recognize the movement as correct, i.e. possessing zero error, when it matches exactly the intended movement. Delay in the provision of feedback impedes learning in the early stages of skill development (Bilodeau and Ryan, 1960) though this effect is lost as proficiency of movement increases. The non-neurologically-impaired process simple motor tasks very rapidly but the time required increases with task complexity. Complex tasks may demand more elaborate cognitive strategies, and hence increase processing time (Weinstein, 1987). (Note the similarity of the process of development of a motor schema to the development of general rules about the world in memory-impaired individuals described in Chapter 10.)

KP and KR occur as a result of feedback. Intrinsic feedback arises from the somatosensory system and vision. Additional auditory, visual and somatosensory feedback may be used to augment intrinsic KP and KR. The therapist can touch or apply pressure or stretch to draw the patient's attention to specific movement parameters. Extrinsic feedback can take the form of verbal feedback about the patient's movement and a description of methods to improve performance on the next trial. Self observation in a mirror or via a video system provides additional external feedback, as do Biofeedback and EMG which are discussed in greater detail below. The more impaired the patient's sensory system (or his ability to attend to it) the more he needs to use extrinsic feedback. The more attentional deficits the patients present with, the simpler the feedback should be and greater the effort required from the therapist to help patients focus their attention on the task.

Withdrawal of extrinsic feedback may produce deterioration in motor performance when the degree of skill acquisition is low or moderate (Bilodeau and Bilodeau, 1958). While the reason for this is unknown, it is possible that when KR is no longer available and perceptual traces are weak (comparisons can only be made with a poorly formed schema) they may be 'contaminated' hence becoming increasingly poor guides for response. A vicious cycle is then set up in which continued practice promotes inaccurate responses with a deterioration of performance. This phenomenon may be particularly marked when the individual is not consciously monitoring his own performance. An implication of this is that poor performance should be followed by a waiting period to allow the most recent (poor) perceptual trace to fade. In addition, following particularly poor performance the therapist may wish to intervene more energetically to control the patient's movement. After a relatively large amount of training, learning can continue when KR is withdrawn or only available intermittently. Adams *et al.* (1972) studied the acquisition of a linear self-paced positioning task using visual, auditory and proprioceptive feedback to aid motor learning. Acquisition was positively related to the amount of feedback given. When feedback was withdrawn those subjects who had had more experience of the task were able to maintain a higher level of accuracy longer than those with less experience of the task. Maintenance of skill after withdrawal of feedback was also positively related to the amount of feedback available during the acquisition phase. The amount of feedback and practice interact to predict the degree of consolidation of skilled performance and its resistance to deterioration.

Practice

Practice decreases the amount of conscious processing required to perform a movement (Bernstein, 1967). Some movements, which initially can only be performed slowly, may be performed more rapidly following practice. Some movements are ineffective when performed slowly, for example postural adjustments in ambulation, and only become effective when the rapidity of execution has increased as a result of practice. Practice schedules are typically not considered in the design of motor relearning programmes, and may be influenced by a number of haphazard factors such as the number of motor tasks the individual is attempting to learn, or other priorities within their overall rehabilitation programme.

A limited number of studies have attempted to determine the practice schedules which maximize learning in the non-neurologically-impaired population (Lee *et al.*, 1985). Considerable work has centered on a prediction derived from schema theory which suggests that increased variability of practice on a task will increase transfer of skill to a similar task. Attempts to validate this hypothesis has however produced inconsistent results (Bird and Riki, 1983; Catalano and Kleiner, 1984; Husak and Reeve, 1979; Johnson and McCabe, 1982). Lee *et al.* (1985) suggest that differences in research design account for the conflicting findings. Studies where the variations in task are blocked together (all of one type occurring at once) do not support the predictions from schema theory, whereas random variable practice on a motor task (interchanging first one task then the other in a way that cannot be predicted by the subject) provides strong support for the schema prediction (Lee *et al.*, 1985). It has been suggested that when practice is blocked together subjects have a memory trace remaining from the previous performances which they can use in the repetition of the task. When different tasks are interspersed, however, subjects are unable to use this strategy and must actively attempt to recall and generate the movement patterns *de novo*, leading to a greater ability to generalize. Other workers have examined similar issues from a different perspective. Shea and Morgan (1979) found that in comparing random to blocked practice, the blocked repetition facilitated acquisition performance but led to poor retention, while random ordering facilitated retention but was detrimental to acquisition. It may be that the difference in performance can, as with generalization, best be acounted for by suggesting that random practice requires subjects to use more cognitively effortful recall strategies. The discussion above indicates two specific ways to enhance learning. Firstly, practice of a task in slightly different ways may result in the subject having greater ability to transfer skills to new areas. In training a patient to transfer from his wheelchair, varying the heights of the surfaces to be transferred to, the distances and angles between the transfer surfaces and so on will make it easier for the patient to use the skill in novel circumstances. Secondly, by interspersing a number of different to-be-learned tasks randomly in one therapy session, long-term retention will be facilitated although at some cost to the immediate standard of performance. Therapists may wish to use blocked trials at first, so that the patient gains an initial level of mastery, and then progress to more variations (in a single task) and randomness (alternation between tasks) in the practice of skills.

The processes of motor skill acquisition can be conceptualized as occurring in three stages: (1) The cognitive stage (verbal motor) involves active attention and maximum cognitive effort. Individuals concentrate on all forms of sensory information to help them understand the task requirements and use language to initiate and sequence the tasks. (2) The fixative stage involves practice and feedback, which are required to learn the motor tasks. Studies of acquisition of even simple motor skills in normal individuals suggest that well over a million repetitions are required to achieve optimum performance. (3) The automatic stage describes a degree of overlearning where controlled attention is not required for action. Language may no longer assist performance.

ASSESSMENT

Formal sensory and motor assessments are completed by physiotherapists and occupational therapists to identify sensory and motor deficits and are supplemented by observation of the patient in functional settings. Local practice determines the style and depth of these assessment procedures and the communication between disciplines prevents unnecessary duplication.

Results of assessment are utilized in the development of treatment plans designed to reduce impairment and handicap.

Sensory assessment

Sensory assessment consists of two components: the application of a stimulus and observation of the patient response. Similar procedures are utilized in the assessment of the comatose patient. In the lower functioning patient (i.e. patients who cannot reliably give yes/no responses or can only sustain attention for very brief periods) formal sensory assessment should not be attempted. However responses to tactile, visual and auditory stimulation can be observed in order to derive an overall clinical picture of the patient. (Assessment of the patient in the acute stage of recovery is more fully discussed in Chapter 8). General principles of sensory assessment include ensuring the individual is comfortable, providing adequate instructions, ensuring sensory compensation is prevented and that stimulus administration is adequately paced. Sensory impairment may result from dysfunction at any point in the sensory system and the possibility of peripheral nerve injury should not be overlooked. As sensory deficits will influence motor performance, sensory assessment should normally be completed prior to formal motor evaluation. Superficial sensation is usually tested prior to testing proprioception.

Before beginning the sensory assessment it is important to determine the patient's ability to reliably give yes/no answers and to follow instructions. It is difficult to carry out a sensory assessment on severely confused and disoriented clients and the therapist is likely to elicit a large number of false positive responses (i.e. find a sensory deficit when none exists). There is little recent evidence regarding the reliability of sensory testing with the neurologically impaired. Kent (1965) reported adequate test-retest reliability using a standard protocol for sensory and motor deficits when applied to adults with hemiplegia. The assessment of simple sensory functions is described here; perceptual assessment is described in Chapter 10.

Pain

The assessment of pain should begin by asking the patient if they are currently experiencing pain. A description of the type, duration, severity and location of any abnormal pain should be recorded on a human figure chart. Type of pain could include sharp or dull aches, nagging or persistent pain, and severity of the pain syndrome can be evaluated by the use of analogue scales from between 0–9 (0 is equal to no pain and 9 is equivalent to severe, unbearable pain). Pain sensitivity is then assessed by a 'forced alternate choice' and tested by using a large-headed pin which has a pointed and blunted end. With eyes closed the individual is asked to respond to the stimulus with 'dull' or 'sharp'. An interval of 1 – 2 seconds between each stimulus must be allowed to prevent summation. In the hands of a trained observer this procedure can determine the sensitivity of the individual to pain, for instance hypersensitivity, normal, or hyposensitivity.

Temperature

Brain-injured individuals may have altered central and peripheral nervous systems which affect their ability to perceive temperatures. An approximate test of temperature sensation involves the patient describing the temperature of running hot or cold tap water with his eyes closed. The therapist needs to ensure that the water temperatures from the taps are stable and in the ranges of cold 5–10°C and hot 40–45°C. Care should be taken to ensure that the water contacts the skin over a sufficient area, for a sufficient length of time. The use of two test tubes, one filled with cold and one with hot water, present the illusion of greater rigour in testing. However, given the problems of maintaining temperature and of achieving contact with an adequate surface area, the advantage of being able to apply the tubes to different body parts is in our view not worth the effort. Performing a test of temperature awareness before allowing patients to bath is essential as a lack of awareness of temperature could result in tissue damage. Some patients are unable to use an awareness of temperature to influence their behaviour (for example wearing heavy winter clothes on a hot summer day). The patient may have undisturbed temperature sensation on testing, so the condition is functionally equivalent to a temperature 'neglect'.

Touch

Sensory losses contribute to abnormal motor control and may result in disuse of the involved limbs. Tactile sensation is essential for normal motoric functioning and any sensory deficits make motor relearning more difficult. Deficits of touch can severely limit functional performance. Most tests of touch rely on forced choice responses. The patients are instructed to close their eyes and asked to respond yes or no, yes if they were touched and no if they were not. As many patients will give random responses it is important to vary the time periods between applying stimulation. Light touch can be assessed by softly touching or stroking the patient's skin with cotton wool. Pressure sensation can be assessed by the application of firm pressure of the end of the eraser end of a pencil applied with sufficient force to indent the skin. A test of the ability to localize touch is to ask the patients to close their eyes and state where they were touched. Patients with language deficits can be asked to point to the place they were touched. Two-point discrimination assessment measures the minimum distance between two stimuli (applied simultaneously and with equal force) that an individual can perceive as distinct. This minimum distance varies considerably over different parts of the body. Nolan (1982; 1985) has published normative data for the head, trunk and upper extremities of young adults.

All of the methods so far described assess the patient's ability to recognize rapid transient touch (which involves horizontal or vertical stretch of skin). Sustained touch sensation may however be equally important for functional activities (for example, holding objects). Dannenbaum and Dykes (1990) have described deficits of sustained touch/pressure sensation in patients after brain injury, and present a method to assess sustained touch. A mechanical touch/pressure applicator was fabricated which consisted of a wooden stand supporting a perpendicular wooden rod. On top of the rod is a platform in which weights may be placed. Below the rod is a padded area on which the supinated hand and forearm may be placed. Assessment is carried out by applying various weights via the rod to the index finger for various durations with the patient instructed to say 'yes' if they think the weight still in place and 'no' if they think it absent. Some patients were shown by Dannenbaum and Dykes (1990) to have markedly impaired sustained touch appreciation. In addition to the above, some therapists test texture sensation, barognosis (recognition of weight), vibration, graphesthesia (the recognition of letters, numbers or designs traced on the hand), the assessments of which are not described here. The assessment of stereognosis, hemi-aesthesia, somatic hemi-inattention and suppression are discussed in Chapter 10.

Proprioception

Proprioception is the awareness of body movement (kinaesthesia) and position in space (position sense). Kinaesthetic sense may be assessed in the following manner. The individual is asked to close his eyes and the therapist holds the limbs or digit at the sides of the joint in order to prevent pressure cues. The person is asked to indicate whether his or her limb (digit) is being moved up or down, and could also be asked the speed or amplitude (it is best to dichotomize these discriminations into fast/slow and a lot/a little). Kent (1965) reported that the number of errors of hemiplegic subjects was lowered when the range of motion was increased from 15 to 30 degrees. In our experience the assessment of joint position sense is difficult in the severely impaired brain-injured patient, due to the rather abstract conceptualization required to test it. The patient may be asked to either describe the position of a joint or limb in space or duplicate the position of one limb with the contralateral extremity. Individuals with proprioception loss often demonstrate 'clumsy' motor performance, but can often use vision to compensate for these deficits.

Vision, hearing, smell and taste

Brain-injured persons frequently have damage to the eye, optic nerves and occipital cortex and it is important for the therapist to distinguish vision from oculo-motor functioning (discussed in Chapter 3). An approximate (screening) test may involve asking the patient to read a standard eye chart or to identify the time from a wall clock. An assessment by a neuro-ophthalmologist indicates the degree of visual impairment and should be read and understood by the therapists.

Hearing deficits may be mistaken for impairments in attention, speed of information processing and language comprehension (or vice versa). Observation of the patient's response to speech of different volumes and tones may indicate the need for specialized testing in an audiology assessment.

The senses of smell and taste are often affected by brain injury. Many individuals feel that loss of pleasure in eating (arising from alterations in the senses of smell and taste) significantly affects their quality of life. There are however only minor effects on function, for example, being unable to smell cooking, rotting food or when clothes need laundering.

Motor assessment

Motor assessment should include the following.

Range of motion

As noted in Chapter 8, prolonged immobility particularly when associated with abnormal tone, can lead to soft tissue contractures and decreased range of motion (ROM). These changes may alter biomechanical alignment and result in abnormal movement patterns. In addition, alterations in biomechanical alignment can increase the amount of strength and endurance required to perform an activity. ROM should be evaluated with slow and even passive movements to minimize the influence of abnormal tone (Duncan 1990). The use of joint ROM-measuring equipment is described in basic physiotherapy and occupational therapy texts (Trombly, 1983; Pedretti, 1985) and is not reviewed here. Accessory joint movement such as the downward glide of the head of the humerus during shoulder flexion should also be assessed as absence of these accessory movements lead to ROM limitations (Duncan, 1990).

Head and trunk control

Severely impaired patients may have difficulty with head and trunk control. This may result from a complex combination of deficits including low arousal, abnormal muscle tone and movement patterns, weakness and alterations in sensation. In the initial stages of recovery, treatment and evaluation are not mutually exclusive as treatment involves attempting to stimulate the patient to maximize postural control in different positions. Alterations in trunk and limb position affect head control and these factors should be kept in mind when assessing feeding and ADL. Assessment at this stage is best accomplished as a joint undertaking of the physiotherapist and occupational therapist. As recovery progresses, assessment involves observing the patient's ability to maintain head and trunk control with decreasing support and increasing demands for dynamic (moving) balance.

Muscle tone

Alteration in muscle tone may occur unilaterally or bilaterally. Tone fluctuates and is influenced by the individual's starting position, temperature, anxiety or infection (e.g. urinary tract infection). Abnormalities of tone are usually assessed by rating the resistance to passive ROM as when the patient has increased tone the therapist experiences a marked resistance to passive stretch. The resistance to movement may depend on the speed of the stretch, and be more evident in some planes of movement than others. Tonal abnormalities are usually distributed within specific muscle groups. As noted by Duncan (1990), however, the tonal abnormality felt by the therapist when moving the patient passively may be different from that experienced by the patient during active movement, and may have a different cause. The resistance to passive movement might, for example, be due to a hyperactive stretch reflex while, in active movement, it is the result of poor timing in the regulation of the neuronal pool with continued antagonistic contraction (Duncan, 1990). Assessment of tonal abnormalities must therefore include assessment of the patient performing active (purposeful) movement. It is difficult to measure the extent of tonal abnormality but it is possible to complete standardized tests of a patient's ability to carry out motor tasks such as the Jebsen Hand Function Test (Jebsen *et al*:, 1969) or the Minnesota Rate of Manipulation Test (1969).

Abnormal movement patterns

All skilled movement relies on complex patterns of contraction, co-contraction and relaxations of muscles. Functionally related patterns of muscle contraction have precise spatio-temporal relationships (Duncan, 1990) and these precise interrelationships are frequently disrupted after severe brain-injury. The abnormal movement patterns are not due to the acquisition of abnormal reflexes, but to the loss of overlearned movement patterns. The primitive reflex patterns displayed by patients are frequently assumed to be the fundamental motor programmes, that are partially suppressed and built upon during motor development. The severely injured patient's movement is often limited to stereotyped patterns of flexion and extension (the upper extremity is flexed and retracted, adducted and internally rotated at the shoulder, and flexed at the elbow, wrist and fingers; the lower extremity is retracted, adducted and internally rotated at the hip, extended at the knee, and plantar flexed and inverted at the foot). Although these patterns may be crudely adequate in the lower extremity they are often non-functional in the upper extremity. Duncan (1990) emphasizes that movement synergies may be a result of movement programming failure and not 'spasticity'. Assessment involves observing the individual's tendency to produce movement synergies in various positions such as free sitting, sitting at a table and standing.

Strength

Until recently the possibility of a primary strength disorder following brain-injury has been largely overlooked (Duncan, 1990). Although marked weakness is frequently observed, it has been accounted for by reference to abnormal tone. Given the role of the motor cortex in regulating recruitment and frequency of motor unit firing, weakness should be an expected consequence of disruption of the cortex or descending motor tracts. As indicated by Duncan (1990) the presence of antagonistic co-activation and impaired reciprocal inhibition contribute to the reduced force of movement but are not always primary in producing weakness. The action of each muscle should be observed separately as weakness may be specific to one muscle or muscle group. The Oxford scale is widely accepted for the assessment of muscle strength.

0 No contraction
1 Flicker or trace of contraction
2 Active movement with gravity eliminated
3 Active movement against gravity
4 Active movement against gravity and resistance
  (4− slight, 4 moderate, 4+ strong resistance)
5 Normal power

(After Medical Research Council (1976) *Aids to the Examination of the Peripheral Nervous System*, Her Majesty's Stationary Office, London.)

Endurance

Many patients fatigue rapidly during activity following severe brain-injury. In addition to the general reduction in fitness which may follow prolonged hospitalization, alterations in biomechanics and/or impaired motor co-ordination may make a fixed amount of work more fatiguing for a brain-injured patient than a non-neurologically impaired individual. Taken together these factors may explain the extreme fatiguability of many patients. Therapists should observe patients closely for signs of fatigue during all stages of rehabilitation. Note should be made of the distance patients can walk in the community without fatigue or deterioration of gait pattern, and the duration of time that the patient can work or engage in other relevant activities.

Initiation and regulation of movement

Impaired initiation of movement may result from arousal deficits or dyspraxia as well as difficulties in initiation *per se*. Parkinsonian deficits are now recognized as being not uncommon following brain-injury and are treated with anti-parkinsonian medications (medications intended to increase the availability of the neurotransmitter dopamine within the nigro-striatal system). The term motor perseveration describes an inability to terminate or inhibit the repetition of a motor behaviour. This disorder is frequently associated with frontal brain damage, which could also impair the patient's ability to organize motor behaviour, resulting in impulsive, unsafe motor activity. Assessment of these disorders is not included in standardized tests of motor dysfunction but is central to understanding a patient's real-world functioning.

Compensatory movements

The evaluation of motor behaviour must include an assessment of the patient's actual performance in functional settings. Patients may spontaneously attempt to compensate for a motor deficit by developing compensatory movement patterns (for example, the typical hemiplegic gait). Observation during functional activities, such as eating and dressing, will establish the patient's habitual patterns of movement. Often compensatory movements are adaptive; however some compensatory actions used spontaneously by patients actually limit physical recovery. Patients need to be taught more adaptive movement strategies.

Patient D.J. (case study 9.2 below) had severe spasticity and ataxia, and frequently dropped items when attempting functional tasks. Due to abnormal tone he had difficulty bending forward in the wheelchair to pick up the fallen articles. To compensate for this, he would slide his feet back under his wheelchair and flex his knees so that when he reached down he did not need as great a hip bend. Unfortunately, without a stable base of support he frequently fell forward out of his chair and onto the floor.

Compensatory behaviours

Patients may engage in a range of other activities in order to avoid motor tasks or physical rehabilitation (Hooper-Roe, 1988). Some patients prefer to ask others for help or passively avoid activities whilst others can be non-compliant, physically or verbally aggressive or scream constantly to avoid activities or therapy. Assessment should include the therapist's evaluation of the patient's best physical abilities and an evaluation of the patient's behaviours which influence motor performance and their likely response to rehabilitation (see Chapter 12). Patients may be genuinely unable to perform the task but do not engage in appropriate compensatory behaviours (for example, asking others for help) due to embarrassment, poor initiation or other cognitive deficits. Only observation of the patient in functional settings will enable the therapist to evaluate the patient's actual, habitual motor performance.

APPROACHES TO IMPROVE SENSORY AND MOTOR FUNCTION

Sensory relearning

Sensory stimulation, whilst appropriate in the acute stage of recovery, may not improve functional abilities in the later stages of rehabilitation. Environmental modification or the overlearning of routines, which rely less on the impaired sense, may be the most appropriate form of therapeutic intervention. Strategies should be developed to work around functional problems caused by the sensory deficits, for example the use of a thermometer to check the temperature of water. Some adapted equipment provides feedback via alternative sensory channels, which helps individuals achieve the functional tasks. For example, an electronic gadget makes a noise when a cup is full of water, for a person with limited sight.

Preventing physical dysfunction

The prevention of contractures, and the resultant abnormal compensatory movement patterns, is required if normal movement is to be achieved. Black *et al.* (1975) have demonstrated that passive movements 10 to 14 times a day enabled monkeys recovering from surgically induced 'injury' to achieve a return of function considerably superior to those not receiving 'therapy'. Brain-injured individuals are more predisposed to contractures and subsequent loss of range of motion. The immobilization of any joint leads to chemical changes and increased density of connective tissue which leads to increased tissue resistance (Woo *et al.*, 1975). The existence of contractures accelerates disuse muscle atrophy, which has been attributed to the loss of the trophic influence of stretch on muscle tissue. The functional effects of these changes are increased atrophy, shortened muscles and tendon lengths and decreased muscular force production. A muscle's size is influenced by its pattern of activity

(Goldspink, 1977) and increased work demands lead to compensatory growth. Muscles restrained in shortened positions lose sarcomeres, become smaller and will in time atrophy. This process does not occur when the tissues are immobilized in a lengthened position, because the loss of isotonic activity is compensated for by certain growth-promoting factors related to stretch. A further problem, caused by immobilization and the subsequent contractures, is the alteration of normal biomechanical alignment. This contributes to the excessive effort involved in movement, altered movement synergies, and increased tone. The prevention of contractures may be achieved by passive range of movement exercises. It is easier to prevent contractures by repeated frequent activity that opposes this natural shortening action of connective tissue than it is to correct them after they have developed (see Chapter 8). Regular changes of position designed to inhibit muscle tone may reduce the development of abnormal postures and pressure sores. The application of stretching and immobilization by splinting can be used to increase the lengths of muscles and tendons, thus preventing or limiting contractures.

Motor relearning

To facilitate motor learning in the brain-injured adult, all approaches (other than compensation training) attempt to overcome physical disabilities by encouraging normal movement. New rules need to be established in the process of motor relearning, as previously used parameters are inadequate as a result of the brain injury impairing the motor control system. To overcome the motor disabilities caused by abnormal tone, sensory dysfunction, and proprioceptive loss, facilitations to retrain normal movement and to inhibit abnormal movement are described. The details of the approaches and the rationales for their use vary widely.

Kottke (1982) identified four phases of recovery, each demanding different therapeutic approaches. First, if the patient is unable to contract his paretic muscles voluntarily, the therapist may assist by using any of the varied cutaneous proprioceptive facilitation techniques (icing, tapping, vibration) by activating reflex synergies or applying direct electrical stimulation to nerve or muscle. Second, once the desired muscles contract, the patient must perceive the contraction. Sensory reinforcement of the movement can be increased through visual or auditory sources, from the therapist or EMG feedback. Third, the patient must learn to inhibit muscles that do not belong to the desired pattern of movement. This training can be accomplished by requiring precise execution of the movement pattern, perhaps assisted by reflex inhibiting patterns or EMG biofeedback. In order to avoid general increases in tone, activities should lead to minimal stress on the patient. Fourth, the patient should increase the ease and fluency and decrease the effortful components of performance. This can only be accomplished by multiple repetitions of the correct movement patterns. These movements need to be co-ordinated into a functional routine to ensure that motor learning generalizes into functional situations.

Many approaches have been developed in an attempt to remediate motor deficits following CNS damage. Approaches include those of the Bobaths (Bobath, 1978), Brunstromm (Brunstromm, 1970), Rood (Rood, 1962), conductive education (Clark-Wilson and Gent, 1989), EMG behaviour therapy and biofeedback. Despite an increasing number of studies attempting to compare treatment efficacy, no clearly superior approach has emerged (Dickstein *et al.*, 1986; Stern *et al.*, 1970; Logigian *et al.*, 1983). Belief in the greater effectiveness of individual approaches remains a matter of faith among practitioners. However the concept of increasing motility by progressing through stages of a neuro-developmental sequence is difficult to support. We will review a number of the available approaches and attempt to highlight elements of a rational approach to treatment. Because of the dearth of studies of treatment for patients with traumatic brain injury, some of the studies discussed below involve patients with non-traumatic injuries but in each case diagnosis is specified.

Neurophysiological approaches (Bobath, Rood and Brunstromm)

Bobath

The Bobaths (neurodevelopmental/NDT) suggest that the use of techniques that normalize sensations and movement, during the acute phase of recovery after brain-injury, can prevent spastic patterns of movement developing. The Bobaths (1978) observed that movement or change in position of proximal joints can reduce spasticity and facilitate normal movement. It was stated that by preventing abnormal movements, previously ineffective synapses concerned with segmental presynaptic inhibition may be activated, or that strengthening of the remaining segmental pathways may occur. Rehabilitation programmes based on Bobath principles attempt to maximize the individual's potential by advocating the use of voluntary movements. The therapist suppresses spastic synergy patterns, by maintaining the patient's limbs in 'reflex-inhibiting patterns'. As control of spasticity develops in voluntary movements, greater mobility can be achieved in functional activities. When more normal movement can be facilitated, retraining in functional activities is considered effective, as long as movement during these activities utilizes the same reflex inhibiting patterns.

Rood

Neurophysiological studies in both animals and man indicate that skeletal muscles are associated with specific patterns of body surface dermatomal representation. The Rood approach attempts to increase reduced muscle tone by the use of cutaneous stimulation. Application of stimulations, such as fast stroking, or brushing over a discrete skin area, facilitates contraction of the corresponding muscle while inhibiting its antagonist. In addition, Rood (1962) advocates proprioceptive techniques as a basis for facilitating progress in a developmental sequence of learned motor control. Goff (1969), in describing the techniques of Rood, suggested that 'her aim is always to obtain as normal a response as possible by applying the appropriate stimuli to produce movement or postural reactions'.

Brunstromm

Brunstromm (1970) suggests therapists facilitate the emergence of flexion and extension synergies in the early stages of recovery after brain injury. By the use of a combination of central facilitations, peripheral proprioceptive stimulation and cutaneous stimulation, the patient is trained to bring the abnormal synergies under voluntary control and to shape voluntary movement patterns. This approach is difficult to generalize into functional retraining techniques.

Proprioceptive neuromuscular facilitation

Proprioceptive neuromuscular facilitation (PNF) of Knott and Voss (1968), emphasizes proprioceptive stimuli, such as muscle stretch; maximum resistance to contraction and traction; or compression of joints as sensory inputs to facilitate muscle activity. These techniques require close therapist involvement as the patient's limbs are positioned and guided through specific diagonal and spiral patterns against resistance. Surburg (1977) has demonstrated the effectiveness of these patterning techniques on the training of normal subjects to improve response time and speed in a movement task. Functional applications are not emphasized.

Conductive education

Advocates of conductive education describe it as rehabilitation through learning (Giles and Gent, 1988; Clark-Wilson and Gent, 1989). It is described at more length here because it is a learning-oriented, functional approach. It is based upon teaching the individual to overcome motor dysfunction by teaching basic motor patterns and strategies to incorporate movement retraining into meaningful function. In conductive education success in rehabilitation is measured by the individual's increased ability to perform activities and to become integrated into the community. The goals of rehabilitation must, therefore, be realistic and meaningful. Knowledge of the functional goal focuses the individual's attention on the activity and increases motivation.

There are many different ways of achieving the same functional goal and these functional goals are identified and analysed into a series of motor tasks (subgoals) and task parts (movements). The methods which could be used to complete the functional task are then co-ordinated into flowing programmes, incorporating facilitations which aid organization, regulation and sequencing of motor activity. These programmes include sensory, cognitive and physical approaches, ensure achievement of the tasks, and allow the individuals to learn to facilitate their own movement.

Rehabilitation takes place in groups and is led by a conductor who is assisted by facilitators. Language is used to describe the motor tasks to be attempted, and aids the planning of the motor task. The conductor leads the group by initiating the motor intentions, before the group repeats the intention. Counting or dynamic speech is used to pace the motor response, either as a slow count to allow relaxation and a reduction of spasticity or as fast, dynamic speech, to increase arousal. Physical facilitations are utilized to encourage stability and accuracy and speed of movement. This retraining helps the brain-injured to learn to control their own movement, take responsibility for their actions and develop a problem-solving approach to find their own ways of achieving goals.

Conductive education incorporates the use of conductors who are trained as 'generic therapists' (teacher, physiotherapist, occupational therapist, speech therapist and psychologist), who lead the groups, organize the programme and direct the facilitations required within the group. Conductive education stimulates active learning and the motor skills learnt are practised to a level of automaticity and transferred into functional situations within the home and community. Ultimately, this approach aims to teach people with motor disorders to acquire skills, to make decisions and to function as independently as possible in the community.

Behavioural retraining and biofeedback

Biofeedback utilizes augmentive feedback systems to facilitate control of movement by retraining the patient to reduce hypertonus and/or achieve stronger contractions of paretic muscles. Biofeedback is effective in training the inhibition of abnormal tone (Swan *et al.*, 1974) and in increasing range of movement in neurologically-impaired patients (Mroczec *et al.*, 1978). Mroczec and co-workers (1978) found that biofeedback and physical therapy were not significantly different in their ability to increase range of motion. The authors conclude that biofeedback could help the patient regain control of an isolated specific muscle, but multiple supplementary instructions would be required to assist him to use his movements functionally. Biofeedback is probably best considered not as a therapy in itself, but rather a modality of therapy that is particularly useful where sensory loss interferes with regaining motor control (Mroczec *et al.*, 1978). Basmajian *et al* (1987) reported a controlled trial comparing the efficacy of two forms of therapy on upper limb function in hemiplegia after stroke. An integrated behavioural and EMG method was compared with a neuro-developmental (Bobath) approach. The behavioural approach recognized the role of the patient's cognition during treatment and was designed to follow the cognitive-behavioural model proposed by Meichenbaum (1977). This consists of four phases: (1) conceptualization, (2) skill acquisition, (3) skill rehearsal, and (4) skill transfer. During phase (1) the patient is converted, as much as possible, from a passive recipient to an active participant in treatment. During skill acquisition, EMG feedback goals are learned and the patient is taught how to direct his cognitive skills. During repeated skill rehearsal, home practice of the skill is emphasized. The final phase is skill transfer. The EMG component was pivotal for precise goal setting and specific feedback.

The comparison approach was based on neurofacilitatory techniques; following Bobath this approach uses facilitations and inhibitions with selected sensory input in an attempt to bring about automatic high quality motor output. The handling skill of the therapist is emphasized and home practice is not included in the treatment plan. The study examined the effect of the two approaches on subgroups of stroke patients using multifunction tests performed by a technician who was blind to the treatment conditions. Results indicated that both forms of treatment resulted in worthwhile clinical and statistical improvement which was maintained at a nine months retesting. There was, however, no significant superiority of one treatment protocol over another.

Wissel *et al.* (1989) treated eleven stroke patients with a modified biofeedback technique in which the patients practised a functional task and not isolated movement. The method described involved connecting not only the patient's paretic limb but also his unaffected extremity (or the corresponding limb of the therapist) to the feedback apparatus. The feedback system converted the muscle activation sequence into an acoustic signal. The patient is therefore assisted in learning the sequences of activity in normal movement. The patient then attempts to reproduce the activity (and thus the same signal) sequence with the paretic limb. All 11 patients were treated at least one year post-injury, and despite ongoing therapy the paresis was stable in each case. Patients received 12–30 treatments for the upper extremity and/or the lower extremity. The upper extremity task involved drinking from a cup and the lower extremity task, gait training concentrating on overcoming flexor and extensor synergies with EMG feedback system electrodes located on the anterio-tibial muscle. Effectiveness of treatment was evaluated by rating the EMG signal, the ability to perform the trained action as measured by a specific grading system and a general increase in movement competency rated on a Bobath movement test. Six patients were trained on each task. Ten patients demonstrated increased strength, four of the six made gains on performance of the upper extremity task and four of the six showed marked improvement in gait. Four patients in each group improved in general movement as rated on the Bobath test. The authors note that directed learning of a useful activity, or physiologic co-ordination in walking in conjunction with EMG feedback, has not been reported by others. Despite this dearth of reports there is increasing evidence to suggest the benefits of physical function when aligned to purposive activity (Mulder, 1985). Wissel and co-workers (1989) suggest that patients perform better because they are learning useful movements for everyday living, and are hence motivated to participate more intensely. Long-term success depends on the integration of increased behavioural competency in everyday life.

A specialized retraining programme for ataxic gait

Balliet and associates (1987) have described a method to retrain functional gait through the progressive reduction of upper extremity weight-bearing in individuals with chronic cerebellar ataxia. They cite evidence that cerebellar function can be affected by learning. They state that since motor control is based on the integration of reflexes as modifiable sub-assemblies, ataxic patients may benefit from neuromuscular retraining. This should allow them to re-establish motor control and associated balance by slow, successively adapted and increasingly demanding task conditions. Although similar to other neurodevelopmental approaches, this approach was specifically designed to reduce reliance on upper extremity weight-bearing, develop co-ordination and balance and integrate these elements into a functional gait pattern. Five ataxic patients were trained:

four patients had motor deficits as a result of traumatic brain injury and one as a result of acute (remitted) leukaemia. Patient ages were between 22 and 63 years and time since neurological injury ranged from 15 months to 12 years (average 5.5 years). Four simple scales were used to establish functional performance and ambulation. Re-education consisted of three increasingly demanding stages. All training was carried out in a quiet minimally distracting environment to maximize relevant sensory feedback. Therapists conducted a one-hour therapy session, twice weekly, for three months, and then once every two months. The first stage involved reciprocal leg movements, thought to approximate the pattern found in walking which the patient performed while seated. The second stage involved training in both static and dynamic balance and the third stage involved integrative ambulation using a horizontal straight cane. All patients improved on all of the evaluations of functional performance. All patients completed the study, being able to ambulate using a single assistive device or better. Three patients made gains significant enough to increase their mobility and safety and reduce their need for attendant care. In the three cases available for follow-up one year following termination of treatment, there was no reduction in functional independence. Of particular interest is that although the approach required very considerable commitment from the patient, only 5% of the actual therapy hours involved a therapist. Therefore, the training methods as outlined are probably not appropriate for use with patients who have severe cognitive impairments.

Compensatory techniques

Brain-injured individuals with unilateral motor impairments may be trained to use the unaffected side to compensate for the affected extremities in locomotion and daily living activities. Inaba et al (1973) have demonstrated the effectiveness of these therapy techniques. Retraining hemiplegics to perform functional activities by strengthening the unaffected limbs and exercising them against resistance, could limit improvements on the affected side, if used in early stages. It could also restrict their opportunities to learn greater motor control of their whole body in functional activities.

Strengthening, exercise and relaxation training

As noted above, patients may be weak and lack endurance following brain injury. These deficits may be addressed directly via strengthening exercises and aerobics training. Jankowski and Sullivan (1990) provided aerobic and neuromuscular training of moderate intensity to brain-injured patients. Although the patients did not increase their locomotor efficiency, they did increase their aerobic capacity and fatiguability was reduced. The authors note that in this case, fatiguability was directly related to the patients' ability to work at a sheltered workshop. While there is little direct evidence supporting the efficacy of relaxation training with the brain-injured it might be beneficial to a subgroup of this population.

Principles for facilitating sensori-motor skills in functional activities

a) Assess sensory and motor deficits with other members of the rehabilitation team.

b) Define priorities of rehabilitation with relevant members of the rehabilitation team, the brain-injured individual and those close to them.

c) Initiate training sessions for learning sensori-motor tasks, with other professionals.

d) Transfer the acquired techniques into functional programmes, thus incorporating the skills used in a training session into a functional setting. For example, in standing and transferring weight in walking and lower extremity dressing.

e) Establish the functional priorities of rehabilitation and design programmes which incorporate reflex inhibiting patterns of movement, thereby retraining individuals to overcome their motor deficits through functional activity.

f) Increase the number of opportunities to learn and use the acquired motor skills throughout the day. This increases the amount of practice and feedback available.

g) Ensure the consistencey and communication of the team involved in retraining the motor and functional skills.

h) Facilitate the retraining and practice within other environments, for example, home, work and social settings.

Case study 9.1
Eating
S.I. (coma duration unknown; three years post-injury) had severe ataxia and hemiplegia with minimal proprioceptive feedback from the right side. Although S.I. attempted to feed himself, his motor disorders were severe enough to make feeding both extremely frustrating and time-consuming. The activity of eating was analysed into motor tasks, and individual and group training assisted S.I. learn how to increase his stability, extend his elbow and use his right hand to form a tripod grasp. S.I. was taught to use visual feedback to check the positioning of his limbs. As S.I. improved in his control of movement, this was incorporated into a feeding programme. He had to sit well, hold the knife and fork, cut the food and place the food in his mouth. Both motor control and speed increased over the three months of the programme to the point where S.I. became independent in eating. Once the positioning involved in maintaining stability while eating had been over-learned, the transfer of the stabilizing position to other skills was rapid, for example, learning to maintain stability while operating an outdoor mobility aid.

Case study 9.2
Wheelchair stability and transfer training
D.I. (coma duration 12 weeks; time post-injury 5 years) had severe spasticity on his left side and tremor on the right. Due to the movement disorder D.I. was unable to carry out functional activities independently. D.I. frequently fell whilst wheeling his wheelchair, or whilst engaging in physical activities. He was unable to plan his motor behaviour, inhibit spasticity, reduce tremor, and co-ordinate motor activity. During motor relearning sessions, D.I. was taught to increase control of his movements and although he could organize his movement behaviour he was unable to do this spontaneously in functional settings. A transfer programme (Table 9.1) and a washing and dressing programme (Table 9.2) were designed to help D.I. control his movement in functional tasks. The same language was used in the programmes as for the instructions in the motor-control training session.

Table 9.1 Transfer programme (Patient required to use specified routine for each transfer on a 24-hour basis. All staff were trained to supervise the patient)

1. Sit well (feet flat, 6–9 inches apart, knees over feet, bottom in the back of the chair, back straight, head up and centred, and hands on knees).
2. Clasp hands together.
3. Stretch elbows.
4. Lean forward: head down.
5. Lift bottom.
6. Stand up.
7. Weight on left leg.
8. Lift right leg out to the side and turn.
9. Weight on right leg.
10. Lift left leg to right and turn.
11. Lean forward and head down.
12. Sit down.

Table 9.2 Washing and Dressing Programme
(D.I. learned the verbal prompts rapidly and was motivated towards his recovery. He learned to keep his feet flat in all tasks in order to maintain his stability. When he successfully completed each prompt, he was given social reinforcement, and a token. If he gained a specified number of tokens he was able to exchange them for a reinforcer of his choice.)

1. Position wheelchair in front of the sink and sit well.
2. Put soap on wash cloth, and wash face, neck and ears, rinse and dry.
3. Put soap on wash cloth and wash chest and underarms, rinse and dry.
4. Put soap on wash cloth and wash hands and arms, rinse and dry.
5. Put soap on wash cloth and wash feet (cross one leg over the other – keeping one foot flat), rinse and dry.
6. Move wheelchair back, apply brakes.
7. Put soap on wash cloth, put wash cloth on side of basin.
8. Hold onto the taps. Lean forward. Head down. Lift bottom. Stand up.
9. Pick up wash cloth, wash between legs, rinse and dry.
10. Sit down slowly.
11. Move wheelchair forwards to basin. Apply brakes.
12. Empty basin. Clean teeth. Dry face.
13. Put on talc and deodorant.
14. Tidy up basin.
15. Position chair in front of towel-rail and apply brakes.
16. Get dressed (to keep feet flat, stand as before holding onto the rail, and crossing legs to put on shoes).

As D.I. improved on these tasks he started to walk with a rollator, and was eventually able to walk moderate distances (e.g. around the local shopping mall) without supervision.

SUMMARY

Overcoming physical dysfunction involves learning methods of controlling and improving movement whilst learning either one or various methods of approaching functional tasks. Techniques are aimed towards teaching normal movement and by consolidating the retraining used with other professions into re-establishing previously learned functional tasks and developing skills to meet new requirements. Functional retraining can aid awareness and understanding of normal movement by providing positions and facilitations to inhibit abnormal movements and establish stability and symmetry (Bobath, 1979; Cotton and Kinsman, 1983). Practical methods of achieving tasks can also be used which inhibit unwanted movements and promote isolated and controlled movements (see case studies). Functional activities can be broken down into the component tasks and each task analysed to identify the suitable methods of teaching the individual to physically achieve each task. Positioning is used to achieve stability and motor control, for example to 'sit well' (i.e. feet flat and apart, bottom back in the chair, hands down, back straight, head up and centred), and can aid performance of activities like eating, writing, and dressing. Many functional activities have similar motor components, therefore, once motor tasks are learned, these can be included in many other functional activities. Functional retraining should involve sufficient practice so that motor skills become automatic in the appropriate functional settings, and become easily transferrable into home or social environments.

10

Improving cognitive abilities in functional settings

The cognitive deficits which may follow brain injury have been the subject of intense study during the 1980s and into the 1990s. There has been a considerable increase in our understanding of memory and attentional disorders, however our understanding of disorders of higher cognitive functioning remains rudimentary. No definite guidelines can yet be presented as to what constitutes effective therapy. Enough evidence, however, has been accumulated to indicate that not all types of treatment are effective in remediating all types of cognitive process dysfunction and treatment is increasingly being seen as process specific. Similarly not all treatments are successful with all different degrees of deficit or at all stages of recovery.

For the discussion in this chapter we have divided interventions, intended to help brain-injured individuals overcome cognitive impairments, into three general categories. The first type of intervention involves retraining the cognitive impairment itself. In the acute stages of recovery, stimulating the individual towards the highest level of functioning may be the most appropriate intervention (see Chapter 2). In the later stages of recovery, some workers have advocated interventions designed to stimulate the recovery of specific cognitive functions (Powell, 1981; Sohlberg and Mateer, 1987). The second form of intervention involves training the patient in the use of strategies (internal or external) to compensate for the cognitive disability. This is most appropriate in the post-acute period and for aspects of cognitive functioning which do not respond to the first approach. For example, there is considerable evidence that memory does not improve by practising to remember in either the non-neurologically (Wagenaar, 1986) or the neurologically impaired (Glisky *et al.*, 1986) (see below). However, there is evidence that certain aspects of memory dysfunction may be ameliorated by training the patient to record the relevant information in a diary. The third type of intervention involves training the patient in specific tasks (rather than cognitive skills). This task-specific training is most appropriate for severely impaired patients who have not developed independence, using the first two types of intervention.

The principles of learning theory should be applied in the design of training programmes (except in non-specific stimulation applied in the acute stage of recovery). Interventions should be individually developed and tailored to the patient's needs. Central to the success of intervention is the performance of the patient in normal activities in real-life environments. Although this chapter can only be considered an overview of cognitive retraining it attempts to stimulate therapists to think about the relevance of the types of intervention they are using (Giles and Fussey, 1988). Wherever appropriate we have divided our discussion into efforts to retrain cognitive function itself, training in compensatory strategies and task-specific training.

ATTENTION

Assessment

Attention should not be confused with alertness. Patients in the acute stage of recovery commonly only remain alert for short periods of time and go in and out of a stuporous state. General deficits in attention should also be distinguished from unilateral attentional deficits (the evaluation of which is described below). Considerable information can be obtained by observing the patient's behaviour in the therapy department or in functional activities. Does the patient lapse into inactivity if he is not constantly redirected towards the task (sustained attention)? Is the patient constantly looking at what others are doing and repeatedly orienting towards noise or activity in the environment (selective attention)? Can the patient intersperse conversation with others while performing a task (alternating attention) or can he perform two simple activities at the same time (divided attention)? Attentional deficits severely disrupt performance in functional activities. Activities which would have been automatic prior to brain injury frequently require conscious effort following injury.

Basic attention can be assessed by asking the patient to repeat strings of digits of increasing length, beginning with two numbers. Natural sequences should be avoided (e.g. 1,2,3) and the patient is given only one trial of each sequence. The digits should be presented at the rate of one per second in a normal tone of voice with no grouping of digits. The unimpaired patient can repeat five to seven digits presented in this manner without difficulty.

Strub and Black (1985) describe an auditory test of sustained attention. The therapist reads a list of letters at one letter per second and the patient's task is to signal the occurrence of the target letters by tapping the table. The average non-neurologically impaired person can perform a test of this type without error. Types of impaired performance described by Strub and Black (1985) include failure to indicate when a target letter has been presented (error of omission), indicating a target letter has occurred when it has not (errors of commission), and continued indication with the presentation of subsequent non-target letters (preservation). Both this test and the digit repetition test are invalid for patients with a marked aphasia.

The Allen cognitive level test (1982) is an attempt to use a routine task to assess cognitive functioning. The examiner provides equipment and specific instructions for leather-stitching and records ability to carry out instructions according to a specific schedule. Many forms of deficits could result in difficulties with performing this task, but this is an interesting attempt to use a quasi-functional task in assessing cognitive function. Many commercial computer programmes are designed to assist the therapist evaluating reaction time and other processes related to attention. Patients who are able to perform these tasks in the standard ranges may none the less have deficits in attention which impair functional performance.

Therapists should remain alert to deficits in attention in higher functioning patients and evaluate attentional performance in domestic and community activities of daily living and during pre-vocational and vocational-assessment. Therapists should be aware of a test increasingly used by psychologists as a measure of attention following brain-injury, the Paced Auditory

Serial Addition Task (PASAT) of Gronwall (1977). The PASAT involves the presentation of digits at a constant rate; the patient is required to add the first two digits and announce the sum, then add the second to the third digit and announce the sum and so on. The digits are presented at four different rates: 2.4, 2.0, 1.6 and 1.2 per second. The PASAT is one of the most sensitive tests of attention and even mildly impaired patients may show deficits which distinguish them from uninjured controls on this test.

The efficacy of attentional retraining

Much of the initial work indicating the effectiveness of attentional retraining failed to take account of confounding variables. Methodological problems included a failure to account for spontaneous recovery, the ubiquitous effect of practice and control of therapist's attention. Despite the enthusiasm, much of the original work only served to demonstrate that people usually get better after brain injury and that if one practises a task, performance usually improves. The improvements in the tasks which were claimed to be evidence of improvements in attention almost invariably had no real-world correlates. More recently a number of studies with better research designs have examined the efficacy of attentional retraining (Wood and Fussey, 1987; Sohlberg and Mateer, 1987; Ponsford and Kinsella, 1988). In most cases the studies have not supported a general effect of attentional retraining. However the studies of Wood and Fussey (1987) and Ponsford and Kinsella (1988) suggest that behavioural aspects of attention (i.e. sitting and watching the screen and engaging in the task) improved in response to reinforcement and feedback. An exception to the generally negative findings was reported by Sohlberg and Mateer (1987). The work of these authors is reviewed below. Although the weight of evidence suggests that the underlying function of attention is not susceptible to currently available interventions, the work of Sohlberg and Mateer indicates that further study is required in this area before a definitive conclusion about the efficacy of attentional retraining is possible.

Remediating attentional disorders

Research into disorders of attention following brain injury has typically focused on the later stages of recovery, because acutely ill patients are too impaired to fulfil the research criteria. As a result, researchers may have underestimated the early disruption of attentional processes. After severe brain injury many individuals have a limited attention span and cannot direct attention to activities for long before becoming distracted or confused. Attention span is highly variable and affected by factors such as medical state, time of day and fatigue. Acute rehabilitation efforts should be designed to tax but not exceed the individual's attentional abilities. As the individuals improve, the duration of tasks can be extended, thus requiring attention to be sustained for longer periods. For a person beginning to attend to functional activities, the therapists can control the environment by limiting environmental distractions such as the activity in the room and the duration of the task. Stuss and co-workers (1989) suggest the ability of the patient to focus attention could depend on the amount of redundant information that needs to be ignored. As the individual's attentional capacity increases, tasks of greater complexity can be incorporated in treatment.

For use in the post-acute stage of recovery, Sohlberg and Mateer (1987) describe a multi-levelled hierarchical treatment programme to remediate attentional deficits in brain-injured persons. Rather than general stimulation (see Chapter 2) they emphasized process-specific interventions to selectively place demands on attention rather than on memory or perceptual processes. The authors reported results of intervention with four patients in a multiple baseline across behaviours design. The independent measure of attention used was the Paced Auditory Serial Addition Test (PASAT) (Gronwall 1977). All subjects showed improvement on the PASAT during the attentional training, suggesting a generalized effect on attention. This increased ability was not reflected in other (untreated) cognitive areas. The intervention programme was called Attention Process Training (APT) and addressed five levels of attention. The researchers developed hierarchies of therapeutic tasks for each of the five levels. The five levels of attention are: focused attention (the ability to respond to specific stimuli pre-

sented in various modalities); sustained attention (the maintenance of a specific behavioural response during continuous or
repetitive activity); selective attention (the development and
maintenance of an attentional set which involves responding to
specific stimuli and the suppression of responses to alternative
stimuli); alternating attention (requiring successive attentional
sets with different requirements); divided attention (the ability
to concurrently respond to two or more tasks, Sohlberg and
Mateer, 1987). Specific therapeutic tasks include commercially
available computer programmes and materials developed by the
researchers and are listed by the authors in an appendix
(Sohlberg and Mateer, 1987).

Verbal control as an attentional strategy

The verbal mediation of behaviour is described in various sections of this book. Verbal mediation has been used effectively
with the mentally handicapped (Wacker *et al.*, 1988), the traumatically brain-injured (Robertson *et al.*, 1988) and with patients
with other types of acquired neurological impairments (Giles
and Morgan, 1989). Verbal mediation can be divided into verbal
self-instruction and verbal self-monitoring (or regulation). Some
types of verbal regulations can be thought of as 'highlighting'
(see Chapter 7) and as an aid in attending to task. Wacker
et al. (1988) conducted two experiments in which moderately
mentally retarded persons were trained first to label information
and then to enter the details into a computer, calculator or
cheque book (label-then-do) in a multiple baseline design. The
individuals were taught to produce a verbal label to make the
relevant aspects of the task more salient and guide their performance. In the first experiment, five young adults were
trained to enter statistical programmes into computers in an
office. Prior to the introduction of the label-then-do approach
none of the clients performed more than 40% of the entries
correctly. Subsequent to training, all subjects scored in an
acceptable range on the task (95% accuracy). Following training,
all subjects used verbal labels and key entry skills and these
generalized across tasks (programmes) and settings (offices and
computer terminals). In the second experiment, three high
school students were taught the key entry task and how to
balance a cheque book. The performance of all students general-

ized across tasks and settings and the use of the labels generalized in two of the students. The student who failed to continue to use the labels did not deteriorate in accuracy suggesting that the labelling procedure need not be either overt or used after mastery of the task has been attained. Self-instruction and self-monitoring are similar to the extent that both guide behaviour through verbal control. With self-instruction, however, the individual states the behaviour to be performed whereas with self-monitoring the client states the antecedent stimulus which in turn guides behaviour. This increases the salience of the stimulus.

Specific task training

Severely impaired individuals may be unable to attend to even basic functional tasks. Behavioural learning programmes can help individuals attend to everyday activities. Feedback and reinforcement schedules can be designed to increase the patient's attention to specified functional tasks.

K.F. (coma duration 3 months and seen 10 months post-injury) wandered the treatment unit apparently without purpose. He wandered into other people's rooms, investigated their personal belongings and in other ways invaded their privacy. He was inadvertently reinforced for this behaviour by the attention he received from staff and clients. A programme was devised to prompt K.F. to sit with other clients in a communal area. If he sat down he was given social attention and praise, and after 5 minutes (if still seated) he was given an edible reinforcer. If he did not respond to the prompt, he was taken to the chair without any social attention. Gradually the time he was expected to remain seated was increased. As a result of the programme, he stopped wandering. A similar programme was used to assist him to remain seated during mealtimes so he could be trained to feed himself.

Three years following herpes simplex encephalitis, B.N. had a severe disorder of attention, which was apparent in all activities. Teaching him to cross the street was targetted as the main goal, because he could live at home with his mother, if he was safe to go out on his own. (Prior to the initiation of the programme, while staying at home he had been hit by a truck and hospitalized for 12 weeks with a fractured right femur). He was unsafe in crossing roads as he did not look before he stepped into the road, and would wander around in the road regardless of traffic. He would not walk close by the people accompanying him. A programme was devised to increase his awareness of road safety. A task analysis was performed and a series of prompts was developed for crossing the road safely. Using these prompts a programme was devised, where small amounts of money were given for correct performance of each of the components of the programme. B.N. practised the task three times a week for twenty weeks, with the staff changing the routes regularly after ten weeks. B.N. steadily improved and the programme was continued in his home environment until he was safe and independent in crossing the street. Table 10.1 shows B.N.'s road safety programme as an example of a programme designed to focus on attention and improve performance on a functional task.

Drug treatment

Psychostimulants, such as methylphenidate (Ritalin), Dexamphetamine (Dexedizine) and Magnesium Pemoline (Pemoline) have been shown to decrease distractibility, disorganization, hyperactivity and impulsiveness. It is widely believed that the best responses occur in patients with mild to moderate impairments (Gualtieri, 1988; Jackson *et al.*, 1984). There is some evidence that anti-depressants may be helpful with patients whose attentional disorder is associated with marked agitation.

PERCEPTION AND PRAXIS

Assessment

Both perceptual deficits and dyspraxia (see Chapter 3) may result in functional impairment. Occupational therapists are recognized as being specially trained to assess and treat individuals with perceptual disorders (Lamm-Warburg, 1988). The underlying disorder must be correctly identified if relevant treat-

Table 10.1 B.N.'s road safety programme

Walk to the grocery store with B.N. Always use the specified route to assist B.N. Learn the basic procedures involved in crossing the street safely. He is given a penny for each stage in the sequence below, if he follows the procedures without requiring prompts. When he reaches the other side of the road, give him the total reward earned and feedback about his performance. If he attempts to cross the street without looking, bring him back and say stop. He also earns an extra five pennies for each of the following if he achieves them without prompts.

a) Crosses the road at an appropriate location, i.e. not when behind a large vehicle, e.g. a bus where he cannot see.
b) Does not walk in the road.
c) Walks with the member of staff accompanying him (not more than 10 feet ahead or behind).

The total amount he can earn is 37 pence. If he earns more than 30 pence, give him 50 pence as a bonus for good performance.

1. At Green Road, turn right towards the pedestrian crossing. B. N. is expected to
   a) press the button for the pedestrian crossing
   b) stop
   c) look right
   d) look left
   e) look right
   f) cross the road only when the light indicates it is safe to do so.

2. After crossing Green Road turn left. Arrive at the road junction (cross Cliff Road)
   a) stop
   b) look right
   c) look left
   d) look right
   e) cross road when safe.

3. Continue along Green Road. Turn right into Worth Road. Arrive at road junction (cross King Road)
   a) stop
   b) look right
   c) look left
   d) look right
   e) cross road when safe.

4. Continue along Worth Road. Turn right into Well Road. At pedestrian crossing
   a) press the button for the pedestrian crossing
   b) stop at road
   c) look right
   d) look left
   e) look right
   f) cross the road only when the light indicates it is safe to do so.

Turn left along Well Road and right into the grocery store.

ment is to be provided. Individuals may demonstrate perceptual deficits while attempting to perform functional activities. Detailed behavioural observation elucidates the nature of the problem and provides the therapist with an understanding of how the individual attempts to compensate. More formal testing may assist the therapist determine the exact nature of the patient's perceptual dysfunction. Psychologists and others, including occupational therapists (Zoltan *et al.*, 1987) have established standardized tests for perceptual dysfunction in adults (Van Deusen and Harlowe, 1987). Many therapists use their own non-standardized tests to assess perceptual problems but may not know whether the tests are valid. The same general principles used for sensory assessment should be used in perceptual testing (see Chapter 9). Retraining techniques can be directed towards improving specific perceptual or praxic abilities, the development of a prosthetic environment, or specific skills training in an attempt to overcome the perceptual or praxic deficit as it affects a specific functional skill.

Body scheme disorders and somatic neglect

Body scheme impairment is a lack of awareness of the relationship of body parts to one another. An individual with body scheme disorder is unable to point to or move specific body parts to command. Body scheme disorders may be evident during physical retraining. For example the patient may have difficulty in following commands during transfer training. Dressing may be disrupted but impairments may be difficult to distinguish from dyspraxia. Assessment techniques for body scheme disorder include asking the patient to complete a human figure puzzle, asking the patient to describe the relationship of body parts to each other (e.g. are your knees above or below your hips?) and instructing the patient repeat movements performed by the therapist. Right-left discrimination disorder is an inability to distinguish left and right on one's own body or that of the examiner. Right-left discrimination disorder may be apparent when asking the patient to perform a unilateral activity, for example use the right arm/leg in dressing. An individual with unilateral somatic neglect disregards one half of his body. Sensation is intact but the individual does not spontaneously attend to it. When testing for somatic neglect, bilateral and unilateral stimulation should be alternated. When performing bilateral stimulation it is important to stimulate symmetrically, as non-neurologically impaired subjects may show extinction to asymmetrical stimulation (Bender, 1952). Patients could be asked to engage in a variety of bilateral activities for their actions to be observed. The individual may demonstrate an inability to sustain bilateral action (akinesia); for example, when requested to raise both arms, the patient may only raise one arm, or may raise both, but let one drop.

Visual neglect

Visual field deficits are common. Whilst hemianopia is the inability to see in one half of the visual field, patients with visual neglect (or inattention) do not attend to stimuli in the affected hemispace. The patient with unilateral visual neglect will ignore stimuli on the affected side when stimuli are presented bilaterally. This phenomenon is called unilateral extinction or suppression of visual stimuli. Visual supression may be tested by moving a finger in both the right and left half of the patient's visual field. If the patient only reports unilateral movement when the movement occurred bilaterally, then in the absence of hemianopia the patient is manifesting suppression. An alternative method of evaluating visual inattention/neglect requires the patient to bisect a horizontal line drawn on a sheet of paper. Patients with left visual neglect typically bisect the line significantly to the right of the true centre point. With successive line length (shortest 20 mm, longest 2000 mm) the extent of the displacement to the right increases. Visual inattention/neglect may also be assessed by asking the patient to draw objects, for example, a clock, flower, or by completing a cancellation task. Patients with unilateral neglect often draw only one half of the object or omit details on the neglected hemispace.

In functional situations, patients make errors as a result of missing environmental cues, miss the food on the left when eating, dress one half of their body, or walk into doorways or people on their neglected side. They may fail to observe traffic coming from the left or tend to make predominantly right turns therefore becoming lost in the community. Wilson *et al.* (1987) have reported a preliminary evaluation of the Rivermead Behavioural Inattention Test (RBIT). The RBIT consists of nine items sampling activities of daily living. The subtests are simulations of the scanning skills needed in: eating a meal (approximated by a life-sized coloured photograph divided into eight sections), dialling a telephone, reading a menu, telling the time (digital and analogue), setting the table, sorting coins, copying an address and following a map. Since these are the types of tasks that a patient with inattention is likely to have difficulty with, the development of this test should provide clinicians with a more precise description of the patient's abilities. The test is valid and reliable for patients below 65. There is however likely to be a ceiling effect. Some patients who score well on this test could still show mild deficits in real-life settings.

Spatial disorders

Figure-ground dysfunction interferes with the individual's ability to distinguish an object from its background. Figure-ground discrimination may be assessed by visual tasks which consist of imbedded or mixed figures, for example the Hooper Figure Ground Test (1958). In functional settings these skills are needed when looking for cutlery in a drawer, or clothes in a closet. Depth or distance may be inadequately perceived leading to difficulty in negotiating kerbs or steps or in judging the speed or distance of approaching traffic.

Agnosia

Agnosia is characterized by a failure to recognize an object using one sensory system, while the ability to recognize the object via other sensory systems is retained. Deficits in the synthesis of visual information (simultagnosia) can be assessed by presenting the patient with a picture which depicts a story or activity and asking him to describe the central features. Deficits in the recognition of faces (prosopagnosia) can be assessed by showing the patient pictures of familiar and unfamiliar faces and asking him to distinguish between them.

Visual object agnosia is the most common form of agnosia and to assess for this, the therapist places an array of common objects in front of the patient. The patient is asked to name an object, point to an object specified by the therapist or to specify its use. Toglia (1989) has proposed a specific evaluation technique for the assessment of visual object recognition. Central to the method proposed by Toglia is the idea that task conditions that influence visual perception should be specified and that tasks can be graded in difficulty. Toglia proposes varying the visual integrative demands of object recognition by altering six parameters: environment, familiarity, direction, amount, spatial arrangements and response rate (Toglia, 1989). Environment refers to the context in which recognition takes place (the object in the setting in which it is normally used). Recognition is easier in context. Familiarity refers to how frequently an object is encountered in daily life. Self-related objects (items for personal use, for example a toothbrush) may be easier to recognize than objects which the individual is unaccustomed to. Direction refers to the verbal instructions given for the task. For example pointing to an object and saying 'what is this?' is easier than asking the patient to list the items on a table with the instruction 'what is on the table?' Amount refers to the number of objects presented at one time and spatial arrangements refers to the way objects are presented during testing. A left to right arrangement (for those who read left to right) is easier than a scattered visually overlapping arrangement. Response rate refers to the speed of response demanded. Toglia recommends beginning with an intermediate level of difficulty and varying the demands of the task according to success or failure (Toglia, 1989). It should, of course, be remembered that this type of table-top testing should be used in an attempt to delineate the way performance breaks down and is not a substitute for evaluation in real-life settings.

Auditory agnosia refers to the inability to recognize and discriminate between sounds, and in assessment the patient can be asked to identify the cause of various sounds. Somatic agnosia, the inability to recognize objects by touch, may be tested by asking the patient who is blindfolded to manipulate an object and name it or state its use.

Praxis

Apraxia is a disorder of skilled movement not accounted for by weakness, spasticity or ataxia and may also be regarded as a collective name for disorders of motor planning. Ideomotor apraxia is the failure to perform previously learned movements and is the most frequently encountered form of apraxia. Apraxia is frequently associated with language impairments and the therapist must ensure that the patient has adequate verbal comprehension to carry out the instructions during evaluation. Deficits may be limited to the mouth and face, the upper extremities or involve the whole body.

Strub and Black (1985) describe a hierarchy of difficulty in performing ideomotor tasks. The most difficult test involves following verbal commands to mime an action (for example, 'show me how you would use a toothbrush') without any non-verbal cues from the therapist. The next level of difficulty involves asking the patient to imitate the therapist and perform the task (again in the absence of the object itself). The lowest level of difficulty is using the object itself.

Buccofacial disorders may be evaluated by asking the patient to stick out his tongue or drink through a straw. Upper extremity ideomotor apraxia may be assessed by asking the patient to comb his hair or demonstrate how to shave or hammer a nail. Failure may be characterized by the patient demonstrating displacement behaviours, using the hand as the object itself, and incorrect hand positioning. Whole body ideomotor apraxia may be evaluated by asking the patient to demonstrate how he would play golf, cricket or baseball.

Ideational apraxia is a disturbance of more complex or sequenced motor behaviours. Patients are often able to perform the individual discrete elements which make up a movement but cannot string them together into a coherent and functional pattern. Strub and Black (1985) describe two simple tasks which may be used to evaluate ideational apraxia: folding a letter, placing it in an envelope, sealing it and placing a stamp on the envelope; opening toothpaste, taking a toothbrush from a holder and placing toothpaste on a toothbrush. In attempting to perform these tasks the patient can usually perform each step of the task but cannot co-ordinate the individual movements to complete the sequence (Strub and Black, 1985).

Perceptual rehabilitation

The area of perceptual retraining is vast and a full review will not be attempted here. During the 1970s much work was carried out attempting to remediate perceptual deficits (particularly neglect) in patients with CVA and traumatic brain injury. The work of Diller and co-workers has been influential. These workers produced a series of monographs of their work with hemiplegic patients which were widely circulated. A report published in 1974 (Diller *et al.*, 1974) indicated successful retraining and transfer of the skills to functional (ADL) activities. A more recent study by the same group of workers (Gordon *et al.*, 1985) showed that a group of patients with right hemisphere brain damage improved more rapidly than a matched control group but that ultimate outcome was the same. However Gordon *et al.* (1985) were unable to find any transfer of training to performance of functional skills. Other workers have not always been as successful in showing a specific treatment effect. Lincoln *et al.* (1985) compared two group approaches to perceptual disorders in a group of 33 patients with CVA and traumatic brain injury. The active treatment group practised perceptual tasks using various types of games (e.g. peg boards, jigsaws), while the conventional therapy group did not practise tasks thought to improve perceptual skills. No significant differences were found between the two groups. Since both groups improved it is not clear whether the nonspecific aspects of the rehabilitation programme or spontaneous recovery account for the improvement. However, taken together these findings may indicate that in the acute stage of recovery of function a stimulatory approach to perceptual deficits may be helpful.

Training in compensatory routines

An example of compensation training is provided by the report of Robertson (1988) who provided successful intervention for visual neglect in a non-hemianopic brain-injured subject. The patient was a 20-year-old student injured in a road traffic accident (GCS score on admission was three and PTA was two weeks). The aim of the training programme, which used a micro-computer, was to 'establish a verbally regulated motor habit for orienting leftwards' (Robertson, 1988). The training method was a simple self-instructional procedure involving the command 'look left'. Initially the command was spoken loudly in the patient's ear immediately before the scanning task appeared on the computer screen, then he was cued to direct his own performance verbally and the final stage was for the patient to instruct himself sub-vocally. In the computer reading task the patient was instructed to fixate on the left side of each word rather than the middle. The patient showed significant improvement on the test of reading and not on the untrained control measures of visuospatial and attentional capacity. The patient was successfully trained to perform a motor routine to compensate for the visual inattention. Although not clearly demonstrated by this study, this motor behaviour might also be applied to other functional tasks which depend on adequate scanning of the environment (e.g. crossing the street).

Specific task training

The third approach specific task training involves teaching the patient to perform in the specific functional tasks compromised by the perceptual impairment. Training methods are described elsewhere in this text. However, in addition to the standard approach, it is necessary to alter the retraining programme to ensure the patient can actually perform the programme despite the perceptual deficits. Techniques could be built into the programme including: descriptive prompting (for example, 'this is your right hand, put your right hand in the sleeve'); discriminatory prompting (e.g. touching or pointing to a neglected extremity, modelling and motor guidance through tasks).

N.C. (coma duration 14 days, seen two years post-injury) was unable to identify body parts. When asked to wash her face, she would wash a part of her body apparently at random. There was evidence of slight receptive dysphasia, but N.C. was able to carry out tasks when instructions did not make reference to a part of the body. When teaching her to wash, she was given a prompt, for example, 'wash your face'. If she did not start washing her face, or was unsure of what to do, the therapist would touch her face and repeat 'wash your face'. If she still had difficulties, the therapist carefully took her hand and guided her hand over her face and said 'you are washing your face'. After approximately four weeks these prompts were no longer necessary.

Apraxia

Although defined negatively (a disorder of skilled movement which cannot be accounted for by other movement disorders), apraxia often occurs in conjunction with other severe motor and cognitive deficits. In apraxic individuals, previously highly overlearned movement patterns maybe disrupted. Alternatively, the individual may be able to carry out automatic action patterns but be unable to perform an action to command or as a result of conscious volition. Mildly impaired patients may simply require more time to work out how to perform the activity. Apraxia is frequently undiagnosed and patients are labelled as 'variable', 'uncooperative' or 'not responsive to rehabilitation'. Observation of automatic functional behaviour on how the patient responds to prompts, assists therapists determining the most functional rehabilitative interventions. Often, patients remain inactive or engage in displacement behaviours. For example, one patient when asked to throw his T-shirt in the dirty laundry basket alternated between shaking it and arranging it in his hand continuously until the behaviour was interrupted. Severely impaired patients may become physically or verbally aggressive when asked to perform a task which they are unable to initiate.

The same hierarchical principles could be used in rehabilitation as are used in assessment. It is most difficult for patients to respond to specific verbal cues. Some apraxic individuals may perform better if instructions are given which outline the goal rather than the method. Instructions often need to be repeated, but in a non-confronting manner to reduce stress, which could exacerbate the patient's difficulties. When patients cannot respond to verbal cues alone (or are only able to do so intermittently) the therapist can mime the activity for the patient as well as giving the verbal instruction. Where the patient continues to be unable to initiate the activity, the therapist may begin the task for the patient (for example, putting the fork in the patient's hand and guiding the fork to the patient's mouth). Since the goal is for the patient to be able to follow verbal commands, these should always be paired with the activity (for example, saying 'fork to mouth'). As in many areas of retraining, frequent practice of correct performance reduces the attentional demands of tasks and results in increased ease and fluency of performance. Motor planning or movement groups may be of assistance to some patients (for example, an oral-motor group). In these groups specific movement patterns can be practised and the patient provided with the cues required to help him perform the movement. The therapist should educate other staff about apraxic disorders as untrained staff may regard apraxic phenomena as evidence of wilfulness.

S.F. (two years post severe brain injury, coma duration unknown) had severe apraxia and was unable to wash and dress himself. When asked to dress he compensated with displacement behaviours, such as pinching, slapping, giggling, and swearing. When given clothes he could occasionally put them on without any difficulty but at other times would appear to be playing the fool, throwing clothes on the floor, or wandering out of the room. He could not maintain attention to tasks, and once distracted only exhibited displacement behaviours. A supportive, non-confronting approach was used, which encouraged S.F. to put on the whole item, with oblique reinforcement if the task was achieved. If he could not do this, the task was broken down, and help was given if needed. Gradually, he learned to dress independently.

In addition to the difficulties described above S.F. was frequently doubly incontinent. He could not initiate finding the washroom or reliably manage his clothing when he went to the toilet. Several continence-related programmes had been tried, which included having regular toileting times, prompting him, helping him with his clothing and onto the toilet, all without success. Finally, a programme was initiated, where a member of staff modelled the behaviour for S.F. at regular toileting times. This intervention carried out over a number of weeks was successful to the extent that S.F. was only very occasionally incontinent.

D.G.M., a severely apraxic patient (coma duration 36 days), was unable to feed himself and became very agitated when food was presented. He would jump to his feet, knock chairs and tables over and throw plates. Although he was able to swallow efficiently and without aspiration, oral apraxia resulted in him being unable to move food to the back of his mouth to initiate a swallow reflex. Initially he would only accept food whilst lying down. A backward-chaining feeding programme was instigated where he was first taught to sit on a chair. He was fed with a fork to the back teeth, to teach him to chew and swallow, and gradually he became less agitated. To teach him to eat independently, he was first taught to take food off the fork, then to hold the fork as this was guided to his mouth. Over time the pressure required to guide his arm decreased until he was independent. The patient was discharged to the care of his parents. Following an exacerbation of the patient's medical condition, his patients were unable to fully redevelop self-feeding, but D.G.M. maintained an appropriate sitting posture and the behavioural disregulation recurred only when he was suffering from an infection.

MEMORY

Most experimental paradigms used by psychologists to assess memory make the task easy, because of implicit or explicit cueing to help the person when he needs to recall something. In most practical everyday situations the information that needs to be remembered may be trivially small and the difficulty comes in remembering to remember it. This remembering to remember has been described as prospective memory (Harris, 1984a). As therapists we are most concerned with how patients can function in their daily lives, and this means prospective memory is of central importance. This type of phenomenon has stimulated some researchers to examine everyday aspects of memory function with increased emphasis on ecological validity (Harris and Morris, 1984; Neisser, 1988). This approach is, however, not without its critics who have suggested that increased ecological validity is gained at the cost of the generalizability of results (Banaji and Crowder, 1989). This criticism is appropriate only when the new approach is used to study memory *per se* rather than the individual's use of memory in everyday settings. The therapist needs to know first how memory functioning breaks down and then how to intervene to help the memory-impaired individual overcome his deficits. Functional impairments caused by memory and information processing deficits may be minimized by training the patient in specific facts (orientation training), by helping the individual to develop methods of mentally manipulating information available in the environment (internal strategies) or by augmenting normally available environmental information (external strategies). In addition, practise of organizing common activities into routines may reduce the demands on the memory system itself. These techniques are discussed following the discussion of techniques of memory assessment.

Assessment

Assessment of memory dysfunction includes structured interviews of the individual and his relatives, standardized testing, and observation of the individual in his daily routines. Standardized testing is usually considered the role of the rehabilitation psychologist but only a combination of methods will allow the therapist to identify areas of real-life activities where memory function breaks down. Deficits may range from total amnesia leading to unsafe behaviour and dependence in basic aspects of self-care to mild memory impairment, compromising work or social functioning but allowing continued independent living. Assessment of memory functioning should include the client's ability to recall written, visual and verbal information at 30 seconds and 30 minutes. Assessment should include an examination of the client's ability to learn novel behaviours (ie. the number of repetitions it takes to learn a new behaviour). We have already mentioned the importance of remembering to do things: assessment must therefore also involve the client's ability to initiate a planned behaviour in the future. The more impaired the individuals the more important it is to assess 'savings in learning' in a variety of functional domains. Assessment should also include an examination of the individual's ability to use strategies which help them remember information.

In patients with severe memory problems, impairment will often become apparent within a half-hour interview as the client forgets things said earlier in the interview. Patients are often aware of retrograde memory impairment (i.e. that they cannot remember things from the past) but rarely of the anterograde disorder (i.e. that they have a problem forming new memories). Techniques that can be used to assess the more severely impaired patient include the following:

1. asking the severely disoriented patient to indicate whether he is in a bus station, an airport, a church, or a hospital;
2. asking the patient if he has met you before, when meeting him for the first time. See if the patient knows where he is (the town) and how he arrived there;
3. informing the patient of your name and occupation and asking him to repeat this information one, five, and 30 minutes later;
4. telling the patient a name and street address and asking him to repeat this to you immediately and then ten and 60 minutes later;
5. hiding a desirable object in the room (ensuring that the patient is observing you) and asking the patient to locate the object after an intervening activity;
6. giving the patient simple directions to see if he can follow them or whether the patient requires further instruction.

Wilson and co-workers have developed a formal test attempting to measure functional memory. The Rivermead Behavioural Memory test (Wilson *et al.*, 1985) attempts to capture aspects of prospective memory, as well as recognition and recall. In our experience, it is best used with the severely impaired as it is prone to false negatives. It however provides a useful adjunct to more naturalistic observations by therapists.

For individuals with moderate memory impairments who are having ongoing difficulties in their day-to-day life, adequate assessment requires a protracted period (days) of careful observation on graded functional tasks. Common problems resulting from mild to moderate memory disorder include forgetting information, like names, or whether an activity has been performed; forgetting where personal belongings have been placed; or repeating phrases or questions. Functional assessment involves asking the patient to engage in complex, dependent action sequences which require the initiation of activities in a set order, at different times of day, or in different locations, for example setting up an appointment. The skilled therapist is able to determine if the patient is able to function in his own environment.

The therapist's task is made more complicated by the fact that brain-injured individuals have difficulty in gaining an accurate view of their own memory impairment (Sunderland *et al.*,

1984). Acquiring knowledge about impaired memory is a learning task and therefore it is not surprising that patients with memory problems have a difficult time acquiring this knowledge. Only highly structured and repetitive feedback provided at the time of the memory failure can help patients develop a more realistic view of their own memory functioning. Involving the patient in his own assessment facilitates the patient's understanding of his own deficits making the task of retraining considerably easier.

Orientation training

Orientation has been defined as including awareness of time, locale, identities of people in the patient's environment, general facts, personal facts and episodic information (Corrigan *et al.*, 1985). Jackson *et al.* (1989) have described the Orientation Group Monitoring System (OGMS), the purpose of which is to monitor the patient's recovery of orientation. OGMS represents a simple and reliable behavioural monitoring system, used in conjunction with an orientation training group. The OGMS can be integrated into the ward or unit routine and is described in more detail in Chapter 8.

Informal reality orientation may be conducted throughout the day and involves prompting the patient to recall information relevant to orientation (Powell-Proctor and Miller, 1982). Increasing contextual cues and placing the information that is to be learnt within a meaningful framework aids the individual's recall of information. The exact wording of a question may influence the patient's ability to elicit a specific answer. For example, we attempted to teach a patient with profound memory impairment, caused by anoxic damage, a few discrete items of information. She would typically and spontaneously produce the wrong answer when questioned. It rapidly became obvious that if she gave the wrong answer, the chances she would give this (wrong) answer when next questioned, were greatly increased. It was essential to formulate the questions so that they always or nearly always led to the patient to produce the right answer. This demonstrates that people learn what they think, not what they are told, and therapists need to be aware of this if involved in memory training.

Fading occurs through the gradual reduction of the cues required to elicit a correct answer and the use of specific instructional materials such as videotapes may also assist learning. Providing patients with an incentive to improve their orientation, for example reinforcement for correctly answering orientation questions, has been found to significantly improve memory for recent episodic events (Langer *et al.*, 1979).

Topographical orientation

Deficits in topographical orientation may be manifested by the patient getting lost on simple routes, being unable to find items in the kitchen, or not being able to learn the location of the switches on a microwave oven. Some patients are unable to form a topographical schema and this may be evident when asking the individual to find the location of his room in the hospital or his way in the local community. Deficits may be only evident in novel environments, however some patients are disoriented in what were once familiar surroundings. General spatial concepts could be disturbed when patients are unable to locate major cities on a map of the country. This would mean that patients would be less able to use maps to help them negotiate their environment. These patients could use lists of instructions, however, with a system for recording when each step is completed. Individuals who experience difficulty locating items in the home may be assisted by labelling the cupboards and drawers with lists of their contents.

K.C. (three years post simplex encephalitis) had a severe amnesic disorder and was taught to be independent in his new environment by using maps. He had retained map-reading skills from before injury, but felt anxious and insecure about going out because of his awareness of the severity of his memory problems. He would look at the map of the local hospital area, which included a number of prominent environmental cues, and in addition followed a set of written instructions which he checked off as he performed them. As he improved, he used the checklist less and explored the area using the map only as a support, in case he got lost. He then started to ride his bicycle and used maps to go around the areas marked on his map. The fact that he could never remember where he had parked his bicycle was only a minor problem, as it was always found locked to a lamppost somewhere in the town.

Memory retraining

Therapy for memory dysfunction can be directed at correcting the defective process or function (restitution) or reducing the effect of the deficit by utilizing intact alternative strategies (substitution) (Miller, 1985). In addition, specific tasks may be over-learned to the point at which they become automatic and introspective remembering becomes unnecessary. Harris and Sunderland (1981) sent questionnaires to rehabilitation units or hospitals working with persons with memory dysfunction. They found that therapists were teaching patients to use external memory aids, internal memory strategies and providing a structured environment or daily routine. The therapists utilized training tasks, including memory games, rote learning, retrained individuals in specific skills, and conducted reality orientation and current events groups.

Many memory retraining programmes have provided practice of memory tasks. Memory programmes have aimed to help individuals increase their memory span and memory capacity by, for example, asking patients to recall previously presented lists of words. Improvements on these mental exercises does not mean that the learning transfers to functional settings (Glisky *et al.*, 1986) and practice on specific tasks may not generalize even to apparently similar tasks. However, Harris and Sunderland suggest that practising educational mental exercises, which are relevant and meaningful, improve the individual's morale (Harris and Sunderland, 1981). Despite the lack of evidence for its efficacy, Harris and Sunderland (1981) found that the practising of remembering was the most widely used form of memory therapy. The popularity of this form of memory retraining does not mean remembering is a thing which is possible to practise. For example, Wagenaar (1986) studied his own auto-biographical memory over a six-year period. One event per day was recorded along four parameters: who, what, where and when. The process of recall itself took one year. The practice of remembering had no effect on his ability to remember, despite structured and persistent efforts. Recognition of the failure of the 'mental muscle' approach to memory retraining has led to attempts to teach internal memory strategies. These have been found useful by people without neurological impairments (Pattern, 1972).

Internal strategies

Internal strategies are methods of manipulating information mentally, to increase its availability to introspection at appropriate times. Everyone uses strategies to help store and access information, although these methods are not always recognized, even by those who use them. Harris (1980) found the principal methods used were (self) cueing strategies. Examples of cueing strategies are mentally retracing a sequence of past events or actions, in order to cue a memory of something that has happened, or finding an object which is lost. People retrace their ideas for weekly menus, to help them remember the items they need whilst shopping (Harris, 1980). Alphabetic searching is used when trying to recall a name or word. An individual works through the alphabet letter by letter to find the initial letter of the name to aid retrieval of the information.

The study of memory and memory failures in the non-neurologically impaired has proved helpful in understanding memory failures in the brain-injured. More elaborate strategies are used by the non-neurologically impaired to recall large amounts of information. It has been suggested that the application of some of these methods could assist the brain-injured adult who has continuing memory dysfunction (Pattern, 1972; Wilson and Moffat, 1984).

Visual imagery

Visual imagery has been found to assist the non-neurologically impaired to learn novel material. The place method (or method of loci) is one visualization method, which involves imagining a familiar or schematized area (such as a town or an office) and 'placing' the to-be-remembered information in a specific location. Luria described a cabaret performer who used this method with remarkable success in 'The mind of a Mnemonist' (1968). When recall is required one 'looks' again in the place where the information was left. Another well-known memory strategy involving visualization is the peg method. First one learns to associate a visual image with each of a series of numbers (e.g. one is a bun, two is a shoe!). In order to remember a list of novel items (such as a shopping list), the person imagines the items in combination with the already-learned peg images. Often bizarre visual images are used to associate the material. In order to remember the list the individual thinks first of the number, the peg image associated with it, and as a result recalls the item, remembered in conjunction with it (Pattern, 1972; Moffat, 1984). Although some neurologically impaired populations have shown greater retention of material when tested in a laboratory situation by using visual techniques (Binder and Schreiber, 1980; Lewinsohn *et al.*, 1977), most studies have failed to show transfer of the techniques to new or everyday situations (Crovitz *et al.*, 1979). Individuals after brain injury may display concrete thinking and difficulty in processing material alien to their immediate situation. In a study by Crovitz and colleagues (1979), patients after brain injury were unable to use the bizarre images advocated for the non-neurologically impaired. In addition, the procedure, despite practice remains effortful and many brain-injured individuals are known to have difficulty in initiating this type of (internal) procedure. Visual imagery techniques have successfully helped individuals learn to remember people's names. Glasgow *et al.* (1977) failed to teach the patient to remember names using a modified peg method, but were successful with a second simpler method. In a group setting, the patient attempted to remember people's names, and any of those he forgot, he wrote down. At three scheduled times a day, the patient was asked to read each name on the list while he visualized the person whose name he read. This procedure resulted in significantly improved performance (Glasgow *et al.*, 1977).

Two-and-a-half years following brain injury (coma duration unknown, but in excess of three weeks) J.E. remained unable to remember the names of those he regularly encountered in his environment, a fact which caused him marked distress. It was noted that the only people he remembered were those with prominent distinguishing features, for example, he could remember the name of a very tall staff member. J.E. was helped to write a list of patient and staff names and their specific discriminating physical features. In group settings and around the unit, staff asked him to state their name. When he was unable to do this, they recited their own physical discriminating features and he attempted to remember their name. For example, one of the authors would say 'dark wavy hair, freckles' and he would say 'Jo'. Over a four week period J.E. was prompted to look at a person's physical features and then to remember their name. After this time he remembered the person's name once he identified the distinguishing features. J.E. was gradually able to build up his repertoire of frequently encountered individuals and had a marked increase in his self-esteem.

Patients often have difficulty in forming novel visual associations and memory retraining techniques requiring this have proved largely unsuccessful. Patients with deficits severe enough to warrant introduction of the procedures usually cannot use them. However, stable associations as face/names may be formed using visualization techniques and could be helpful for some patients.

Verbal elaboration

Some verbal elaboration methods are similar to the visual methods described above except that they use words to form associations. There are a number of well-known variants of the word association technique. A chaining-mnemonic format can be used to sequence information together in the form of a story to aid recall of the material, for example the aeroplane list (Crovitz, 1979). However, the application of this type of procedure to novel information is even more cognitively demanding than the visualization techniques described in the previous section, and is therefore not recommended. First letter mnemonics (e.g. Richard Of York Gave Battle In Vain, for the colours of the rainbow) and rhymes (e.g. In fourteen hundred and ninety-two, Columbus sailed the ocean blue, for the recall of a date) can be used to help patients learn fixed pieces of information. This type of technique may be particularly useful in work places where fixed routines must be followed. Much of what has recently been labelled 'vocational memory retraining' is the application of this type of method to the job site

(Parente and Anderson-Parente, 1989). Other methods encourage patients to process the material in more depth (a procedure influenced by the depth of processing model of Craik and Lockhart, 1972). The depth of processing internal methods are used to increase the amount of attention/rehearsal devoted to the material that needs to be remembered (most frequently written material). The PQRST (Preview, Question, Read, State, Test) method is a well-known example (Table 10.2) (Giles and Clark-Wilson. 1988b).

Table 10.2 PQRST method

Preview:	Skim the material to learn the general content.
Question:	Ask yourself about the central features of the content.
Read:	Read actively with the goal of answering the questions.
State:	Repeat to yourself the information that you have read.
Test:	Test yourself by answering your own questions.

Crosson and Buenning (1984) describe an individualized memory retraining programme for a young man following severe brain injury from a motor cycle accident. The patient was trained on a variety of methods to improve recall of passages extracted from magazines. Strategies included the PQRST method and questioning by a friend. The patient showed improvement over the first fifteen day trial period which could not be accounted for by spontaneous recovery. Unfortunately, and in line with reports from other workers (Cermak, 1976; Gianutsos, 1980, 1981), the use of the strategies did not become part of his daily life. Like the more complex visualization methods, verbal elaboration techniques require intensive mental manipulation of the to-be-remembered information and (since they require the initiation of complex internal behaviours) may not be used by the severely brain-injured.

Glasgow *et al.* (1977) compared three different techniques to help a student remember written assignments: a control condition, a rehearsal strategy and the PQRST strategy. The PQRST strategy was superior to the rehearsal strategy, which in turn was better than the control condition, on all performance measures. All three techniques required different periods of processing time, with PQRST needing three times the amount of time of the control condition.

Many difficulties encountered by patients with frontal pathology are failures to spontaneously mentally review new information. Interventions which encourage this type of internal review in patients could be of assistance, but the patient must learn to review materials spontaneously for it to be helpful. The difficulty encountered by patients in doing this suggests the adoption of external strategies to accomplish the same end may be more successful. The fact that many external strategies involve motor routines may make it easier for the patient to develop the use of these as habits.

External strategies

The non-neurologically impaired use external memory strategies more often than internal memory strategies (Harris, 1980). External strategies include asking someone to remind you to do a task, or leaving objects in relevant places so they will be encountered when needed. For example, placing important work papers by the front door, so they will be picked up the following morning before going to work.

The effectiveness of internal versus external strategies in the non-neurologically impaired population is examined in a study by Harris (1984a). Harris found older subjects were more likely to remember to do things than younger subjects. Younger subjects were more confident about their memory ability than older subjects, who were more likely to use external memory aids, such as writing lists or making notes on a calendar (Harris, 1980, 1984a). Although many different types of external strategies may be useful with memory impaired brain-injured adults, here we will discuss check-lists, posters, timetables, diaries and memory books. This will be followed by an extended case study of a person learning to use an electronic diary, the Psion Organizer.

Check-lists
Many amnesic patients believe that they have performed activities which they have not performed (for example, personal hygiene activities) or that they have not done things which they have (for example, eat lunch). Memory impaired patients who do not remember whether they have performed a task have difficulties with either repeating the activity or refusing to participate on the grounds that it has already been performed. A

prominently placed check-list which the patient marks off or signs may be invaluable for increasing patient orientation to these activities and in reducing non-compliance. Patients need to be helped to learn to tick off each instruction/activity on the check-list once it has been performed. Following check-lists can be taught as a 'meta' procedure so whatever needs to be learned can be designed as a check-list. Patients often accept a printed check-list more readily than following instructions (which they are liable to forget) from a therapist. A number of patients have been trained by the authors to sequence washing and dressing activities with a check-list and as the patient learns the routine, the check-list is no longer needed.

Patient S.A. remained confused two months after a severe brain injury (coma duration seven days). Damage was particularly marked in the right frontal area. The patient was fully ambulatory but loquacious and non-compliant. On transfer to the transitional living centre from the acute rehabilitation facility S.A. appeared not to have bathed for several days. Once showering was initiated she was able to perform the activity independently. Unfortunately it was very difficult to help S.A. to participate in the activity as she would always claim to have just showered, to have showered the night before or not to need to shower. Attempts to find a time of day when she would be more likely to respond to prompts were unsuccessful. A large colourful chart was designed which included the patient's name, the time when she was to shower (7:30 am) and had a place for a check mark each day. S.A. reviewed the chart in individual and group sessions. She was instructed that she was the only person who could write on the chart, and that she should do so with a staff member immediately after taking her shower. The chart was posted in the group room where Unit therapy took place, so it could be reviewed frequently and attempts to write on it could be monitored. S.A. was prompted to shower at 7.30 each morning and supervised by staff until the shower was underway. S.A. frequently stated that she had showered the night before or at another time, but the use of the chart helped to redirect her into showering on all but the third and sixth day after the introduction of the chart. After four weeks staff felt that S.A. had developed her daily routine sufficiently automatically to get out of bed and shower independently. Use of the chart was therefore discontinued and S.A. was able to maintain her morning hygiene behaviour without difficulty.

Posters and timetables

Prominently displayed posters may be used to help a patient learn needed information. For example we have used posters as an adjunct to other methods to teach one patient that she must not leave the facility unaccompanied and another patient that he must not take cigarettes from his co-workers. Patients must be able to read to make use of this intervention. The poster should be large and eye-catching and it may be helpful for the patient to sign it to show he has registered agreement. Some patients will read the poster every time they notice it (i.e. have an orienting response) to it. Changing the look of the poster and changing its position will prevent the patient from habituating to it before he has learned its content. Patients can be directed by staff to go to their room to check the poster many times per day. Behaviourally disregulated or non-compliant patients may more readily accept material presented in poster form. (Similar methods have been used to help train staff in new treatment programmes – putting colourful posters around the treatment facility).

A timetable is a simplified version of a diary. Most institutions have a set routine which can be presented in the form of a timetable. The timetable may include wake up time, an appropriate time to wash and dress, lunch, dinner, laundry time and regularly scheduled individual and group therapy times. A version of this timetable may be posted in the patient's room and also in the patient's memory book.

Diaries and memory books

A diary or memory book may be used at many stages of recovery from brain injury. A diary or daily planner is more applicable to prospective memory (remembering to do things in the future) while a memory book is best used as an aid to remembering the past. In the initial stages of recovery a memory book is most appropriate for staff and family to write in. The book, most often a loose leaf file, should be clearly divided and marked into separate sections (although not all sections need to be used at one time). The sections could include the following.

1. An orientation section. This should include the person's name, where they are and what happened to them. A calendar with previous days marked off and a schedule of events at the hospital or rehabilitation facility should also be part of this section.
2. A therapy section. The individual could be encouraged to write down his therapeutic programme and staff comments on his performance.
3. A visitors section. Visitors could be asked to write down when they came to the hospital, and what they and the patient talked about.
4. Two prospective memory sections could be included, consisting of 'Things I need to ask' (this section may have subheadings such as 'Questions to ask Mother', 'Questions to ask the doctor') and things to remember to do.

Part of the routine in the morning could involve reviewing the memory book. The patient should have the memory book with him at all times and should be encouraged by all staff to use it at regular intervals to check information. The memory book is very useful in encouraging staff to interact with the patient around a limited set of orienting information. As the patient recovers, they learn to review the book spontaneously and make entries about events in their day. Effective use of the prospective sections of a memory book usually occurs later.

When it becomes evident that the rapid stage of spontaneous recovery is slowing, the patient should be assessed to determine whether he will need a memory aid to function in his daily life. The patient's needs are assessed with consideration being given to the severity of memory deficits, vocational and living environments. Since training to use a memory aid is effortful and time consuming, it is important that it actually addresses the patient's real-world requirements. Memory aids, for example diaries, are more likely to be accepted if they match the individual's pre-injury lifestyle. To use a day-at-a-glance diary efficiently an individual must be able to read and write and able to extract the essential components of a plan or action in order to write them down. In addition he must be able to initiate the use of the diary at the appropriate times, both for entry and retrieval of information. A three-stage behavioural approach has been found to be most effective in training patients in the use of memory aids. The first step involves daily cognitive overlearning. On a sessional basis, the therapist and patient review the patient's deficits, the reasons for using the memory aid and the specific techniques which need to be used for the system to work. The second step involves specific practice sessions in the use of the memory aid. The patient could be set real-world tasks which require use of the memory aid and supervised in the use of the aid. The third step involves the patient using the memory aid on a twenty-four hour basis. All staff in the treatment facility and the patient's family need to be aware of the purpose of the memory aid and the methods being taught. Sohlberg and Mateer (1989) have described a variant of this approach for use with a memory book. Patients who have difficulty in initiating behaviour would initially need prompting on a twenty-four hour basis to use the diary, record relevant information and check the diary frequently enough for it to be of use. One method to overcome this last problem is to provide the patient with a wrist-watch which bleeps on the hour or half-hour. The patient can be trained to respond to the bleep as a cue to look in the diary. Recently a number of reasonably priced pocket computers have become available. With some machines, an alarm can be set to sound and remind the patient to check the aid to see pre-programmed instructions which appear on the screen.

L.C., a 25-year-old woman, experienced a massive subarachnoid haemorrhage with bleeding into the ventricles. She underwent a number of surgical procedures over the following four months. Medical recovery from the procedures was uneventful. L.C. was admitted to the Transitional Living Centre 18 months after the final surgery. L.C. suffered a significant memory disorder with neuropsychological test results showing memory impairment in the moderate range. In functional settings her memory impairment resulted in, for example, missing or mistaking the time of appointments. L.C. remained of average intelligence and was interested and enthusiastic about learning how to use the Psion Organizer.

Method

On admission to the TLC, L.C. was taught to use a Day-at-a-Glance diary (Sheaffer *et al.*, 1986) which she carried with her at all times. Quantifiable data about function was gathered by asking L.C. to perform ten normal household activities at specific times, when at home over the weekend. Although the activities were similar, they were varied, as were times of execution, to limit a practice effect. All activities were related to L.C.'s daily life and were generated with her help prior to initial testing, and included watering plants, feeding the cats and performing other household chores. Instruction in the tasks was given on the Friday and results collected on the Monday. Baseline information was gathered on two occasions and two experimental conditions were employed such that an ABAC experimental design was used (Kazdin, 1982). L.C. was asked to record separately if the task was performed and, if it was not performed within a half-hour of the appointed time, to record when it was performed. The first baseline (A) was followed two weeks later by the first experimental condition (B) (Day-at-a-Glance). One month later the second baseline recording (A) occurred and one month after that the second experimental condition (C) (Psion). The baselines and experimental conditions were widely separated in order to minimize practice effects and to allow a comparable period between all conditions. During both baselines L.C. was prevented from recording the instructions in any way. In the first experimental condition L.C. used the Day-at-a-Glance which she had previously been using for two months. Immediately following the second baseline, training in the use of the Psion Organizer was begun. Four hours of individual training was followed by L.C. using the manual and practising with the Organizer for a further six hours (with help from relatives). After one month she felt comfortable with the machine and used it constantly. The second experimental condition using the Organizer was then carried out.

Results and discussion

During baselines one and two (recording not permitted), L.C. did not perform any of the assigned activities. She reported that she had forgotten about the instructions until reminded the following Monday. Experimental condition B (diary recording) resulted in eight out of ten items being performed, six at or within a half-hour of the time. In experimental condition C (Psion Organizer) nine out of ten activities were performed all within the half-hour time period. Two years later L.C. continues to use the Organizer and states that she prefers it to a diary. She is observed to use the Organizer effectively in daily life. L.C.'s improved performance with the Psion over the diary may be accounted for by the interactive (alarm) function which she uses regularly. This supposition is supported by the reduced number of timing errors when using the Psion. L.C. was in many ways an ideal candidate for training in this kind of equipment. She had insight into her deficits, memory disorder produced functional impairments but occurred against a background of IQ in the normal range and only mild difficulties in initiating behaviour. It is unlikely that improvement over the course of the study was a result of spontaneous recovery as L.C. was 18 months post the neurological event. Also the nature of the study and the widely separated baselines with identical results argue against this explanation.

The Psion Organizer presents a considerable advance over earlier memory aids (reviewed by Harris, 1984b) and may be helpful to patients similar to L.C. Although a number of newer machines are now available, for example the Sharp Wizard and Casio Boss pocket computers, these are more complex to operate and offer no additional advantages. The following criteria are recommended for determining the usefulness of a electronic memory aid for a client.

1. Average or near average intelligence.
2. Retained or mildly impaired reasoning skills.
3. Insight into deficits.
4. Adequate ability to initiate behaviour.
5. Functional disorder as a result of significant memory impairment.

Specific task training

Analysis of the demands of the individual's daily life allows some activities to become routine and ultimately habits. The degree to which activities become automatic mean the demands on the individual's memory is reduced. Procedures involved in specific skills training are discussed below and elsewhere in this book.

A preliminary retraining model

While there has been increasing interest in memory over recent years, there has been very little effort devoted to applied studies of learning. Research into memory has been of little practical assistance to those involved in training the neurologically impaired. Considering the theories and evidence in attention and memory, outlined here and in Chapter four, it is possible to suggest a retraining model with practical implications for therapists. We rely particularly on the procedural declarative (episodic semantic) typology, the work of Shiffrin and Schnieder (1977) on automatic and control processing, and the increasing evidence that learning requires attention but not understanding of what is to be learned.

As an example of this we will discuss how an individual could be trained to cross the street. Crossing the street safely consists of stopping at the kerbside, looking in both directions and then walking directly across the street, when there are no motor vehicles within a certain distance (depending on the patient's speed of ambulation, the velocity of the vehicles and so forth). The first time this retraining occurs is an 'episode'. It is processed and the specific to-be-learned activity is associated with the specific street intersection, the traffic which was passing and other incidental information. This episode may not be available later for introspection (due to hippocampal damage), but a certain priming effect will have occurred. In amnesic individuals, this information will undoubtedly be sub-threshold for recall. On the second occasion retraining occurs, only certain aspects of the situation will have been held constant, such as the specific instructions given. As this street-crossing routine is repeated, always in exactly the same way, the street crossing episodes are not retained (or at least are not recallable). The street crossing memory becomes an abstraction of many specific memory traces, all inevitably slightly different, that eventually produces the generalized memory structure of 'crossing streets'. This experience becomes prototypical and part of semantic memory. In optimum cases the patient no longer chooses to cross the street in a certain manner, the patients just 'knows' that this is how they cross the street. As we have pointed out elsewhere (Giles and Morgan, 1989) it is not clear that either procedural or semantic memory fully describes the process taking place and the information may or may not be available to introspection. The use of the patient's intact learning abilities is central to the work of the therapist and is also discussed in Chapter 7.

Drug treatments

Many drugs have been advocated for use with patients with attentional and memory disorders. Psychostimulants are thought to improve long-term memory in attention deficit-hyperactive disorders, and are recommended in relatively high functioning, mild to moderately impaired patients with deficits in attention, memory, organization or initiative (Gualtieri, 1988). Neuropeptides have been shown to facilitate learning in animals and more recently to improve short-term memory in healthy adults. Vasopressin-like peptides appear to improve the initial acquisition of information and facilitate memory consolidation. Jolles (1983) has suggested that vasopressin may only benefit patients with mild amnesia though well-controlled clinical trials are necessary to elucidate this further.

LANGUAGE

Speech and language problems influence an individual's ability in a vast number of functional areas. Not only does verbal performance in everyday settings need to be assessed by the speech and occupational therapists, but reading and writing must also be evaluated to judge its adequacy in meeting environmental demands. Considering their social environment and analysing performance in functional settings, in conjunction with standardized assessments performed by the speech therapist, facilitates an understanding of the language deficits affecting the individual's ability to communicate.

After severe brain injury many patients have receptive language deficits (see Chapter 4). These deficits should be taken into account when designing and grading functional retraining programmes, with respect to the mode of presentation and expectation of the patient's performance. This applies to the type of verbal prompts, written instructions and non-verbal communication used with the patient.

For patients with expressive language disorders , a co-ordinated therapeutic approach can help with the treatment of specific deficits or the use of compensatory strategies. In functional situations there are many opportunities to encourage participation in language-based activities, for example in reading, writing and talking. Structured interventions in functional activities could help the patients learn to generalize skills which have been taught in individual sessions by the speech and language therapists, for example in reading, the recognition of familiar words (reading labels in shops), sequencing letters (filing) and sentences and prose (reading letters/newspaper articles). Levels of difficulty can be varied, as in writing, from signing a name to writing addresses and more complex activities like filling in forms and writing reports. Asking for items in shops/restaurants, using social routines and making social conversation can all be facilitated by using specific strategies to overcome the deficits, whilst performing and learning the functional skills.

Communication aids such as letter-boards and electronic equipment and over-enthusiastic interpreters can reduce the individual's chances of learning to communicate verbally. Compensatory strategies should only be used when they assist the patient's recovery of language and communication or if further recovery of language function is unlikely.

D. T. (2 weeks coma, PTA unknown) suffered from a severe receptive and expressive dysphasia and visual-object agnosia after a road traffic accident. He had difficulty recognizing and understanding the meaning of words and misinterpreted visual information. In the shops, he could identify food items which had distinctive colouring or features, like bread and eggs, but could not read labels on pre-packed foods or bottles. Initially he worked with the speech and language therapist on recognition of letters and on matching words with pictures of food items. In the shops he took cards with the names of food items (one word) typed on them. He was requested to match each card with the food items. As D. T. progressed in language therapy and when he was finding the correct items whilst shopping, this approach was increased in complexity. This was done by increasing the number of words on the card, developing more difficult grammatical constructs, including non-food items, and by using a shopping list instead of individual cards.

PROBLEM SOLVING/REASONING

Most individuals encounter situations which require novel (non-routine) behaviours. Many brain-injured people have difficulty with the normal problem solving and planning activities involved in everyday life. Patients often fail to appreciate the consequences of their actions (i.e. if they spend all their money they will be unable to pay their bills). The Los Angeles Head Injury Survey (Jacobs, 1988) found 80% of survivors were independent in basic self-care, but 63% were dependent in higher-order self-care tasks which involved problem solving, such as maintaining personal safety or purchasing clothes.

A problem refers to a specific situation or set of related situations to which an individual must respond in order to function effectively in the environment. Problem solving can be defined as a behavioural process of selection of the optimum response from a set of possible responses. Reasoning refers more to internal consistency and logic than goodness of fit with the environmental contingencies. Patients have difficulty with both inductive and deductive reasoning. Induction is the discovery of a general rule from the observation of several instances, thus patients may be unable to learn that a way of approaching a task or problem does not work despite constant failure. The deduction process refers to the drawing of specific conclusions from a general set of statements or principles and patients may be unable to apply general rules to specific instances. Cognitive deficits, such as attention and memory deficits, may contribute to the problems encountered by patients in novel situations, however many believe that there are primary deficits in higher cognitive functioning which can be called problem solving and reasoning deficits.

Introspection regarding normal mental processing suggests that mental organization, planning and problem solving are effortful for non-neurologically impaired subjects. Failure to perform these activities could result in deficits analogous to deficits in initiation. Many problems which have been classified as impairments in problem solving and reasoning, could result in the individual not participating in the planning of complex sequences of actions. In many individuals, the components involved in these skills are preserved, because with external prompting or questioning they are able to produce the respective activities. What the brain-injured individual is not able to do is to construct a mental representation of an action sequence and initiate component actions at the relevant times. Many lines of evidence suggest that these deficits result from frontal lobe impairment.

Therapists may attempt to stimulate the patient into improving their reasoning skills by setting them tasks which require problem solving/reasoning. Some authors have produced cognitive rehabilitation exercises which include reasoning tasks (Dougherty and Radomski, 1987). The Cognitive Rehabilitation Workbook of Dougherty and Radomski (1987) provides materials for cognitive retraining exercises in specific domains relevant to occupational and speech therapy, such as using the telephone directory. Practice and repetition of the exercises should increase the patient's awareness of the factors involved in the content areas, such as scheduling, meal planning and balancing a cheque book. Practical activities involving problem solving and reasoning could also be utilized.

As a compensatory procedure brain-injured individuals can be instructed in a problem-solving strategy. The aim is to teach the patient ways to think about problematic situations that confront them in day-to-day living in a routine way. The therapist, therefore, is attempting to teach the patient to externalize (and make routine) a behaviour which is typically performed spontaneously and internally. Adoption of this type of approach does not imply that all non-neurologically impaired individuals actually follow these procedures either consciously or sequentially, but it helps patients learn to structure methods of approaching new situations. One method of problem solving training involves consideration of the following steps.

Training in problem solving

a) Attitudes towards approaching a problem

Many brain-injured individuals experience frustration in their daily lives but do not recognize the situations which cause frustration as problems which can be solved actively. Individuals could have difficulty in accepting that problematic situations constitute a normal part of life. In order to solve the problems and cope with the situations effectively, individuals need to recognize problematic situations when they occur, and inhibit automatic responses of, for example, anger, passivity or impulsive urges to deal with the situation without thinking about it. Discussion of these facts with the patient and demonstrating to the individuals that they can in fact solve many problems themselves may be helpful in itself (see the discussion of learned helplessness, Chapter 2).

b) Definition of a problem

Individuals after brain injury can learn to define problems by asking questions, of themselves and others, about the nature of the frustrating or difficult situation. Asking individuals to examine real-life situations, and extract the problems they have within that setting, help define the issues they find difficult in everyday life. Role play of family and work situations may be helpful as well as the processing of situations which arise naturally in the treatment setting.

c) Generation of alternative methods of approaching a problem

Training could be required to help patients think about ways to solve problems. Therapists aim to teach and facilitate the individual's ability to 'brainstorm' ideas of approaching the problem (Osborne, 1963). Initially the quantity of ideas is more important than the quality. The more alternatives the individual can generate, the more likely he will arrive at the potentially best ideas for a solution.

d) Decision making

Once the brain-injured individual has generated ideas, he needs to decide how to solve the problem. He may not always be able to accurately identify the best of the alternatives he has generated. This requires an estimate of the probability that each alternative will achieve the preferred outcome. The patient's previous experience and the suggestions of 'significant others' influence decisions. Factors to be considered could include cost, time, effort and comfort to the individual or short-term and long-term benefits for himself and other family members and friends.

e) Feedback and verification

Once the individual has decided which approach would be the most effective, encouragement should be given to him to act on the decision. Outcome evaluation is necessary in order to re-assess the situation or take any further action. Verification helps to teach the person to observe and record the consequences of his actions.

Specific task training

When patients after appropriate acute rehabilitation are unable to develop novel actions, plans or solve problems independently, the goal of therapy may be externalization of the procedures to reduce the effort involved. Rather than the general compensatory strategy described above, therapists may prefer to teach domain specific compensatory strategies as routines. Specific activities can themselves be practised, reducing the demands of problem solving. The overlearning of behavioural routines will reduce the patient's need to problem solve and may be helpful to patients with profound impairments in higher cognitive functioning. Patients could, for example, be taught the specific steps they need to plan a meal by determining the list of items to be purchased, transport required to go to the shops, the amount of money needed, method of cooking and so on, then shopping. The use of a check-list or instruction list could be included initially to direct the patient's thinking towards the requirements of the functional activity.

SUMMARY

In this chapter we have described methods which have been used in an attempt to improve cognitive functioning. The most appropriate measure of success is not whether the patient improves on 'cognitive tasks' but whether the patient's ability to function in the real world is increased. Making this judgement is made more complex by the fact that brain-injured people, particularly early after injury, have a natural tendency to get better. For the purposes of discussion we have divided cognitive deficits into attention, perceptions and praxis, memory, language and problem solving and reasoning. It should be remembered however that these are only constructs developed in an attempt to understand human behaviour. Our constructs will change as our knowledge of the factors which influence human behaviour expands. We have divided attempts to redress cognitive deficits into three general categories. The first type of intervention attempts to address the cognitive dysfunction directly (W.H.O. 'impairment'). The second type of intervention attempts to train the patient to compensate for the impairment (W.H.O. 'disability'). The third type of intervention we describe attempts to train the individual in the functional behaviour disrupted by the cognitive impairment (W.H.O. 'disability'), especially those of specific importance to him (W.H.O. 'handicap').

Much of the research which has studied attempts to directly address disorders of attention has been methodologically inadequate. Newer studies with the exception of that of Sohlberg and Mateer (1987) have shown only limited treatment effects. The contradictory findings suggest further research is warranted. Attentional compensation strategies have been shown to be effective in some populations. Training in the functional skills impaired by the attentional deficit is effective for some patients. Training may however need to be prolonged and intensive as attentional processes are so fundamental to the process of learning itself.

The remediation of perceptual deficits was studied intensely in the 1970s. Although results have been mixed, standard approaches conducted in occupational therapy departments in Great Britain appear to be ineffective. Many perceptual deficits are difficult to develop compensatory approaches to. Compensatory visual scanning training does however appear to be effective in patients with hemispatial neglect as it is in hemianopia. Tasks specific compensation training for perceptual disorders is common (e.g. reading and street crossing).

Attempts to redress memory functioning as a cognitive skill have proved to be largely ineffective. General stimulation may be helpful in the early stages of recovery but beyond this point an alternative method for assisting the memory-impaired must be utilized. Available methods may be divided into internal and external strategies. Internal strategies designed to increase the recall of novel material have not usually proved effective among the brain-injured population. However internal visualization or verbal association strategies used to help brain-injured people learn fixed items of information often prove effective. External strategies are the type of strategies most often used by the non-neurologically impaired and are the most useful for those with acquired brain injury. Use of a pocket computer system was described in an extended case study but use of a memory book or diary will be the most important type of memory aid used by most patients. Training in specific skills (which previously relied on recall) so that they become habits reduces the demands on the memory system. It should be remembered that previously automatic behaviours may have become disrupted. Unless these are retrained they may place excessive demands on the memory system.

Language skills are the specific area of expertise of the speech and language pathologist. However functional language retraining usually requires an interdisciplinary team effort. Problem solving and reasoning present complex problems for those who wish to address the deficits directly. Although we can challenge a brain-injured person to solve novel problems, our understanding of how the non-neurologically impaired solve problems is rudimentary. We contend that much of what is called a problem-solving deficit is more commonly a planning deficit. A prosthetic problem-solving system is presented. This is a checklist of stages of thinking about a problem. This system can be taught as an internal or an external strategy. The use of this kind of system does not imply that a covert version of this procedure takes place in the non-neurologically impaired. Most patients' difficulties revolve around novel problems – to an extent that for a situation which is overlearned, new problem solving is not required. Practising specific behaviours can reduce the need for problem solving and reasoning skills. In the next chapter we discuss strategies for working with the behaviourally disordered and non-compliant client.

11

Enhancing behavioural control in functional settings

Behavioural control, like other skills, can be compromized by brain injury and part of the therapist's role is to help patients with brain injury re-establish behavioural control. The behaviour of brain-injured individuals may be so socially unacceptable that it precludes independence. Maladaptive behaviours which could be demonstrated include physical or verbal aggression, disinhibition (social and sexual), lack of drive and motivation or psychotic behaviour. Psychiatric disorders which may follow brain injury and the pharmacological agents used either singly or in combination with behavioural interventions are discussed in Chapter 5. This chapter focuses on interventions based on learning theory which may be used to help patients increase their behavioural control.

Cognitive deficits, such as attention and memory impairments, perceptual disturbances, language and problem-solving disorders, can influence an individual's ability to deal with his new self after brain injury. Behavioural control can be influenced by the frustration involved in coping with new environmental constraints and adjusting to changed roles. Discussion of these cognitive disorders is included in Chapter 4 and their treatment is discussed in Chapter 10. A more general discussion of the impact of role changes is included in Chapters 2 and 6. Supportive psychotherapy is indicated to help patients through the life changes associated with severe injury and prolonged hospitalization. In this chapter we are concerned with behaviours severe enough that, were they to continue, they would be profoundly handicapping. We will review the brain-injured individual's social presentation and social skills in Chapter 12.

In the acute period following brain injury, many patients go through a time when they are confused and agitated. For many individuals, the duration of this disturbed behaviour is brief and they emerge from this state without displaying further behavioural abnormality (see Chapter 8). The patient at this stage is often best managed environmentally, for example, with the use of a Craig bed, reduction of stimulation, a calm and reassuring approach and orienting statements. An initial step in the management of disturbed behaviour in acutely and seriously disturbed patients is to attempt to eliminate environmental precipitants (e.g. pain, a full bladder or bowel, alien surroundings, or insensitive and authoritarian handling). Where this type of sensitive handling fails and the patient is at risk of injuring himself, alternative methods may be considered. If physical restraints are used, for example posy vests, these should be fitted according to manufacturer's instructions to limit the risk of possible injury to the patient (Berrol, 1988). In some cases, medication could be necessary.

The individual with behavioural disturbances, which persist into the acute rehabilitation stage, can be assisted to improve his control of inappropriate behaviours, and the staff assisted in their management of the patient. Adequate behavioural management at this stage may also prevent the development of later behavioural disturbances, for example, when the patient learns to avoid unpleasant activities by screaming, shouting or pinching staff.

Over the last ten years the work of Brooks and his colleagues at Glasgow (Brooks and McKinlay, 1983; Brooks *et al.*, 1986) has demonstrated that a significant proportion of traumatically brain-injured people display behavioural disturbance continuing into the post-acute stage of recovery. The behaviour disturbance could become worse as time from injury increases and there is continuing stress on the patient's family. Serious behavioural disorders could result in prolonged periods of hospitalization, and in the less severely impaired the behaviour disorder may result in significant social isolation. When knowledge is insufficient or when the rehabilitation setting is not organized to provide the patient with suitable behavioural interventions, therapists may be unable to provide therapies relating to other domains (for instance, cognitive or motor impairments). For example, the realistic goal of ambulation may not be obtained because the patient becomes physically aggressive whenever an attempt is made to teach him to stand.

This chapter will review the principle techniques developed in experimental and clinical psychology and adapted for the treatment of behaviour disorder in brain-injured adults. Due to the cognitive deficits found in this population some types of behavioural interventions, used with other populations, may be inappropriate. Whilst some patients will display very severe behavioural disturbances that require interventions in a specialist behaviour management unit, many patients' problems can be addressed adequately in more general acute and post-acute head injury rehabilitation settings. This will, however, only be the case if adequate resources are provided for staff training and other organizational issues in the rehabilitation setting are addressed (see below and Fussey and Giles, 1988).

THE AIMS OF BEHAVIOURAL INTERVENTION

Behaviour disorders could jeopardize the future quality of life for the injured individual and their family (Gloag, 1985a, 1985b). Behavioural training helps individuals change their established automatic behavioural responses by the manipulation of reinforcement. The therapeutic environment ensures that the consequences of the individual's actions increase the probability of appropriate behaviours and decrease the probability of inappropriate behaviours (Eames and Wood, 1985a, 1985b). Various procedures can be employed to decrease or increase the probability of the patient engaging in the targeted behaviours. Programmes are individually designed according to the type and frequency of the behaviours exhibited by the patients and the patient's neuropsychological status. In addition, an adequate therapeutic environment includes a practically designed physical environment, trained staff and any pre-arranged system to ensure the availability of reinforcers, for example in a token economy.

ASSESSMENT AND RECORDING

Treatment goals should be determined co-operatively by the brain-injured individual, his family and the treatment team (see Preface). Assessment should involve talking to the patient and the family about the problem and the 'cognitive' method of asking the patient to stop the offensive behaviour should be tried before more elaborate and intrusive methods are adopted. For example, a patient was referred to one of the authors because he repeatedly groped therapists during physical therapy. It was privately explained to the patient that the therapists did not appreciate it and that the behaviour had to stop. To the surprise of the therapists the behaviour did not recur.

Behaviour can be defined as the directly observable activities of another individual. Since behaviour is the result of a dynamic interrelation of the individual and his environment, behavioural assessment should consider not only the behaviour, but its antecedents, consequences and the context and environment in which the behaviour is exhibited. These factors should be described accurately, avoiding inferences, subjective interpretation or evaluation which could bias observation. Assessment of physical aggression is often compromised by staff anxiety. For example, patients who are confused and non-compliant may wander around the treatment facility, shout and interfere with other people or property. Unfortunately, staff could describe this confused wandering as 'aggression', possibly leading to inappropriate treatment or placement.

The initial process of observing and recording behaviour is usually referred to as behavioural baselining. Baselines record the type, frequency, and duration of behaviours allowing a comparison of an individual's behaviour before and after treatment. Behavioural baselines are not usually used in an attempt to capture the full range of an individual's behaviour for practical reasons. There are several ways to structure behavioural baselines. Time sampling is used to establish the timing of behavioural observations, with staff either making general notes of the individual's behaviour or counting the frequency of previously specified behaviours. ABC recordings (Antecedent, Behaviour, Consequence) are valuable to record inappropriate behaviours exhibited by the individual at any point in his daily routine. Behavioural baselines are most often used to record the frequency (the rate at which the behaviour occurs) and specific features of a certain class of behaviour, which have already been specified and noted to be problematic.

C.H. (coma duration six weeks) frequently touched other

patients and staff members in ways that were unwanted and experienced as intrusive. A behavioural baseline was used to establish who he touched, how often he touched, where he touched, and the circumstances of the behaviour. This information was essential before designing a treatment programme which specified the meaning of 'inappropriate touch'.

Specificity is important in selecting target behaviours as many types of behaviour are complex responses showing subtle variations. Unless there is adequate operational specificity when structuring behavioural baselines and designing programmes, treatment team members will become unsure how to implement reinforcement contingencies. An outline of basic methods of behavioural observation and baselining can be found in most introductory psychology textbooks.

A number of structured observational systems have been developed which focus, at least in part, on behaviour disorders. Levin *et al.* (1987a) reported on a neurobehavioural rating scale (NRS) used to rate the sequelae of brain injury. Many of the items on the scale are adapted from the Brief Psychiatric Rating Scale (Overall and Gorham, 1962). The neurobehavioural scale is made up of 27 individual items which can be scored on seven levels of severity ranging from not present to extremely severe. The assessment emphasizes the particular deficits likely to arise after brain injury and a principle component analysis was performed which revealed four factors. Factor I (cognition/energy) consisted of items assessing cognition, memory, motor retardation and emotional withdrawal. Factor II (metacognition) reflected knowledge of one's own cognitive processes, reflecting inaccurate self appraisal, unrealistic planning and disinhibition, unusual thought content, and excitement. Factor III (somatic concern/anxiety) included physical complaints, anxiety, depression and irritability and factor IV (language) was made up of scales of expressive and receptive language. Factors I, II and IV showed a pattern of greater disturbance as severity of injury increased. Factor III (somatic concern/anxiety), however, showed no such relation. Levin *et al* (1987a) pointed out that their mild brain-injury group expressed greater somatic concern than the severely injured group. A scale such as the NRS could aid clinicians in monitoring behavioural changes during initial hospitalization and in in-patient and out-patient rehabilitation.

The Overt Aggression Scale (Yudofsky *et al.*, 1986) is a 4-point rating scale that measures aggressive behaviour in adults and children. The scale is divided into four categories: verbal aggression, physical aggression against objects, physical aggression against self, and finally physical aggression against others. Specific interventions related to each aggressive event can be recorded on the scale and can be easily completed by staff or family.

A behavioural assessment described by Wood (1987) includes 11 categories of inappropriate behaviours seen frequently after brain injury. These include aggression, lack of arousal, and types of manipulation. The behaviours are rated by staff on a scale of 0–9.

The Adaptive Behavior Scale (Nihira *et al.*, 1975) was developed for the mentally handicapped population and has two sections. The first part allows the rating of adaptive behaviour in the domains of independent functioning (basic self-care activities), physical development, economic activity, language development, numbers and time, domestic activity, vocational activity, self-direction, responsibility and socializ-ation. The second part allows ratings of inappropriate behaviours in the domains of violent or destructive behaviour, antisocial behaviour, rebellious behaviour, untrustworthy behaviour, withdrawal, stereotyped behaviour and odd man-nerisms, inappropriate manners, unacceptable vocal habits, self-abusive behaviour, hyperactive tendencies, and sexually aberrant behaviour. Although the Adaptive Behavior Rating Scale's focus is on mental retardation it provides detailed infor-mation for post-acute rehabilitation settings and has good stat-istical characteristics.

The purpose of behavioural analysis is to enable the develop-ment of an effective intervention plan. The following, however, should be noted. Detailed neurological examination of the patient is important in determining any neurological substrate to the behaviour, as the nature of any organic contribution to the disorder profoundly influences treatment. Some behaviours are so dangerous (e.g. physical aggression, self mutilation) that a period of observation prior to intervention cannot be war-ranted.

DEVELOPING A BEHAVIOURAL MILIEU

Philosophies which emphasize an educational approach encourage brain-injured individuals to become aware of deficits, control behaviour and improve social skills (see Chapter 12). A behavioural framework within the rehabilitation environment ensures clients and staff know what is acceptable conduct, and understand the consequences of anti-social behaviour. A number of measures allow an assessment of programmes. The Ward Atmosphere Scale and the Community Oriented Programs Environment Scale of Moos (1988a; 1988b) have scales pertaining to order and organization, programme clarity and staff control.

An interdisciplinary team approach is a prerequisite for consistency in behavioural assessment and programming. All staff should understand the purpose of treatment, be involved in programme development and work at maintaining good communication to maintain consistent intervention with the ultimate end of helping the patient learn. Staff require training in behavioural interventions, the consequences of brain injury, the types of behaviours which can be seen following brain injury and their specific role in reinforcing appropriate and not inappropriate behaviour. Adequate opportunities for communication and agreement in planning behavioural intervention strategies are essential components for the development of consistent individual patient programmes. Unit managers need to understand that an interdisciplinary team approach requires ongoing treatment planning and staff training time.

Positive goals should be established for each individual patient. The maintenance of an emphasis on positive reinforcements and recording the success of each patient helps staff retain an enthusiastic and reinforcing approach to this group of patients. Behaviour management requires attention to both the problem behaviour, and the clinician and environmental variables involved in the maintenance of such behaviour (Wood, 1987). The therapy staff have a central role with the unit psychologist in the design and execution of behavioural interventions as overcoming behaviour disorders is essential for functional independence.

Behavioural interventions need to be specifically designed for the individual's behavioural deficits and defined so that all staff understand the procedures involved. A thorough grasp of principles of assessment, measurement and recording will aid the staff's analysis of the behavioural problems. Control of potentially haphazard and overlapping interventions, such as multiple behavioural and pharmacological interventions, is necessary to determine the causes of behavioural change and prevent the continuation of ineffective treatment methods.

IDENTIFICATION OF REINFORCERS

A reinforcer is any event following a behavioural response which increases the likelihood of that response being repeated. The mechanism of behavioural change is associative. The individual pairs the specific behaviour with a pleasant feeling or directly with the reinforcement. For any individual there are many different potential reinforcers (see Table 11.1). The most commonly used ones include social attention (for example, paying attention when someone talks), social praise, tangible reinforcers (such as chocolate), and participation in preferred activities. Knowledge of results can be a reinforcer when the person is motivated towards the task which needs to be learned. Often the most powerful reinforcers cannot be applied because of temporal, moral or financial constraints.

In developing intervention programmes the most valid method of determining what is reinforcing for an individual is to offer a range of options and observe the rate and duration of responding. Green *et al.* (1988) evaluated a systematic assessment technique for determining reinforcers for the profoundly handicapped. The approach and avoidance behaviours of seven severely mentally and physically handicapped students were systematically observed with twelve different stimuli. Results indicated patients had different stimulus preferences and showed the outcome of the systematic assessment did not coincide with the more traditional care-givers' methods for determining preferences. A second experiment evaluated whether the stimuli that were determined to be reinforcers using the systematic assessment would function as reinforcers in skill training programmes. Results indicated that stimulus items selected did operate as reinforcers, and that those items selected using the more traditional method did so only if those stimuli were also preferred on the systematic assessment (Green *et al.*, 1988). Unfortunately, this procedure is very time-consuming and asking the individual what he would work for or observing him in free choice situations is a practical alternative. The more time-consuming technique could be reserved for the most handicapped, the habitually uncooperative, or where previous attempts to find reinforcers have failed.

In some cases with the severely brain-injured, it is possible to identify environmental reinforcements that have caused the individual to develop or maintain undesirable behaviours. Patients may be able to get what they want and avoid non-preferred activities, if, for example, they scream loud enough. The contingencies of reinforcement that act to support normal social behaviours no longer operate in hospital settings and attempts to reimpose them may be strongly resisted by patients. For instance in the majority of households, breakfast is typically only available after one gets out of bed.

Reinforcing behaviours incompatible to those demonstrated by the patient may help to extinguish inappropriate behaviours. High frequency behaviours may be used to reinforce low frequency behaviours when more standard reinforcement techniques are less effective (the Premack principle). For example, when an individual who is given free choice consistently chooses to rest in his room, this is likely to act as a reinforcer for other activities. A brief period of behaviour that needs to be extinguished can be used as a reinforcement for periods of appropriate behaviour. For instance, an individual who constantly asks questions could be given reinforcement of five minutes questioning as a consequence of not asking questions for an hour.

In practice, operant conditioning for the brain-injured individual is an attempt to introduce or remove reinforcement contingent on certain behaviours. These can be divided into a 2 by 2 grid shown in table 11.1.

Table 11.1 Basic paradigms in behavioural intervention

Technique:	Positive reinforcement	Negative reinforcement
Aims to:	Increase frequency of behaviour	Increase frequency of behaviour
Form:	Present something desirable	End something undesirable

Technique:	Positive punishment	Negative punishment
Aims to:	Decrease frequency of behaviour	Decrease frequency of behaviour
Form:	Present something undesirable	Remove something desirable

While all of these types of intervention may be used from time to time, the most important are positive reinforcement and negative punishment. In addition strenuous attempts may be required to remove hitherto existing reinforcements for certain types of behaviour. Learning characteristics of the brain-injured individual are discussed in Chapter 7.

REINFORCEMENT

Positive reinforcement

We discussed the role of positive reinforcement in functional skill building in Chapter 7. It is used in a similar way to help patients eliminate inappropriate behaviours. Programmes can be designed to reward behaviours which are incompatible with, or alternatives to, the inappropriate behaviours that need to be eliminated. For example, reinforcement can occur for periods of time where these behaviours are not displayed.

In programmes which are constructed to help the patient reduce inappropriate behaviour, it is important to 'start where the patient is' and not to set unrealistic goals. Small reinforcement which is frequently applied for goals the patient can achieve (with some effort), are preferable to large rewards which the patient is unable to earn because the earning requirements vastly outweigh the patient's abilities. The difficulty in generating immediate rewards can be minimized in higher functioning patients by the use of secondary reinforcement.

Reasons for using rewards to help patients develop behavioural control include:

1. rewards assist the patient to focus on the behaviours that need to be eliminated;
2. rewards increase compliance;
3. rewards help the patient retain a positive attitude towards the behavioural intervention programme;

4. rewards help the staff maintain a positive (non-punitive) attitude towards more difficult clients.

It is not inconsistent for a programme to have positive reinforcement and extinction components which operate in tandem.

The reinforcement of every instance of the desired behaviour is the most efficient way of establishing a preferred response pattern. However in order to increase the endurance of behavioural change, an intermittent schedule of reinforcement for criterion behaviours may be more successful. The increased resilience of criterion behaviours, which have not been continuously reinforced, can be understood as the result of persistence (also known as the partial reinforcement extinction effect). Failure to receive reinforcement when it is expected is functionally equivalent to punishment. Persistence refers to the ability of a learned behaviour to survive a protracted period of non-reinforcement. Training schedules, which include reinforcing and non-reinforcing events, produce greater resistance to extinction than 100% (or continuous) reinforcement schedules. When a patient does not have experience of non-reinforcement, the newly developed behaviours are likely to be rapidly extinguished in the natural environment, when reinforcement is no longer available all of the time (Nation and Woods, 1980). Behaviours developed with social reinforcement are likely to be more readily maintained in the natural environment. This will however only be the case where social praise acts as a reinforcer for the individual. See also below, p. 300

Positive reinforcers can be divided into two categories, primary and secondary. Primary reinforcers are inherently rewarding and are most usually attention, praise or consumables such as chocolate, soft drinks and cigarettes. Consumables should be used with social reinforcement (attention, praise or encouragement). Severely handicapped brain-injured individuals have difficulty in understanding subtle social cues and staff may have to exaggerate their social praise. The positive social reinforcement can be directly linked to the behaviour or skill exhibited, for example, 'you have worked hard in your meal-planning session this morning'. Individuals often find this type of praise less patronizing than the more generic 'Well done'. The therapist must judge the ability of the client to make use of subtle social cues. Secondary reinforcers, for example, money, tokens or stars, have no inherent reinforcing characteristics and rely for their value on the meaning attached to them. The selection of primary or secondary reinforcers should be based on the cognitive and behavioural characteristics of the patient. Feedback is important in helping individuals discriminate which responses are being reinforced, thereby increasing the power of the intervention in changing the target behaviour. This knowledge can be supported during the actual execution of the programme each time a reinforcer is provided and on charts and graphs to which the client has frequent access. The law of effect (Herrstein, 1970; McDowell, 1982) represents an advance over Skinner's view of reinforcement in that it allows a theoretical consideration of not only reinforcement obtained for responding but also reinforcement obtained from all other concurrent sources. Simply stated, the law of effect suggests that a constant rate of reinforcement results in a higher response rate in an environment with low ambient reinforcement. The law of effect proposes that we take into account sources of reinforcement other than the ones (temporally) associated with the behaviour. Four types of intervention strategies are suggested by the law of effect: two methods for reducing inappropriate behaviour and two methods to increase appropriate behaviour. All methods involve environmental manipulation and can only be implemented as a whole unit approach. Firstly inappropriate behaviour can be reduced by increasing reinforcement for a concurrent (but not incompatible) behaviour. Secondly inappropriate behaviour might decrease as a consequence of increasing the rate of non-contingent ambient reinforcement. In both cases the effect of the unchanged reinforcement attached to the unwanted behaviour is reduced (hopefully to the point where it no longer maintains the unwanted behaviour). The same logic is turned on its head to assist clients to increase the display of an appropriate behaviour. Here one reduces the reinforcement available for all behaviours other than the desired response (staff might time-out-on-the-spot all but a single to-be-reinforced response). Alternatively one might attempt to attach previous ambient (non-specific) reinforcement to a to-be-reinforced response (this approach might be particularly appropriate in a reinforcement-rich environment). Consideration of the law of effect may be an important factor in assisting clients to increase the frequency of appropriate and decrease the frequency of inappropriate behaviour. However this type of sophisticated intervention is only possible in mature specialist systems where the environmental contingencies are deliberately arranged.

Token system

A token system is one way to systematically deliver reinforcement to a group of people, and provides a method to structure the environment to promote adaptive social behaviour. Even a unit-wide token economy can be adapted to meet the reinforcement needs of individual clients. The token system can be varied on the parameters of the reinforcement period, token exchange, and reinforcer. A token economy can be adapted to support individualized behavioural programmes. Token economies which incorporate adequate measurement and recording methods can be used to evaluate a response to therapy over time. There are three essential components in setting up a token system. These include the medium of exchange, the back-up reinforcers and the rules which describe the interrelationship between the token and back-up reinforcers.

Established token systems have different time-based reinforcement schedules (15, 30, 60 minute intervals); many kinds of back-up reinforcers (attention, food, activities) and different types of currency such as money, tokens or stamps. Savings of tokens can be limited through either control of prices, enticements to spend, or the dating of tokens so that, if not used, they lose their exchange value. Individuals with behaviour disorders after brain injury usually require rigid systems at the start of their rehabilitation, but as they improve they can learn to become more involved in learning higher-level skills, such as negotiation.

B.L. (coma duration two weeks) had severe memory deficits and behavioural disorder; he would argue about situations which he could not remember, repetitively asking questions, and not follow instructions or cues to help him remember information which was essential for his independence. He started to write a weekly timetable of his work requirements and requested leisure time activities. With supervision, he set his own criteria for earning leisure time activities. This was dependent on his behavioural control and work performance which was recorded on a points sheet and marked by the staff.

Self-administration must be carefully monitored as individuals tend to become too lenient or too stringent in the delivery of their own reinforcement. Careful evaluation of the system is required to ensure that it fulfils the criteria for helping patients extinguish inappropriate behaviours and learn adaptive skills.

Token economies incorporating a privilege level system

A token economy used in conjunction with a privilege level system allows a hierarchy of privileges through which the patient may progress. Maintenance of higher privilege levels usually requires longer durations of appropriate behaviour. Reinforcers available at higher levels take into account the patient's greater behavioural control and are often community-based to encourage independent activities. Once a certain percentage of token earning has been attained at the highest level of the token system the tokens themselves may be withdrawn. The individual may be expected to maintain appropriate behavioural control as measured by an alternative criterion such as points or by more subjective criteria. Alternatively the individual may just be required to avoid major behavioural infractions (such as physical aggression). Privilege level systems provide a means of shaping complex behaviours and provide a structured way to withdraw the support of the token economy. The behavioural expectations developed for progress through the hierarchy, the reinforcers and the treatment activities which occur within the system, should be relevant to the individual and related to their discharge goals and future environment.

From the staff's perspective a token economy is helpful in providing the background against which therapeutic activities can take place. As clients are motivated to earn tokens, money or points, any lack of intrinsic motivation to perform in therapy becomes less problematic. As therapists have a built-in method of responding to situations in which an individual is non-compliant the therapist experiences less stress than in settings without a token economy. (This assists therapists in not reinforcing patients with attention when the patient is behaving inappropriately).

The systematic withholding of reinforcement as a result of inappropriate behaviour is referred to as negative punishment (Wood and Burgess, 1988). A level system can be arranged to provide negative punishment, as privileges are withdrawn contingent on the production of inappropriate behaviour. For example, an individual on level 3 can go to the movies once a week. However, as a result of an incident of physical aggression, his privilege level could be reduced to level 2 and the privilege is lost, until he can earn his way back up to level 3.

There is little evidence that a fixed interval token economy is effective with the profoundly cognitively impaired population. It is most likely to be effective amongst patients who are operating at a high cognitive level and who require contingency management. Turnbull (1988) has described other difficulties in applying the token economy system with the brain-injured adult.

Control of aggressive behaviour with a programme including antecedents

The control of behaviour by antecedents was discussed in Chapter 7. Recently Burke, Wesolowski and Lane (1988) have reported a positive approach to the treatment of aggressive brain-injured clients. Intervention included antecedent control as part of an operant programme (see discussion of the law of effect). The following techniques were used with each of five clients for whom data is reported.

1. Increased density of reinforcement. Reinforcement was provided for all pro-social client behaviours, for example, clients were paid special attention, provided with special dinners or dessert and so on.
2. Reinforcement sampling. A special menu of reinforcement was determined for each client for use in future programmes.
3. Antecedent control. A generally low level of stimulation with few demands was provided. The clients were fully oriented to their new surroundings and continuous

reinforcement was available for appropriate behaviours. They were frequently reinforced for being calm, speaking in a low tone of voice and generally demonstrating behavioural control. No negative consequences are applied for aggressive behaviour and if clients appeared to become agitated, an attempt was made to redirect them to a task at hand. If a client became aggressive, punches were blocked, and the client was redirected to the activity again.

4. Appropriate response selection. During the first 24 hours in the programme, ten things which the client did well were identified. This exercise was done to reinforce activities incompatible with aggressive behaviour. In addition, it was thought that if clients maintained positive self-statements this would be inconsistent with aggressive behaviour.

5. Inconvenience review. After the first 48 hours clients were taught how aggressive behaviour was inconvenient for them. This inconvenience review was repeated following any act of aggression.

6. Self control training. An attempt was made to teach problem-solving techniques and relaxation.

7. Self monitoring. Clients were taught to record their daily programmes.

Prior to treatment the average number of aggressive behaviours (sexual assaults, physical assaults and damage to property) was 20.2 per week. During the first week of treatment, the number of such incidents is reported to have fallen to an average of less than one per client and to have subsequently fallen further. The precipitous change does indicate that a change in environment (setting events; environmental conditions) can, in some clients, result in a dramatic alteration of behaviour. Similar reduction in aggression as a response to being placed in a highly reinforcing environment has been reported in other populations (Mace *et al.*, 1983). The rapidity of the change in behaviour suggests that operant learning may not account for the change in behaviour. The risk with this type of approach is that the reimposition of demands on the client's behavioural control could result in deterioration.

Differential reinforcement

Variants of differential reinforcement procedures can be used in the treatment of behaviour disorders. These procedures are advantageous because they provide a positive approach to patients with seriously disturbed behaviours.

DRO (Differential reinforcement of other behaviours)

For patients who display a very high frequency of inappropriate behaviours and a low frequency of appropriate behaviours, a DRO procedure may be indicated. In this approach, any instances of any appropriate behaviour are reinforced.

DRA (Differential reinforcement of an alternative behaviour)

DRA is the reinforcement of a specified behaviour (different from the targeted inappropriate behaviour's). The behaviour targeted need not be important from a rehabilitation perspective. DRA is easier to define and operationalize than DRO procedures.

DRI (Differential reinforcement of an incompatible behaviour)

This approach reinforces behaviour which is incompatible with those behaviours which are to be extinguished. The approach is especially helpful for patients who demonstrate self-injurious or aggressive behaviour. For example, one patient was taught to apply the brakes on his wheelchair as a DRI to wheeling after people and hitting them. The patient was taught to respond to a verbal prompt and a mime of putting the brakes on; and given social reinforcement for achievement of the action. More complex paradigm stimulus control procedures incorporate aspects of DRI.

STIMULUS CONTROL

Stimulus control procedures, used to help patients develop behavioural control, have a mixed theoretical paradigm. The aim of these procedures is to interrupt the progression from patient frustration to physical aggression. Since patients often fail to notice their heightened state of arousal, intervention involves the administration of a discriminatory stimulus; for instance, a verbal instruction or physical prompt, for example making a stop sign with the hand. They are then taught to participate in a behaviour which is incompatible with the aggressive behaviour. This could involve the patient going to his room (or other designated location) for a specified period of time. Patients can be reinforced for responding to the staff cue and going to their room (essentially a DRI procedure). Replacing the inappropriate strategy behaviour can then be instigated.

The aims of training is for the patient to notice his or her level of arousal and respond to this, as a cue to leave the situation. The patient is taught reasons why the aggressive behaviour is dysfunctional for him and how to respond to the verbal and/or physical cues. He can also learn appropriate verbalizations (which could parallel the cue) like 'I am getting angry – I need to take time away from the situation'. The individual is then cued in all situations in which he becomes angry or over-aroused. Variants of this procedure have been successfully used with numerous patients, particularly those whose behavioural-control difficulties involved over-responsiveness to normal frustration (affective aggression).

Extinction

Extinction procedures are customarily used to decrease severe behaviour disorders, and are a set of highly effective clinical procedures for which the theoretical underpinnings are rather obscure. The term extinction refers to the process when a behaviour is not being reinforced. Typically many reinforcers are naturally occurring and produced spontaneously by people in the individual's environment (for example, attention for swearing loudly in public). The process of extinction is the weakening of the previously established associations between a behaviour and its (reinforcing) consequences. Four of the major theories which suggest this process occurs with the brain-injured population are reviewed by Wood and Burgess (1988).

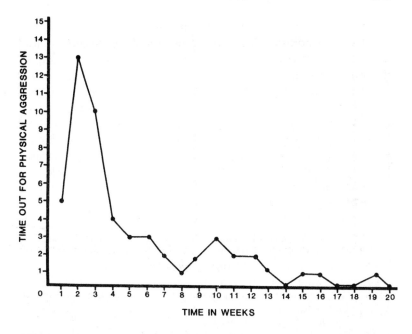

Figure 11.1 Response of a patient with severe paroxysmal aggressive outbursts to a programme of five minutes in a time-out room contingent on physical aggression. The patient was concurrently receiving carbamazepine. Note the extinction burst phenomenon immediately following the introduction of treatment.

Time-out

Time-out is often considered an extinction procedure and designed to remove the individual from reinforcement, which happens as the result of inappropriate behaviour (Ullman and Krasner, 1969). Time-out, as it is currently used, has a number of different forms.

Time-out room

In specialist behavioural units, the time-out room is most frequently (and appropriately) used following episodes of physical aggression. This involves taking the patient to a bare room, where he can remain (under close though discrete observation) for a period of between 2–5 minutes. At a practical level, this

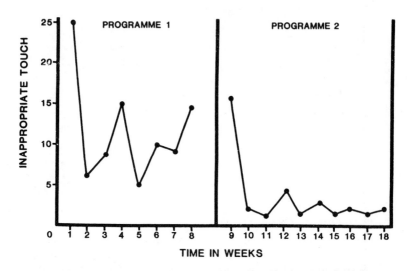

Figure 11.2 Response of a single patient to two programmes designed to help him reduce the number of times he inappropriately touched others. The first programme involved disengaging the individual's hand. The second and more successful programme involved placing the individual in the time-out room for two minutes with the statement 'Don't touch'.

technique gives all staff a response to situations which could be dangerous to both staff and patients. As noted by Wood and Burgess (1988), it is agreed by many that time-out in the time-out room relies for its effectiveness on its aversive qualities. Therapists should note the patient's response to time-out as a small number of patients will seek the time-out room as an avoidance behaviour (e.g. the patient may prefer to be in time-out than participate in physical therapy) (see Figures 11.1, 11.2).

Situational time-out

Situational time-out has the same rationale as that of the time-out room. The goal of situational time out is to remove the individual from positive reinforcement. When a special room is not available, staff can place patients in a corridor or at the other end of the room if it is safe to do so.

Time-out-on-the-spot

Time-out-on-the-spot (TOOTS) also involves not reinforcing an individual for inappropriate behaviour. The method is similar to time-out in a time-out room except that the programme is carried out *in situ* (Wood and Burgess, 1988). One method is to not pay attention to the individual (for about 20 seconds) contingent on the production of inappropriate behaviour (this can be done by moving away or talking to someone else). This 'time-out to person' is most effective when the patient is attempting to engage in interpersonal interaction. A second method is to continue to pay attention to the patient but to ignore the inappropriate behaviour. This latter method is most suitable when therapy is underway and should not be interrupted. Time-out to behaviour may be less successful in reducing the undesirable behaviour due to the fact that many patients do not realize what is being ignored. Time-out of a behaviour does have the advantage of preventing the patient from derailing therapy. This dialogue occurred when teaching an individual with brain injury to wash and dress and demonstrates the use of a TOOTS procedure.

Therapist: Put soap on the wash cloth
Client: Am I going to die? (performing the task)
Therapist: Good, well done, you did that very quickly, now wash your face.
Client: Are you going to kill me?
Therapist: Wash your face (the therapist reprompts the activity at hand and this time the client complies). Well done, you're doing a great job this morning.
   The therapist ignores the patient's inappropriate verbalizations and concentrates on teaching the task, being very rewarding of on-task behaviour.

After the initiation of any of the extinction procedures described above, the rate of the inappropriate behaviour often shows a transient increase; this is called an 'extinction burst' phenomenon, first noted by Skinner in 1938. Some behaviours (e.g. severe head banging, lip biting) are so harmful that even a brief exacerbation is to be avoided and an alternative type of intervention should be adopted.

Discriminatory paradigms

Individuals with cognitive deficits may need help to associate their inappropriate behaviours with time-out procedures. For example, the individual who excessively touches others could be verbally cued 'touch' on admission to the time-out room.

RESPONSE COSTS

Response cost approaches are designed to approximate the deterrents which occur in everyday life for inappropriate behaviours, for example a parking ticket is a response cost for parking in a no-parking zone. Response cost programmes are valuable for interrupting continual behaviours which are potentially dangerous, self-reinforcing, or disruptive of the therapy process. Since the response cost system allows reinforcement and punishment to be administered along the same dimensions, it can be combined with a token economy. Tangible or secondary reinforcers, for example tokens, may be lost as well as gained.

G.H. (coma duration 4 weeks) swore continually during his waking hours. A thirty-minute sessional retraining programme was begun to assist G.H. reduce his swearing. At the beginning of the session G.H. was given his daily allotment of cigarettes and the purpose of the programme was reiterated. For every two minutes that G.H. did not swear, the number of cigarettes which would be available to him during the rest of the day remained the same, but one cigarette was taken away for each two minute period in which swearing occurred.

Restitutional over-correction

In our view the use of over-correction is rarely indicated for the brain-injured adults. It has, however, been reported to be successful with the behaviourally disturbed and the mentally handicapped.

PROBLEMS WITH BEGINNING AND/OR MAINTAINING
BEHAVIOURAL PROGRAMMING

The organization of the rehabilitation system to facilitate communication between staff, and develop the consistency of
approach required to help the individual gain control over his
behavioural deficits, is a complex task. Treatment centres which
specialize in different stages of an individual's recovery are
organized in ways which may either facilitate or hinder the
application of a behavioural approach. For example, in acute
hospitals and acute rehabilitation settings, staff are often organized into multi-disciplinary teams with each discipline focusing
on different goals. This type of team organization makes the
implementation of consistent behavioural interventions
extremely problematic.

The number of staff working with the individual, the movement of staff to other units and reliance on contract or agency
staff, make consistent intervention more difficult to establish
and maintain. Structure and consistency help individuals with
brain injury make sense of their environment, and assist the
staff in their identification and analysis of the individual's
behavioural disorders.

An effective intervention must be feasible, and supported by
the staff who have sufficient expertise to apply it. Behavioural
programmes place considerable demands on the staff members'
memory capacity as the staff have to know exactly how to
respond immediately to a set of behaviours emitted by each
patient. One solution to this problem is to have only a limited
number of staff responses which can be applied to a wide
range of patient behaviours. For example, TOOTS could be the
response to all behaviours labelled as 'inappropriate' and time-
out in the time-out room can be the automatic overlearned
response among staff for physical aggression.

This approach lacks flexibility, but an overall balance needs
to be maintained between the staff's limited ability to learn
novel behavioural programmes and the patient's need to have
individualized treatment. When a programme does not need to
be initiated immediately, staff should be provided with in-ser-
vice training prior to its implementation. This reduces the cognitive demands on the staff of operating the programme and
assists staff in overcoming their 'stage fright'. On-going moni-

toring of staff compliance with the programme should also be established.

In order for consistent behavioural management to be achieved, the behaviours requiring intervention should be clearly defined, the reinforcers identified and guidelines regarding intervention made explicit. It is virtually impossible for a group of up to 25 rehabilitation staff, who may be in frequent contact with a patient, to produce identical verbal or nonverbal responses but it is possible to bring the specific responses required by a behavioural programme within acceptable limits.

Behavioural interventions can go awry for a number of reasons other than the demands of the behavioural system on staff and inadequate programme design. Behavioural programmes may not be perceived as successful because of over-inclusiveness. This can be manifested in two ways. The first is, the programme successfully modifies the behaviour, but as the individual improves, the staff unconsciously increase their expectation and scope of the programme. Recordings will thus show little improvement even though the programmes have been successful.

On admission C.P. (coma duration 2 weeks) swore exuberantly, made obscene gestures, shouted, and banged her fist on herself or on an object. Treatment included a two-minute time-out procedure in the time-out room for any of the above behaviours, swearing, shouting and banging. At six weeks the patient was still being timed-out frequently and the programme had not been revised. In practice the behaviours which were eliciting the time-out programme had changed considerably. The patient was still shouting, but for shorter periods of time and she was only making covert obscene gestures, usually behind her back. The staff responded rapidly to these behaviours, therefore the frequency of the behaviours were the same but the behaviours were less extreme and disruptive than prior to intervention.

Whyte (1988), in another context, has recently drawn attention to the tendency of staff to concentrate on continuing problems rather than areas of improvement. In most cases, success in treating inappropriate behaviour should be judged by the frequency or extent of the behaviour and absolute criteria (all-or-none) are only occasionally warranted. The second manifestation of over-inclusiveness is when a patient is placed on a specific behavioural programme for a target behaviour, for example time-out for physical aggression. Staff then include other non-targetted behaviours in the programme (e.g. shouting) because they are unable to generate an alternative management procedure. If left unchecked, this is likely to have detrimental consequences on the programme.

Problems can be associated with the practical application of token systems. In a time-based token system, if the client behaved in a way that is not acceptable briefly at the beginning or the end of the targeted period, then withholding the token will mean that no reinforcement is given for the longer period of appropriate behaviour. However, if the token is given, there is a danger of reinforcing the inappropriate behaviour. When an individual has not earned a token, there are questions of whether he should be told the reasons for not earning. Attention to the individual could reinforce inappropriate behaviours (by recognition that he was behaving inappropriately), but patients with cognitive defects may be unable to associate the reasons for not earning with the inappropriate behaviour. Procedures for giving out tokens, recording them and taking them back in exchange for reinforcers, should be designed for each individual.

Undetermined behavioural criteria causes staff dissension and 'negativism' within the behavioural system. Staff may not support the programme because they believe that behavioural programmes will 'never work'. This belief is frequently the result of a failure to understand that the introduction of the programme does not lead to the immediate cessation of the behaviour. Egotistical behaviour by staff, for example the belief that they can 'talk the patient out of his behaviour' or feelings that only their love and attention will significantly improve the individual's behaviour, will adversely affect their role in the rehabilitation team and the patient's ability to develop adaptive behaviour. Manipulating the environment to prevent the individual from demonstrating the behaviour by, for example, not asking him to perform activities is likely to lead to behavioural deterioration. Alternatively, the staffs' views that individuals with brain injury are 'wilful' or demonstrating behaviours that are designed to 'get' them, can foster negative feelings and hatred towards the specific patients (Gans, 1983).

Staff involved in a behavioural system need a clear understanding of the theoretical principles of behavioural techniques and a commitment to use them. Factors such as staff stress and fatigue influences their approach to patients and appropriate reinforcement for staff is a prerequisite for good patient treatment. An emphasis of positive aspects of patient progress by focusing on improvements is essential. Some staff, however well trained, simply cannot commit themselves fully to the practice of behaviour modification, and can unwittingly sabotage the patient's learning. Visitors, family and friends often innocently bring gifts and impede the patient's progress, by reducing the individual's incentive to earn such items. Discussions with the family to explain the intervention programmes, and helping family members develop positive methods of dealing with difficult situations, are necessary to gain their co-operation in future aspects of the rehabilitation process (see Chapter 13).

TRAINING FUNCTIONAL ACTIVITIES WITHIN A BEHAVIOURAL SYSTEM

Programmes designed to help patients improve functional skills can be established alongside behavioural management programmes. An individual's behaviour affects his functional performance, but his ability to function also affects his behaviour. Increased control over his environment, like deciding when he wants to go to the toilet or by getting to the bathroom independently, reduces the chances of the patient developing 'learned helplessness' (Seligman, 1975). The functional skills retraining programmes should be designed taking into account the individual's behavioural deficits. The structuring of the programme, for instance the type of prompts (verbal, mime or behavioural shaping), the procedures and the reinforcement schedules need to be carefully defined after assessment has determined (as far as possible) the patient's ability. Realistic expectations of the individual's performance should be defined and solutions to anticipated problems written into the programme. The staffing required for the programme should be specified (especially if the individual is aggressive or needs physical assistance) and the most appropriate setting chosen (for example, near a time-out room if the patient is aggressive).

Programmes should address the behavioural difficulties of the individual in the functional skills activities. Careful assessment of the individual is needed, as many people who present with severe behaviour disorders also often have severe cognitive deficits (see Chapter 4). For example, in writing a programme for individuals with arousal deficits, the therapist should take into account the amount of time the individual takes to perform each activity. A realistic time-based programme can then be defined and assistance only provided when appropriate. Most individuals with arousal deficits require behaviour to be broken down into small steps and frequent re-prompting to help them initiate activity. The degree of effort needed to maintain attention on the task can be great, and social and tangible reinforcements are often required to encourage them to maintain their effort.

Individuals with positive behaviour disorders, for example aggression or disinhibition, could require programmes which increase their participation in the functional activity. Inappropriate behaviours which are exhibited in functional situations can be timed-out-on-the-spot (see above) and appropriate behaviours reinforced. Reinforcers can be defined and linked to the patient's degree of participation and co-operation within the set criteria of the functional programme (these criteria may be independent of the ongoing behaviour management programme). The type of prompts and schedule of reinforcements is specified according to the individual's abilities. Reinforcement could initially be given whenever the individual completes the task following a prompt, and later progress to the stage where they are reinforced for performing without the prompt. The individual who, as a result of non-cooperation, does not perform an activity when requested can be physically assisted. This should be done in a manner free of both positive and negative affect by the therapist, therefore, neither social approval nor disapproval should be shown and the patient assisted in a value-free manner. Therapists should be hesitant in attributing poor functional performance to behaviour disorder. The combination of a tendency among staff to develop ideas of reference when faced with the very difficult patient and the tendency for dyspraxia, poor attention or memory to mimic lack of co-operation, indicates that only experienced clinicians well versed in the presentation of these disorders in functional settings should assess them.

Time-based programmes can assist individuals to initiate tasks (with or without prompting). Time requirements can be established for the activity relating to a single prompt (e.g. wash your face) or alternatively for complete activities (washing, transferring from wheelchair to toilet). A large clock in clear view helps patients and whenever the patient completes the tasks in the specified time, reinforcement is given. Gradually reducing the time allowed for the completion of each task can assist patients to accelerate their performance to an acceptable duration.

Individuals who deny existence of deficits, or their inability to perform functional activities, make the task of the occupational therapist extremely difficult (see Chapter 5). Patients and their families could adopt paranoid belief systems, and misperceive the statements and actions of others. These patients are frequently less successful in rehabilitation. Progress is more likely if a balance of positive supporting statements and confronting statements is achieved. Talking about the patient's present abilities rather then mentioning the past or future could also prevent further denial. The therapist should however avoid supporting the patient's erroneous self-statements.

FADING THE BEHAVIOURAL SYSTEM

Functional programmes can be written which encourage the individual to learn strategies in order to be independent and take the steps to full independence. Many individuals find the process of weaning off the behavioural system difficult as they are having to retake responsibility for themselves after a possibly long period of dependency. During functional retraining programmes, prompting is used to ensure the performance of the desired functional task. Fading is a training procedure in which a prompt is gradually withdrawn so that the functional behaviour can continue without the supporting stimulus. For example, an individual who is learning to transfer independently could learn certain descriptive prompts, which enable him to perform the skill independently. As he learns the prompts and is able to sequence the tasks independently, he relies less on the prompts and thus consolidates the learning of the skill. To encourage the fading of prompts, therapists can wait for the desired action to occur and when it does, reinforce the performance of the task. Alternatively, asking the individual to say what he is going to do next can increase his participation in the task. Reinforcement of the independent behaviour is essential, even after the prompts have gradually been withdrawn. Reinforcement schedules can be gradually altered to ensure they are less intrusive in the activity, mimic those available in the natural environment or used as systems which can be maintained within the discharge setting.

> N.S. (coma duration four weeks, nine years previously) had pronounced attention-seeking behaviours and, although he had learned to wash and dress independently, he would not perform the skill without supervision. He was asked to state what he would like to have as a reward if he performed the skill independently for five days. He chose a trip to his favourite radio station. After three weeks, he achieved the criteria. The programme was discontinued, and he was rewarded each time he looked well-groomed or was known to have showered independently. He needed occasional prompts for his personal hygiene (about once a month) to maintain his awareness of the importance of the task.

Individuals with severe brain injury often rely on added reinforcement for maintenance of their skilled performance and are unable to generalize the skills learned into other settings. Expectations of the individual to participate, provision of the opportunities to practise in all situations and with other staff, and appropriate feedback as to his performance, increase the chances of the individual's consolidation of the skills. Teaching the individual's families or carers in the discharge situation in the retraining routines helps the individual to transfer skills learned in one setting to another. Unless these procedures are utilized, generalization is difficult if not impossible to achieve.

SUMMARY

There are now numerous single case reports in the literature of brain-injured individuals being helped to develop behavioural control (Horton and How, 1981; Wood and Eames, 1981). In addition, many reports of functional skills training also address issues of behavioural control, as the individual unable to perform functional skills can become combative or abusive when confronted. Examples of this latter include the report of Giles and Clark-Wilson (1988a) on washing and dressing training and of Cohen (1986) describing behavioural treatment for incontinence in a profoundly impaired adult. In addition, Eames and Wood (1985a) have reported follow-up data from the Kemsley unit, a unit specializing in the treatment of the behaviourally disordered brain-injured adult. Time since discharge ranged from 6–39 months with a mean of 18.8 months. The principal outcome measure was a hierarchical scale of placements ranked in terms of quality of life for the patient. There was no trend towards relapse as time from discharge increased nor was length of time since injury a factor which reduced the individual's response to treatment. The methods of intervention on the unit are described in Eames and Wood (1985b) and include a fixed interval token economy, time-out in a time-out room. TOOTS procedure, discriminatory time out, and a wide range of other behavioural interventions.

Individuals with brain injury frequently have difficulty in maintaining behavioural control and exhibiting appropriate social behaviours. Behavioural interventions can help individuals develop these skills. The learning principles outlined here are not, however, only limited in their usefulness for the elimination of behaviour disorders. The use of highly structured learning techniques in developing cognitive, functional and motor skills are described in other chapters of this book. In this chapter some of the fundamental procedures of learning theory with wide applicability have been stressed. The importance of maintaining a positive attitude is emphasized and positive reinforcement for appropriate behaviours is regarded as central to helping the individual learn behavioural control. The difficulties many staff experience in accommodating the behavioural system have also been examined.

12

Social skills retraining following severe brain injury

The cognitive, behavioural and physical deficits which frequently follow brain injury are likely to interfere with the development and maintenance of social relationships (see Chapters 4, 10 and 11). More severe deficits may affect multiple domains and be evident in all social interactions, whereas less severe deficits may only become apparent in complex social situations.

In this chapter the patient's difficulties, whatever their cause, are considered from the perspective of interpersonal behaviour. There are many definitions of socially skilled behaviour (Hargie, 1986; Bellack and Hersen, 1978; Trower *et al.*, 1982). Here a person is accepted as being socially skilled if he or she can develop appropriate social goals and pursue these in intended and socially acceptable ways. The neurofunctional framework of assessment outlined in Chapter 6 helps therapists evaluate the impact of deficits on social behaviour. Individuals should be evaluated with reference to their social context, to determine the specific social behaviours they need to demonstrate. Following Argyle (1981) socially skilled behaviour can be viewed as hierarchically organized, with complex social behaviours made up of smaller behavioural units. Social skills retraining, therefore, helps people to master the elements of social behaviour and build these elements into larger patterns of skilled social behaviour. By increasing the individual's awareness of appropriate social goals and developing the patient's repertoire of skilled social behaviours, social skills retraining facilitates successful social interactions and the development and maintenance of interpersonal relationships. In this chapter some of the cognitive and behavioural changes which may impair social functioning are briefly mentioned. The way these changes affect the interpersonal life of brain-injured adults is reviewed and reports of treatment efficacy with this population are discussed. Assessment issues will be reviewed and treatment strategies outlined.

COGNITIVE CHANGES

Despite the difficulties encountered in attempting to relate global social skills performance to specific cognitive deficits (Godfrey *et al.*, 1989), the degree of cognitive impairment significantly impacts social performance. Severely impaired individuals could have inappropriate social goals, but even when the goals are appropriate, many brain-injured individuals find it difficult to generate strategies to develop interpersonal relationships. Attention and memory deficits affect social interactions, as individuals fail to maintain the flow of conversation, due to forgetting information (for example, names or conversational topics) or as a result of repeating statements and questions. For those people with severe memory disorder, developing new social contacts is impossible as they cannot pursue relationships through time. Disorders of expressive and receptive language affect social communication. Even mild receptive language disorders can cause difficulties in understanding the subtle nuances of individual or group discourse. Expressive language disorders can result in paucity of language, word-finding difficulties, or difficulty in constructing conversational statements. Speech can be tangential and circumlocutary and in extreme cases, the patient's verbal output may be totally incomprehensible. Patients who are aware of their difficulties become frustrated or anxious as a result of these problems, and some avoid social situations. Perceptual disabilities affect recognition of facial and bodily expressions, and cause difficulty in understanding interpersonal cues. The dyspraxic individual may be unable to produce facial and body movements intentionally and not be able to make use of facilitating actions such as imitation (Pizzamiglio *et al.*, 1987).

PERSONALITY, BEHAVIOUR AND PSYCHIATRIC CHANGES

Egocentricity is a well-recognized sequelae of severe brain injury (Lezak, 1978). Inability to tolerate frustration (irritability) or to delay gratification as well as lack of interest in the activities, thoughts and feelings of others impact social acceptability. Deficits may range from subtle emotional immaturity and 'gauchness' to marked physical and verbal aggression. Behavioural aspontaneity may result in reduced participation in social behaviours. After mild injury individuals may be able to return to work but due to a fatigue or initiation difficulties do nothing but watch television at night. Psychiatric problems such as obsessional themes, ritualistic behaviours and paranoid ideas interfere with successful social interaction (see Chapter 5).

Behavioural changes

The brain-injured individual may be disinhibited and unable to modify behaviour in the light of changing environmental and social factors. The individual may be insensitive to the effect of his or her behaviour on others and in extreme cases individuals attempt to intimidate others or be physically aggressive in order to achieve their ends. The very severely impaired individual may have a very limited range of social goals which could be sexual in nature and may be pursued indiscriminately.

Physical changes

Obvious physical impairments are socially handicapping in Western society. Oral motor disorders may be particularly handicapping. Interpersonal communication may be impaired by difficulties in conveying non-verbal information to others, e.g. facial expression, gestures and posture. Environmental barriers continue to exist to social integration for the motorically impaired.

The difficulties experienced by the severely brain-injured adult in maintaining social connections are well documented. Thomsen (1974 1985) showed that brain-injured adults retain serious psychosocial deficits and problems in establishing social contacts fifteen years after injury. Weddell, Oddy and Jenkins (1980) followed 42 young adults (mean age 24.4 years) admitted to a rehabilitation centre after very severe brain injury (mean duration of coma 4.2 weeks). Patients were compared with a control group on neurological examination, neuropsychological tests and interview. The brain-injured group had experienced marked changes in work, family life, leisure activities, and contact with friends. They had fewer friends, made and received fewer visits, and dated less frequently. Twenty-one of the brain-injured subjects studied had no friends or acquaintances at all. The brain-injured group were, not surprisingly, rated as being significantly more lonely than the comparison group. The difficulties of the brain-injured in social adjustment have been compared to the problems of the unemployed person, i.e. time is unstructured, limited network of friends, few goals to strive for or opportunities to show his competence and reduced sense of identity and status (Oddy 1985). Brain injuries occur predominantly in young people who may have few well-established friendships. Many friendships may be lost during the enforced withdrawal from social contact of the acute recovery phase. Opportunities to make new friends are limited as social contact is reduced – many brain-injured adults spend the majority of their time at home (Thomsen, 1974, 1985).

Weddell *et al.* (1980) showed that brain-injured adults with personality change maintained contact with friends from before the accident significantly less often than those brain-injured without personality change. There was no difference between the two groups on their absolute number of close friends, but the relationships had become more superficial (Weddell *et al*, 1980; Oddy, 1985). Elsass and Kinsella (1987) investigated the interpersonal relationships and vulnerability to psychiatric disturbances of severely closed brain-injured subjects. Self-report by the severely injured individual was compared with relatives' reports. Fifteen brain-injured adults were individually matched with non-brain-injured controls. The brain-injured group differed significantly from the control group in the quantity of interaction but not in the perceived quality of interaction. The groups differed significantly on behavioural change. The brain-injured showed increased impulsivity; increased fatiguability; greater tendency to sudden mood change; and decreased ability to approach people, e.g. start a conversation. The brain-injured also showed increased tendency to be upset by criticism, experienced memory problems and reduced concentration, had decreased initiative, greater difficulty in becoming interested in anything; and increased stereotyped responses (even when they were clearly inappropriate). The brain-injured were more attention-seeking, slower in doing things and became more easily upset when their needs were not immediately met. These personality changes occur at a time when the individual needs all his personal resources to cope with the changes in lifestyle following a severe injury. Brain-injured individuals suffer severe frustration and lowered self-esteem and self-assurance. Anxiety is very common and probably occurs at least partially as the result of the struggle to cope with the social demands for which the individual is no longer adequately equipped (Tyerman and Humphrey, 1984).

THE EFFECTIVENESS OF SOCIAL SKILLS TRAINING WITH BRAIN-INJURED ADULTS

Social skills retraining has been shown to improve the social interactional skills of patients in both psychiatric and non-psychiatric settings (Plienis et al, 1987). Evaluative studies of social skills retraining with the brain-injured are few and results have been inconsistent. Johnson and Newton (1987a) examined 11 severely brain-injured patients attending an occupational therapy day centre. The brain-injured patients demonstrated a high level of social anxiety, poor social performance and low self-esteem. The authors suggest that these are important contributory factors in the poor overall social adjustment of these patients. Johnson and Newton (1987b) attempted to remedy specific problem areas in social interaction by providing social skills retraining once a week for two hours, over a one-year period. The brain-injured group were assessed on a range of measures at the beginning of the study, at six months and at one year. Measures used included the Katz adjustment scale (1963); a questionnaire of social anxiety; Rosenberg self-esteem scale; neurophysical scale and Wechsler Adult Intelligence Scale. In addition a social performance measure was designed which included videotaping standardized conversation, which was then rated by two observers on 12 aspects of verbal and non-verbal social behaviours. Each training session included a review of the previous meeting and the week's activities, then introduction of the main theme of the meeting, discussion, role play and feedback. Adjunctive procedures included printed handouts, posters, diaries of activities and a video system for immediate feedback. After one year the changes of the assessment scores were not statistically significant, but the authors suggested that their approach may be a useful starting point from which occupational therapists can develop more effective rehabilitation programmes.

Gajar and co-workers (1984) describe the use of feedback and training in self-monitoring on two brain-injured adolescents. Feedback involved providing light signals corresponding to a positive or negative social interaction. Positive responses were those where the client added to a previous group member's statement by making a relevant comment, agreed or disagreed (and provided a rationale) or asked a relevant question. Negative responses were silences following another person's question or statement, statements of three words or less or if a comment was off the topic, mumbled or a joke or interruption. An A1-B1-C1-A2-C2-B2 design was used in which the feedback phase (B) and the self-monitoring phase (C) were alternated to control for order effects. The study demonstrated the efficacy of both types of intervention. Helffestein and Weschler (1982) describe the use of Interpersonal Process Recall (IPR) in the remediation of interpersonal and communication skills deficits in the newly brain-injured. Sixteen 17–35-year-old brain-injured adults were randomly assigned to an experimental and a control group. The experimental group received 20 one-hour IRP sessions while the control group received non-specific attention. The experimental group showed greater improvement in interpersonal skills as assessed by professional staff ignorant of group placement.

Brotherton *et al.* (1988) described a sessional social skills training approach to social interactional deficits after closed brain injury. The four patients treated were two years post-injury and were in coma for at least seven days. They were non-aphasic, capable of following three-stage commands and were not physically violent. A multiple baseline across behaviour design was utilized. The behavioural training package was most effective when applied to simple motoric target behaviours, e.g. self-manipulation or posture. Only the improvements patients made in these domains were retained at one-year follow up. Patients were unable to improve or retain improvement on more complex verbal behaviours, possibly because these areas require more linguistic processing ability than was actually present, or because they would only be responsive to long-term behavioural intervention.

THE IDENTIFICATION OF SOCIAL SKILLS DEFICITS

We have found it useful to consider socially skilled behaviour as verbal, including all aspects of speech, e.g. tone of voice, rate of speech, accent, volume and intonation; and non-verbal including facial expressions, gestures and body movements. The aim of social skills training is to alter social behaviours in ways which increase social opportunities. The needs of individual patients are highly variable so accurate assessment is necessary to ensure a realistic retraining programme. Bellack and Hersen (1978) formulated four questions for guiding social skills assessment.

a) Does the individual manifest some dysfunctional interpersonal behaviour?
b) What are the specific situations in which the dysfunction is manifested?
c) What is the probable source of the dysfunction?
d) What specific social skills deficits does the patient have?

Different causative factors may result in the same disorder. Assessment needs to determine the causative factors, as different treatment methods may be applicable depending on the cause of the impairment. In addition, assessment should both provide the therapist with information about what is appropriate social behaviour for that individual and indicate the environmental demands for social behaviour. For example, one patient referred by a group home for treatment could return there if he could stop screaming and not sit so close to the television because he blocked the view of other residents in the home. A higher-functioning patient would be able to return to live with his wife and family if he could stop shouting and criticizing his children. Only a limited number of formal testing procedures are available for assessing the social skills of brain-injured adults (e.g. Prutting and Kirchner, 1987). Assessment most frequently involves informal observation, behavioural observation, interviews and rating scales. Social behaviour must always be considered in an enviromental context.

1. Informal observation data

Any social situation can be a source of informal observational data, and may be used to assess the brain-injured person's non-verbal and verbal skills. Assessment of the brain-injured in their home environment or in functional social settings, e.g. shops and restaurants, may provide the therapist with an invaluable amount of data on the individual's social behaviour.

2. Behavioural observation and role-play tests.

Behavioural observations employ a more structured approach to data collection by observing the person in natural settings, the ward or unit environment and in structured interactions (role-plays). A variety of recording methods can be utilized, e.g. ABC recordings, frequency-ratings and behavioural sampling techniques.

Although naturalistic observation is the assessment method most advocated by behaviour therapists (Bellack, Hersen and Lamparski, 1979), role-play tests are frequently used as they are less time-consuming. Role-play tests may be more or less structured. Representative of role play tests is the Behavioural Assertiveness Test – Revised (BAT-R) of Eisler *et al.* (1975). The subject is seated next to an interaction partner and the interactions are usually videotaped. An interpersonal situation/ encounter is described, the interaction presents a naturalistic prompt and the subject is expected to respond as if the situation were a natural social encounter. The subject's response is rated on both general characteristics (e.g. anxiety) as well as component behaviours (e.g. eye contact, response duration). Unfortunately it is not clear that the data gained using role-play tests provides an accurate representation of naturalistic performance (Hersen and Turner, 1978; *et al*, 1979). Role-play tests should therefore be used to augment assessment procedures which should include at least some naturalistic observation and other sources of data.

3. Interviews

Interviews provide information about the brain-injured patient's interpersonal history and provide a setting for informal observation. Interviews can explore the patient's views of his background, family history, social contacts and understanding of social norms; his own evaluation of his behaviour in social interactions, and his view of his present social situation. Henderson *et al.* (1978) developed a measure of social interaction – the Interview Schedule for Social Interaction (ISSI). This schedule provides a structured method to investigate the intensity, quality and extent of the patient's interactions over the preceding week. For the more severely injured group of patients it is probably more appropriate to interview a close family member about the patient's interactions.

4. Self, peer and family reports, ratings and check-lists.

Ratings and check list data can be used to categorize patients' social skills deficits. The purpose of scales range from an attempt to chart subtle variations for use in treatment to screening (present or absent) scales (see discussion of types of rating scales Chapter 6). Moderate to severely impaired patients are unlikely to be able to rate their own performance accurately. It is not known if degree of insight is related to ability to improve social behaviour and this could be a fruitful area of study. To assess the brain-injured individual's level of social contact, patients and/or their relatives/friends can be asked to record specific social activities or interactions in a diary, e.g. the number of friends that visit or the number of times the patient went out socially during a specified period. A number of more general check-lists or rating scales have sections for rating social skills. For example, the Adaptive Behaviour Rating Scale developed for the mentally retarded population has a social/behavioural skill section which provides a screening. For many in the moderately-impaired range of deficit a ceiling effect will be evident. Ehrlich and Barry (1989) have reported a rating scale on communication behaviours for use with the brain-injured. Preliminary reports of its use indicate that it may be reliable and valid. Six separate items were considered relevant to functional communication in the brain-injured and were included to be rated on scales of 1–9. The six items are intelligibility, eye gaze, sentence formation, coherence of narrative, topic, initiation of communication. This scale may contribute reliable information in content areas otherwise restricted to general clinical impressions. Prutting and Kirchner (1987) have described a protocol for screening pragmatic aspects of communication. The pragmatic protocol is designed to be completed after observing individuals engaged in spontaneous unstructured communication with a partner. Thirty aspects of behaviour are rated as appropriate (if they facilitate the communicative interaction or are neutral), inappropriate (if they are judged to detract from the communication or penalize the individual) or 'no opportunity to observe'. The 30 categories of behaviour assessed cover verbal and non-verbal aspects and include turn-taking, interruption and overlap. Inter-rater reliability for trained assessors is good. Validity is not assessed in the study but the authors do note a difficulty caused by the interaction itself. Some partners may facilitate communication more than others. The aim of the assessment is functional: it does not focus on cognitive deficits and the patient's performance is rated as inappropriate only if it detracts from communication. So, for example, a patient with a dysfluent dysphasia would not be rated as deficient in turn-training if they could compensate for a delay by interjections. Although its use with the traumatically brain-injured is not described (Prutting and Kirchner, 1987) it could be of considerable use as a screening device with this population.

COMPONENT SKILLS: DEFICITS AND TREATMENT STRATEGIES

The complex social behaviours required for adequate social performance are built from many non-verbal and verbal skills, e.g. facial expressions, tone of voice and the ratio of self-statements to questions. Retraining may be required for some or all aspects of skilled social behaviour following severe brain injury. The more severe the injury the more likely the individual is to have social skills deficits (see below, this chapter). Type of skill deficit may vary with severity of injury. Discussion emphasizes a skill-building model in which retraining of non-verbal and verbal skills is followed by more complex skills training, and the generalization of these skills to use in the community (Trower, 1987). Even the presence of basic social behaviours does not ensure effective social skills performance. The brain-injured individual must know when and where to make various responses as well as how to make them. Utilizing assessment techniques (Chapter 6) and learning strategies (described in

Chapter 7), individual and group treatment programmes can be devised. Whenever possible, social skills retraining programmes should incorporate the following:

1. Sessions highlighting the way the individual's performance is inadequate and the way this inadequate performance will impair the attainment of interpersonal goals.
2. Analysis of social performance by breaking the skills into the component features required for appropriate social interaction. For example, attracting attention incorporates language suitable for the interaction ('Excuse me please' or saying the person's name), gaining appropriate eye contact, ensuring adequate social distance and orientation and maintaining appropriate facial expression.
3. Specific behavioural or cognitive learning techniques adapted to the individual's abilities and deficits.
4. Practice of the component features and of the overall skill in sessional role-plays and in settings in which the skills are to be used. Role-plays simulate interactions needed in the real world. Role-playing may be done in individual or in group sessions.
5. Feedback of the individual's performance can be provided by the group leader and the group (when skills are improving, feedback can be a powerful social reinforcer). Videotapes of the social interaction may also be used (given that confidentiality issues are adequately addressed). As retraining continues, feedback occurs through KR in social interaction.
6. Where the social skills retraining occurs in an in-patient or day-patient unit, a whole unit approach can be utilized. In these settings feedback or reinforcement can be provided for every instance of a to-be-acquired behaviour (this type of intervention is described in more detail below). Family members may also be taught skills so that they can support the generalization of new social behaviours (McKinlay, 1988).

In the next sections of this chapter we discuss the parameters of normal social behaviour, the retraining of component skills and methods of building these into appropriate social behaviour.

NON-VERBAL COMMUNICATION

Non-verbal aspects of communication play a significant role in social interaction. Birdwhistell (1970) demonstrated that in a typical dyadic encounter the verbal components convey one-third and the non-verbal two-thirds of the social meaning. Mehrabian (1972) stated that the most important component of emotional recognition is non-verbal communication, estimating that 93% of the affect of a message is conveyed to the recipient non-verbally. Similarly Zaidel and Mehrabian (1969) found that people are more likely to believe what they see than what they hear. Non-verbal communication may a) replace speech, b) complement the spoken word, c) add emphasis to important parts of verbal messages, e.g. the stress of words, pause, tone and speed, d) initiate and sustain communication by providing sources of feedback and e) help regulate the flow of communication between speaker and listener, e.g. hand gesture, drop in voice, eye gaze. We can divide non-verbal skills into seven areas (Giles and Clark-Wilson, 1988b):

1. Facial expression.
2. Gaze.
3. Gesture.
4. Posture and orientation.
5. Interpersonal space
   – proximity
   – physical contact.
6. Language-free elements of speech.
7. Appearance.

These seven components of non-verbal social skills will be discussed in relation to norms of social behaviour, the deficits which underlie the brain-injured individual's inability to meet normative expectations, and retraining of the appropriate use of non-verbal social skills.

1. Facial expression

Brain-injured individuals may have difficulty controlling the muscles of facial expression as a result of central damage or cranial nerve injury (see Chapter 3). Some patients have apraxia for control of facial muscles. Although some lines of evidence suggest a right hemisphere or right frontal focus for disorders of facial expression of emotion (Borod *et al* 1983), others have found no relationship (Pizzamiglio *et al*, 1987: Mammucari *et al.*, 1988). Severely impaired patients may be unable to recognize facial expressions of emotion. Trower (1978) analysed factors involved in recognizing the emotional content of facial expression. For example 'happy' was defined as head up, mouth pointing at each end, lips slightly apart, eyes open and wrinkles at the corners of the eyes. There is considerable regularity in components of expressions of happy, sad, anger, shock and surprise, fear, blank, and disgust. However not all non-neurologically impaired individuals can reliably distinguish between them. Jackson and Moffit (1987) found that a non-neurologically impaired control group could distinguish happy, frightened, surprised and self-satisfied but not disgusted, thinking, neutral, angry, sad and bored. These authors also examined changes in recognition of facial expression of emotion following brain injury (Jackson and Moffit, 1987). Subjects with significant perceptual impairment or impairment of facial recognition (prosopagnosia) were eliminated from the experimental group. Two sets of test stimuli of facial expression were presented and brain-injured subjects had significantly more difficulty in recognizing facial expression of emotion than a matched set of orthopaedic control subjects. The brain-injured subjects were also less likely to identify negative than positive emotions. When patients are unable to appreciate facial expression of emotion they are deprived of the subtle feedback available for the 'success' or failure of social interactions which is likely to impede social learning. We are not aware of any studies specifically addressing the ability of brain-injured individuals to deliberately express emotional states. It is known however that in the non-neurologically impaired the ability to be deliberately facially expressive is associated with spontaneous emotional expressiveness. Brain injury has been consistently found to reduce expressiveness (Mammucari *et al.*, 1988), presumably impeding social interaction.

Social skills retraining for the brain-injured involves increasing the awareness of their deficit by teaching the expectations of other people and constructing methods to overcome deficits. When training the brain-injured to recognize and display facial expressions, it is first necessary to assess their ability to recognize expressions through the use of pictures in magazines, photos, and videos. An examination of the components which form facial expressions within group and individual teaching sessions may be helpful. The practice of facial recognition and expression with appropriate feedback is essential. Integration of improvements into higher social behaviours can be accomplished by prompting and reinforcement in group and whole-unit settings.

2. Gaze

The identification of normative eye gaze behaviour is problematic because of its variation across situations. Eye contact is longer if emotions are more intense, e.g. love or anger. Avoiding eye contact is associated with avoiding social communication. Expectations of eye gaze also differ for strangers, friends and acquaintances. Kendon (1967) found eye gaze duration during conversation was longer during listening than talking. Eye gaze came in short bursts, and shortly after its initiation by the speaker it was ended by the listener. For example, at the end of A's speech, A looks to B which is a signal for B to speak. As B responds, he looks away. If the speech is long, the listener looks at the speaker intermittently. This pattern of gazing has a monitoring function to synchronize and control the flow of conversation between individuals. It eliminates the need to verbally state whose turn it is to speak and inadvertent interruptions.

Many brain-injured individuals do not use appropriate eye contact when communicating, i.e. eye contact may not be initiated or maintained. This may result from arousal deficits, attention disorders, neuropsychiatric or behavioural problems. In the latter case there may be little eye contact with a refusal to communicate or alternatively staring as a component of aggressive posturing. Gaining eye contact may be difficult for those with anxiety disorders following brain injury and those who lack confidence in social situations.

Methods used to retrain brain-injured individuals in appropriate eye contact depends on the cause(s) of the disorder. Measurement of the individual's level of deficit by recording the duration of eye contact establishes a baseline against which response to training may be compared. Teaching the patient to become aware of their use of eye contact in different social situations through video recording and feedback from peers can establish acceptable durations for gaze in social conversations. We suggest that three seconds is adequate time to gain eye contact, but longer than five seconds is experienced by others as staring. Some brain-injured who are unable to look into the eyes of others, can be taught to look at their conversational partner's forehead or nose. Practice on the use of appropriate eye contact in individual and group sessions with feedback should be incorporated into more complex social skills, e.g. initiating and maintaining the flow of conversations and attracting other people's attention.

3. Gesture

Two types of gestures may be distinguished; gestures which replace speech (autonomous gestures) and those which complement speech (illustrators). Examples include outstretched hands communicating an appeal and shoulder shrugging conveying lack of knowledge. Many gestures are included in a social repertoire and are described by Trower and co-workers (1982).

Many brain-injured individuals cannot interpret the meanings of gestures accurately as a result of attention, cognitive and perceptual deficits. Perceptual deficits influence their ability to recognize and understand gestures, attention disorders affect concentration on the communication. Difficulties may result in the inappropriate use of gesture, i.e. too little or excessive use of gesture or the use of inappropriate gesture. Physical disabilities affect the patient's ability to use gestures to replace or complement speech. For example, one patient with severe receptive and expressive dysphasia used gesture to complement his affected speech. He had increased tone in his right side and used his left hand to gesture. When excited he shook his fist above his head; individuals who did not know the patient found this behaviour disconcerting and social skills training involved the development of alternative methods of expressing excitement. Many brain-injured individuals are unable to coordinate their gestural expression with verbal language, thus giving contradictory information to others.

Retraining the brain-injured in gesture is directed towards

teaching the normal meanings of gesture and by practising and co-ordinating the use of gesture with language to enhance communication.

4. Posture and orientation

Patterson (1983) has identified five basic functions of body posture in social communication: information giving, regulating interaction, expressing affective states, indicating social control and facilitating task goals. Individuals use combinations of postures and orientation in social communication. Postures, i.e. positions in standing, sitting, and lying, can signify positive, neutral or negative attitudes. For example, in sitting, leaning forward gives the impression of being positive and interested, whereas leaning back appears negative and lethargic. In addition, emotions may be displayed through posture, e.g. a downward oriented head and slumped pose may convey depressed mood. The angle at which one person interacts with another affects communications patterns. Sommer (1969) showed that side-by-side positioning was considered co-operative; face-to-face positioning suggested competitiveness and a 90% angle facilitated conversation. Cook (1969) replicated these findings and concluded that the relationship between the individuals involved and the location of the social encounter influenced posture and proximity. Jackson and Moffit (1987) found that brain-injured individuals were less able to interpret the emotional meaning of posture and orientation than an orthopaedic control group. In addition physical deficits such as spasticity and tremor impede the brain-injured's spontaneous use of posture. Social communication is affected as others are less able to understand and interpret the meaning of the patient's non-verbal behaviour.

5. Interpersonal distance

Personal space is the space immediately surrounding an individual and if this personal space is invaded they may feel angry or uncomfortable. Proximity refers to the interpersonal distance that people maintain when they are involved in interaction. Acceptable distances depend on the situation. Hall (1959) classified social distances into four main zones: the intimate zone of

18 inches or less; the personal zone 18 inches to four feet; social or professional consultative distance nine to 12 feet; and public speaking twelve feet or more. When these social distance rules are violated people change their position accordingly. Status differences should be considered when observing interpersonal distances: an equal status means a closer interpersonal distance is more acceptable than when the status is less equal. Physical contact is complicated by social norms regarding who has permission to touch whom in what context. Social touch includes hand shaking, arm-linking, or a comforting touch on the arm.

Brain-injured individuals frequently have difficulties in determining appropriate interpersonal space. Difficulties may be associated with psychiatric disturbance or disinhibition. Problems may be related to either invading personal space with excessive touch or alternatively the opposite, of appearing aloof as a result of maintaining an extended social distance. Patients with difficulty in maintaining appropriate interpersonal space can be taught distances accepted by their culture. In conversation, distance of 'arm's length' is a concrete term which can identify an accepted distance of about three feet.

J. E. was severely injured in a motor vehicle accident (coma duration 14 days) which resulted in serious attention and memory deficits, disinhibited behaviour, and an inability to recognize faces. He wandered continually, approached people in a disinhibited manner, stood too close and touched excessively. Treated at an intensive in-patient unit, J. E. was given the prompt 'arm's length' by all staff whenever he was felt to be too close and reinforced when he moved away. He gradually allowed more distance when he initiated and maintained a conversation with others.

Practice and feedback about touch are essential for the brain-injured who have difficulties in this area. Education about body areas which may be touched, and situations in which touch is appropriate, increases their awareness of this form of social contact. Some patients may require an extinction programme to help them eliminate intrusive touching (see Chapter 11).

6. Language-free elements of speech

Language-free elements of speech include the vocal cues which help carry the impact of a verbal message, for example, the rhythm of speech, the use of silence and pauses, stress on individual words, rate, pitch and volume (Mehrabian and Ferris, 1967). These non-verbal facets of speech assist understanding and promote interest in the speaker's social communication.

Rehabilitation depends on the type and degree of deficits. Techniques used in speech therapy to overcome these deficits need to be identified and used in many functional and social situations. These skills can be practised in sessions, games, role-plays and then transferred into everyday settings in which the individual needs to function.

Individuals with very severe speech deficits may need to rely on these language-free elements of speech with other non-verbal social skills to communicate. Specific compensation for speech can be accommodated for in social skills retraining.

After severe brain injuries (coma duration 1 month), I. D. and S. C. were unable to successfully interact with others, because they could not express their needs verbally or use communication aids. They could understand simple statements without difficulty and in social skills retraining they learnt to attract people's attention by voicing, looking at the person concerned, smiling and then pointing and gesturing their needs to the person they were interacting with. This became their main approach when communicating with others, and was developed to be socially appropriate by a whole unit approach and emphasis on the 'naturally occurring' reinforcement of social attention.

APPEARANCE

Judgements are made about individuals on the basis of their physical appearance, facial characteristics, hair, body shape and clothes (Hargie, 1986). These factors influence 'attractiveness' and the likelihood of others starting and maintaining social interactions. After brain injury altered appearance as a result of physical, cognitive or behavioural problems frequently interacts with the individual's ability to recognize the way their appearance affects social situations. The patients with severe physical deficits have to expend great effort to maintain personal hygiene. Psychiatric disorders can lead to the person wearing bizarre and unsuitable clothing, refusing to wash or change clothing regularly, taking little interest in his appearance, and refusing to participate in any activities directed towards improving appearance (e.g. shaving).

Methods to improve the brain-injured's physical appearance can be incorporated into techniques for retraining washing and dressing (see Chapter 7 on learning). Social skills retraining can increase the individual's awareness of how others perceive him, develop methods to improve appearance, and to alter his appearance according to social situations. Group sessions are especially instrumental in enhancing awareness of these issues. Brooks *et al.* (1987) have discussed the subtle social barriers created by inadequate personal hygiene and dressing behaviour among brain-injured patients which may be best addressed via peer pressure.

CONVERSATIONAL SKILLS

Conversation management involves a vast range of behaviours. Appropriate behaviour depends heavily on context. Variables include subject matter, time available, location, personality and socio-economic background. Recently a number of workers have examined aspects of social interaction and narrative discourse following severe brain injury (Mentis and Prutting, 1987; Godfrey *et al*, 1989). Ehrlich compared his subject's (mean coma duration 9.7 days) descriptions of 'the cookie theft' picture from the Boston Diagnostic Aphasia Examination (Goodglass and Kaplan, 1963) to descriptions given by non-neurologically impaired adults. The brain-injured adults, all of whom were at least six months post-injury, were found to be similar to the control group in the amount of pertinent content expressed and rate of speech. Brain-injury subjects were however slower in the rate of information communicated. The subjects produced lengthier verbal output resulting in reduced communicative efficiency. Ehrlich (1988) notes that the brain-injured appear to talk past the point of diminishing return in terms of communicative efficiency yielding a diffuse texture to their discourse. Godfrey and co-workers (1989) examined social interaction following very severe brain injury (PTA in excess of 7 days). These researchers were also interested in the relationship of speed of information processing to social interaction skills. While Ehrlich (1988) found that brain-injury subjects spoke for longer (but less substantively) than controls, Godfrey and co-workers found a global reduction in behavioural productivity (we describe more general aspects of this negative symptomatology in Chapter 11). The difference in findings may be accounted for by the severe nature of the injuries in Godfrey and co-workers' sample. When compared with non-neurologically impaired controls on global social skills measures, the brain-impaired group in Godfrey and co-workers study were rated as significantly less interesting, less likeable and less socially skilled. The brain-injured group spoke significantly more slowly, were less spontaneous, spoke more monotonously and (unlike Ehrlich's 1988 patients) spoke for shorter duration. Godfrey *et al* (1989) note that ratings on four 'micro-behaviours', speech duration, speech speed, spontaneity and pitch, were strongly associated with 'global' ratings of 'skilful', 'interesting' and 'likable'. The general findings suggest that the severely impaired are not reinforcing to interact with. Although the brain-injured group were significantly impaired on a visual information processing task, contrary to Godfrey and co-workers' expectation there was no consistent relationship between reaction time and social presentation. The authors suggest that the simple reaction time task may have been a poor analogue for social interaction where sustained and complex information processing is required.

Mentis and Prutting (1987) examined cohesion in the discourse of brain-injured and non-neurologically impaired adults. In order to keep both narrative and conversation cohesive, various types of links or 'ties' were used. Mentis and Prutting found that the brain-injured displayed both a qualitative and quantitative difference from controls. Most notable was the high proportion of incomplete ties used by brain-injured subjects. Incomplete ties resulted in semantic confusion and ambiguities leading to requests for revision by the subject's conversation partner. All the brain-injured patients studied had difficulty in establishing inter-sentence semantic relationships (Mentis and Prutting, 1987).

Lewis *et al.* (1988) examined the effect of three separate feedback contingencies on the inappropriate verbalizations of a patient with anoxic damage. The socially inappropriate talk was defined as any unintelligible, foolish or absurd statement not fitting the context of the conversation (e.g. 'Oh it's the cute one' 'do you love me yet?') The patient was two years post-injury and had been treated in both psychiatric and rehabilitation hospitals. In an alternating treatment design administered in random order across three therapists, the patient was provided with four types of responses to his verbalizations (a baseline and three treatment conditions). The baseline involved redirecting the patient to a suitable topic. Treatment conditions involved an attention and interest condition (in which the therapist responded to an inappropriate remark and smiled, maintaining eye contact and responding verbally with phrases such as 'you're too much!' or 'you're too funny!'); a systematic ignoring condition (in which the therapist broke eye contact for three seconds and then initiated a conversation on a suitable topic); and a correction condition (in which the therapist stated in a neutral tone 'You're talking nonsense when you say [repeating the inappropriate remark], people can't understand you. Now start again and tell me about something which makes sense'). Irrespective of therapist variables the correction contingency consistently resulted in the greatest diminution of social inappropriate talk. Systematic ignoring was somewhat less effective while the attention and interest condition, as expected, greatly exacerbated the problem and demonstrated how the high rate of inappropriate talk observed in the natural environment was maintained by social reinforcement (Lewis *et al.*, 1988).

Behavioural learning methods are the most appropriate for training basic social routines to the severely impaired brain-injured person. To-be-trained behaviours should be objectively definable, small, highly motivating and often-repeated. For the less severely impaired, cognitive-behavioural methods can assist patients learn how to analyse and formulate strategies to overcome social skills deficits. Both approaches can be used for fundamental skills; the appropriate intervention depends on the patient's degree of difficulty in new learning and their ability to cognitively drive behaviour.

a) Social routines

Social routines include phrases used in social interactions, for example, 'please', 'thank you', 'sorry' and 'excuse me' which are habitual in nature and expected as basic social etiquette. The brain-injured may need to be retaught to use these routines.

b) Attracting attention

Three behavioural phases are involved in both greetings and partings between friends (Kendon and Freber, 1973). The distant phase which incorporates hand waving, eyebrow raising, smiling, and direct eye contact. Social conversation is initiated at a medium distance with 'arms length', eye contact, and smiling with appropriate verbal communication. The close phase involves the individual's engaging in direct contact, e.g. shaking hands, kissing, eye contact, smiling, with the appropriate verbalization. The actual content of each phase depends on the roles, status and function of interaction, and the location and sex of the interactors.

Retraining of the brain-injured individual incorporates the practice of the individual skills and their integration into an acceptable sequence of social behaviours. For example, the skills of attracting attention could include making appropriate verbalizations to attract attention, e.g. 'excuse me' and/or stating the person's name, establishing eye contact, smiling, and then initiating appropriate conversation. The brain-injured individual's non-verbal and verbal social skills deficits should be identified, his awareness of his deficits increased and skilled social behaviour practised and incorporated in varied social situations.

c) Initiating, maintaining and closing conversations

The ability to initiate and maintain conversations is affected by physical, cognitive and behavioural deficits. Lack of confidence can result in social anxiety, further impeding social performance. Patients with lack of insight may be unable to monitor and adequately structure their verbal interactions. In a study by Sunderland et al. (1984), 'rambling on', as reported by relatives, discriminated between individuals with mild and severe brain-injury. We have noted above that the patients with very severe injuries may have the opposite difficulty and demonstrate poverty of behaviour. Retraining attempts to improve the clarity, fluency and audibility of speech using techniques established by the speech therapist. In addition, retraining aims to increase appropriate conversational content and increase the organization of information. Therapy also attempts to assist the patient to identify the non-verbal and verbal social cues in social interactions which aid an appreciation of the needs of others. In the following sections we will discuss techniques for training conversational management under the following headings; initiating conversation, maintaining conversation, listening skills, questioning, responding and exiting.

Initiating conversation

In most novel social encounters the conversation begins by 'breaking the ice', i.e. talking about non-specific information such as (in Great Britain) the weather, the environment, time; finding out or reviewing general and relevant information about the other person (job, preferred recreational activities). Brain-injured individuals may have difficulty generating appropriate conversation starters so that they say nothing or select inappropriate, personally invasive or bizarre conversation leads (one patient would relentlessly pursue strangers in order to ask how old they were, where they lived, if they were married and if they had children). Developing and practising the use of specific lead topics may enhance the patient's ability to initiate conversation. Some patients will be unable to independently generate novel ways to open conversation but will be able to master a limited number of generic ways to do so.

Maintaining conversation

Conversation requires a co-ordinated exchange between speaker to listener. Listening, questioning and responding provide the basis of communication. Speech and language deficits, slowed information processing, and difficulties in forward planning associated with frontal lobe impairment encumber social performance. Memory problems may affect the flow of conversation; conversational topics and questions may be repeated continually.

Retraining of conversational skills should incorporate the following: appropriate speech volume; co-ordination of verbal and non-verbal communications, conversational reciprocity, obeying appropriate social conventions, attracting attention, listening, questioning and responding skills. Some individuals after brain injury learn strategies to identify the social cues inherent in communication and formulate statements and questions relevant to the flow of conversation. When they have difficulty in learning these strategies, a more arbitrary rule could be taught to increase social acceptability. For example, one post-acute patient with marked temporal lobe dysfunction (resulting in circumstantial and continuous speech) was taught to speak for no more than 90 seconds at a time. This allowed her conversational partner an opportunity to speak and increased her social acceptability.

Listening skills

Wolfe and co-workers (1983) defined listening as the process of hearing and selecting, assimilating and organizing, retaining and correctly responding to aural and non-verbal stimuli. Social skills retraining helps patients to identify those non-verbal and verbal cues which convey the impression of listening, and learn to demonstrate their listening skills during conversation. Indicators of interest in a conversation can be non-verbal and verbal (Duncan, 1972; Hargie, 1986). Non-verbal responses which indicate listening include smiling, eye contact, facial expressions, attentive posture, head movements, for example, nods, shakes or tilt of the head, and using appropriate language-free elements of speech, for instance, 'mmm', ah ah.' Verbal behaviours which indicate listening include verbal reinforcers, for example, 'yes' and 'really'; using language similar to the speakers; sentence completion; requests for clarification or reference to past statements; appropriate questioning; coherent topic shifts; and reflecting and summarization.

Listening skills (which incorporate the behavioural element of attention) can be addressed in tasks which involve following directions, and maintaining conversation via appropriate social cues and on-topic questions. However, in our experience, individuals with severe brain injury have profound difficulties in 'reflective listening', incorporating emotional context and attempting to teach them this skill is often unsuccessful.

Questioning

Questions (requests for information) may be verbal or non-verbal but are most frequently verbal with gestural illustrators. These verbal and non-verbal questions serve a function in conversational management. Vocal inflection, head movement or eye contact at the end of questions provide cues important to conversational turn-taking. Different types of questions can be used in social communication. In closed questions the response is circumscribed and dictated by the nature of the question, for example, the question may require a yes or no response. These types of questions are easy to answer and although it is easy to use them to include someone in an interaction, they also can be restrictive and impose limitation on an individual's possible responses. They give the questioner a high degree of control in the interaction. Open questions can be answered in a number of ways, the respondent deciding on the kind of response. They are broad in nature, and require more than one or two words for an answer. Open questions allow the respondent to talk, allowing further exploration.

Many brain-injured have difficulty formulating appropriate questions because of their poor language skills, rambling speech or a failure to attend to the other person. Non-verbal messages may not complement the verbal questioning, thus providing contradictory information. Individuals can be taught to maintain conversations by using questions. The cognitive element of the intervention involves teaching the different types of questions and utilizing these in a co-ordinated manner. An 'inverted funnel sequence' (Kahn and Cannell, 1957) involves beginning with closed questions and gradually opens out to embrace wider issues. This provides the brain-injured with a degree of structure and organization in their questioning and conversational skills. Patients practise these skills on a sessional basis and then in social situations.

Responding

Inappropriate responses to questions include silence; rambling, disorganized and unconnected responses; jokes, critical comments, confabulations or flagrantly untrue responses. In retraining, individuals can be assisted to investigate social situations in role-plays, and experiment in performing inappropriate and appropriate responses with feedback about the benefits of positive responses in conversation. For example Gajar and co-workers (1984) describe a successful programme for the self-monitoring and shaping of conversational responses (discussed above).

Closure of conversation

Closure (or parting) behaviours draw attention to the satisfactory completion of an interaction sequence. Closure behaviours depend upon the number of participants involved, the purpose of the encounter, location, time of day, as well as the personal characteristics of the individuals such as personality, experience, and socio-economic background. Parting behaviours may be routine conversational behaviours, for example, 'so long', or be at a more complex level of 'terminal exchanges' which pinpoint a series of physical manoeuvres and positioning related to structured closure and leave-taking procedures (Goffman, 1961).

Retraining aims to overcome social deficits by practising the procedures involved in conversational closure. A number of types of closure have been defined (Hargie, 1986), some involve verbal behaviour only but closures are usually accompanied by specific non-verbal behaviours. Closure markers could include factual statements which summarize or reflect aspects of the conversation, or relate to activities or personal relationships of the participants (see Knapp *et al*, 1973). Simple verbal closure statements, such as, 'all the best,' 'see you', are usually linked with non-verbal markers such as a hand-shake or wave. An array of more subtle cues may signify the interaction is drawing to a close, for example changes in body posture or looking at a watch. It is important that non-verbal behaviours support verbal statements and that specific closure markers are used to avoid embarrassing those who are not quite sure whether to carry on talking or terminate an encounter.

D. P. was 17-years-old when involved in a road traffic accident (coma duration four weeks). Among his many social skills problems, when seen two years post-injury, was an inability to terminate conversations. D. P. would follow staff and other clients around the treatment facility and was unable to make use of cues provided by others to indicate their wish to terminate interactions. D. P. was instructed how to use these cues on a sessional basis. Once he understood and could use these cues on a sessional basis, staff began to use them with increased emphasis. For example, saying 'Well goodbye then' especially loudly (a highlighting procedure). D. P. was rewarded (with social attention and praise) by another staff member if he made use of the cue.

ASSERTIVENESS TRAINING

For some less cognitively impaired brain-injured adults assertiveness training may be indicated and is particularly appropriate for patients with anxiety-based disorders and low self-esteem. Assertive behaviour enables a person to act in his or her own interests, to stand up for herself or himself without undue anxiety, to express honest feelings comfortably, or to exercise personal rights without denying the rights of others (Alberti and Emmons, 1982).

Group observations, audiovisual aids and discussions provide feedback to the individual about his performance in specific role-plays and social situations. Verbal and non-verbal behaviours are analysed with regard to whether they are aggressive, assertive or passive and alternative behaviours and strategies to approach social situations are discussed and practised. Keeping an assertiveness book could help identify and evaluate behaviour. Like most other social skills, assertiveness is culturally relative.

A number of studies have examined verbal and non-verbal behaviours which could be categorized within the aggressive, assertive, passivity profile (Lazarus, 1971; Alberti and Emmons 1982; McFall 1982). Aggressive individuals exaggerate eye contact (glaring) and talk loudly (over 84 decibels). In contrast, passive individuals express themselves in an apologetic manner, aiming to appease others and avoid conflict at all costs. The non-verbal behaviour associated with a passive interaction style includes little use of gesture, reduced eye contact, and a marked hesitation before responding to others (16 seconds or longer). In conversation, non-assertive individuals speak softly, below 68 decibels, avoid issues and make self-effacing statements.

Lazarus stated that assertiveness is comprised of four main components. These are being able to initiate, continue and terminate general conversations, express positive and negative feelings, ask for favours and make requests and finally to refuse requests. Assertive non-verbal communication includes controlled, steady, smooth and purposeful body movements, audible voice of about 76 decibels, and speaking without hesitancy, for instance, about a three to four second delay before responses.

GROUP TRAINING PROCEDURES

Group social skills retraining has specific advantages over individual teaching. The group setting provides the opportunity for maladaptive behaviours to be observed and highlighted and for patients to learn and practise adaptive behaviours. The social skills group helps the therapist facilitate the reacquisition and refinement of the basic skills needed for interpersonal communication and social interaction.

Groups can provide a sense of belonging, and a safe environment in which to work through problems. The practice of some social skills, for example getting to know someone by asking appropriate questions in conversations; conveying verbal and non-verbal interest and attention to a group member; disclosing appropriate information about one's own interests, hobbies and background; and talking about topics that are likely to be of interest to peers, all establish group cohesion. The use of behavioural rehearsal, practise and role plays is facilitated by the group setting. Group rehearsal and practice is more stimulating and may be more successful in maintaining the individual's attention, than individual work. As in individual sessions the group requires consistency to ensure learning.

Group facilitators and group members can provide modelling

of appropriate social skills and provide guidance and feedback but other group members can also be encouraged to fulfil this role. Patients can work together to identify the real-life situations which prove difficult in a process which encourages conversational skill development and assertive behaviour.

The overall aims of retraining need to be reviewed regularly and the skills practised within the environment where they are needed.

Individual programmes using a 24-hour approach

Social skill groups are frequently used to address the social interactional deficits of brain-injured adults. However, a 24-hour intervention programme may be of particular benefit to those patients unable to learn from group interventions. Giles, Fussey and Burgess (1988) suggested that 24-hour intervention programmes should involve three components:

1. a cognitive overlearning element to ensure that patients know the nature and likely implications of poor social performance;
2. sessional practice of appropriate social interactional skills;
3. a 24-hour unit operant conditioning procedure.

Without additional (highlighting) cues, patients frequently do not appear to attend to their social performance. Severely injured patients almost uniformly lack the ability to adopt alternative viewpoints, so that it is not surprising that patients often do not understand the impressions they create in others. We advocate multiple methods to increase the salience to the brain-injured individual of his own social performance, including unit based events and reinforcers. Bizarre or funny tokens may be used, for example on one occasion, in order to highlight to the patient a problem of speaking without pauses, the staff and the client all wore orange-coloured joke digital watches to time the patient and (with specific cues and reinforcers) limit her utterances to 90 seconds duration. This 24-hour directed attention to an area of which the individual was not habitually aware could account for the extremely rapid and durable changes observed in her social behaviour.

In the same way, as in Chapter 7 we emphasized not setting physical goals beyond the individual's ability. In social skills

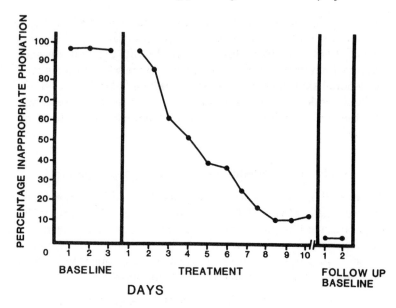

Figure 12.2 The rapid response of patient 7 to a programme to draw attention to her habitual high-pitched whisper. By day 10 of the programme this had been replaced by a forceful voice with good air support.

training, goals should be selected that the individual is cognitively capable of performing. Targets should be concrete, operationalizable, and within the patients cognitive capacity, for example, many patients may find it impossible to learn reflective listening but are capable of learning to put pauses in their conversation to allow their conversational partner to speak.

The results of twelve individual unit programmes are summarized in Table 12.1. Patients from a consecutive series of 37 clients with traumatic brain-injury, who had social/interactional skills deficits severe enough to warrant behavioural intervention, were treated using behavioural methods at a transitional living centre. The average duration of coma for the social skills deficit group was 26.4 (SD 22.8) days and for the non-social skills disordered group 16.4 (SD 19.2) days, suggesting that the former group had more severe injuries. Only three (25%) in the social skills disordered group (N=12) had coma duration under 2 weeks, whereas 21 (57%) of the entire group

(N=37) had coma for that period of time. The problems most frequently experienced by patients were speaking for too long without pausing, being overly critical of others and speaking too softly. In the first two of these problems, treatment outcome was variable. In the three cases of speaking too softly, there was a good recovery and in two cases responses to treatment was immediate. Rapid response to treatment is demonstrated by the pattern of learning of patients 4 and 7 shown in Figures 12.1 and 12.2 respectively. Patient 4 responded to programmes designed to help reduce inappropriate posture, poor phonation and 'giggling' and patient 7 to a programme addressing poor phonation.

Table 12.1

Patient number	Coma duration (in days)	Type of skills deficit	Symptom reduction
1	35	A1, B2, B3	25%
2	28	A2, B1	100%
3	28	A4	50%
4	90	A2, A6, C1	75%
5	1 (focal)	A1	50%
6	1	A3	25%
7	42	A2	100%
8	28	A1, B1, B2, C1, C2, C3	50%
9	14	A5	75%
10	14	A5	75%
11	14	A5	0%
12	8	B2	100%

Patients 2, 6, 7, 11 and 12 were treated six months post-injury; Patients 1, 3, 4, 5, 8, 9 and 10 were treated at least 18 months post-injury. All patients received one or more of a range of behavioural interventions described in the text. Percentage symptom reductions are an approximate average of the overall reduction of a patient's display of the target behaviours from standard behavioural recordings.

A1 Speaks too long without pauses/rambles
A2 Speaks too softly
A3 Speaks too loudly
A4 Speaks too fast
A5 Does not initiate conversation
A6 Has inappropriate laughter

B1 Has repetitive themes/statements
B2 Is overly critical of others
B3 Uses foul language

C1 Has inappropriate posture/mannerisms
C2 Touches others inappropriately
C3 Stands too close.

Case Report 12.1
The patient (S.K.) suffered a severe brain injury as the result of a road traffic accident in July 1983. Initial CT scan showed an extensive comminuted depressed fracture of the right side of the skull vault; midline structures were shown to be moderately displaced towards the left and there was reduction in density in the depth of the parietal lobe. Evacuation of a moderate-sized haematoma on the right side was performed on the same day as the accident. S. K. was discharged from neurosurgical intensive care 13 days after the accident and at this time was only minimally responsive. S. K. gradually made a moderate recovery but remained severely ataxic with a severe left-sided hemiparesis. In addition S. K. displayed both aggressive and manipulative behaviours, was significantly impaired in memory but had reasonable preservation of intellectual ability. Progress in rehabilitation was limited because of the severe aggressive behaviour directed towards rehabilitation staff. As a result S. K. was referred to a specialized unit for the behaviourally disturbed brain-injured adults. It was noted that S. K. was explosive and attention-seeking and would often shout at others. He swore excessively and showed inappropriate responses to frustration and criticism.

S. K. attempted to engage rehabilitation staff in empty conversations. He had a mild scanning dysarthria, but also day-to-day conversation showed marked circumlocutions and an inability to get to the point. S. K. frequently attracted attention and interspersed his conversation with phrases such as 'well the thing is', 'it seems to me'. The phrases would convey no content and their frequent use made S. K. unpopular. An observational assessment measure used on the unit to help staff highlight problem areas showed staff rated S. K. as using this type of communication 52% of the time.

Procedure
Baselines were transcribed from separate recordings of 5 minutes structured, 5 minutes semi-structured and 5 minutes unstructured conversation with a person not involved in the

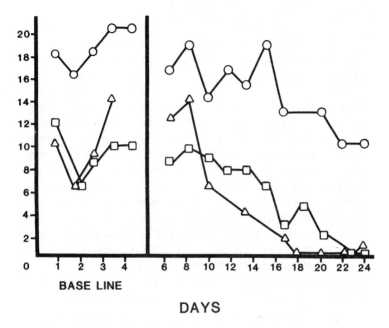

Δ INAPPROPRIATE POSTURE
□ POOR PHONATION
○ "GIGGLING"

Figure 12.3 The response of patient 4 to programmes designed to address inappropriate posture, poor phonation and giggling. These behaviours were grouped together by staff as they resulted in the patient appearing highly immature. Inappropriate posture describes the patient's tendency to lean forward and to one side in his wheelchair and rock (particularly while giggling). Poor phonation describes the patient's high pitched, whining voice which had inadequate air support. Giggling describes a high pitched, rapid and prolonged laugh. The cause of these behaviours is unknown, however the patient's prolonged hospitalization may have resulted in infantilization. Alternatively, the reinforcement contingencies of the hospital could have led to behavioural continuation of originally neurologically mediated behaviour. Both poor posture and poor phonation responded to intervention very rapidly. Response to the intervention for giggling was slower and more limited.

treatment programme. The structured conversation involved asking direct closed questions, such as 'Can you tell where you were born?'. The semi-structured conversation involved questions such as 'Tell me what effect the accident has had upon you?'. The unstructured conversation was commenced with the comment 'I want you to tell me as much about yourself as you can so that I can understand how you feel'. The conversation was sustained by reflective repetition of the themes.

Treatment
It was explained to S. K. that people liked him but found him boring, and it was important for him to make what he wanted to say shorter and to get to the point faster. However, it was also made clear to S. K. that if he needed time to think of an answer a delayed response was acceptable. The programme involved five half-hour sessions per week. Consistently throughout the programme the phrase 'short answers' was used as a prompt to encourage clear, concise statements and the importance of giving short answers was explained to S. K. on at least two occasions per session with the fact that it was permissible for him to take time in responding.

Three separate types of task were set in each session.

1. S. K. was prompted to give one-word answers. S. K. would then be questioned, with one-word answers being required. The questions posed were well within his capacity to answer and related to his immediate environment, for example, 'What month is it?' 'Is it raining?'; 'What colour is the table top?'. Alternatively, props such as cards with photographs of objects were used and the patient asked to name them.
2. S. K. was asked closed questions with highly specific content but which required more than one word answers, for example, 'What is the weather like?'; 'What did you do this morning?'.
3. S. K. was engaged in unstructured conversation. S. K. was required not to wander from the point and not to speak for too long at any one time, which was arbitrarily determined to be 90 seconds.

Successfully completing the task led to social attention and praise, and to intermittent tangible reinforcement in the form of chocolate (which the patient liked). Failing in the task led to S. K. being timed-out-on-the-spot (TOOTS) (see Chapter 11). After a delay of 20 seconds S. K. would be re-prompted with the phrase 'short answers' and a new question would be asked. Conversational themes and questions varied during treatment and the questions used in assessment were not used in treatment.

S. K. understood the purpose of the sessions, and was friendly and co-operative throughout. At the same time as the period covered by the special programme, staff were instructed to TOOTS all speech where the point was not immediately apparent. At the end of one month S. K. was re-baselined using the procedure described above. This involved a repetition of the questions originally used in the baseline measures. At one month S. K.'s conversational style in regard to empty conversation was felt to be within normal limits and the programme was therefore discontinued. Two months after the completion of the programme the patient's verbal performance was re-baselined.

Results and discussion
The treatment resulted in significant improvement, the greatest improvement overall being in the structured questions. Continued progress was shown after the end of the formal treatment sessions, resulting in significantly fewer words per minute in all question types when compared with pre-treatment. To give an indication of the improvement found, it is useful to give a verbatim example. Before the programme S. K.'s reply to the question 'Can you tell me the name of your favourite food?' was 'Basically, no. Taste-wise I like oriental-type food, Indian-type food, English-type food, just about every-type food to a certain extent, but the Indian, no the Chinese – I can't think what it was I was going to say, something I'd like, but with the Indian – no the Chinese – one thing I do not like is beansprouts but I can't remember why'. The answer to the same question one month later was succinct: 'Sirloin steak'.

Structured conversation showed the greatest initial improvement. Prior to the programme S. K. was never able to give one-word answers whereas after treatment he was frequently able to do so. Semi-structured conversation showed the smallest overall improvement possibly because the scope for improvement was less. Unstructured conversation showed the second largest improvement. The TOOTS procedure continued throughout the treatment and follow-up period and is likely to have had its biggest effect in this area. It is not possible to ascribe any particular proportion of the improvement to the special programme. The approach to the problem was clinically biased and therefore multi-faceted, attempting to maximise all chances for success. Elements of the programme included the teaching, practice and reinforcement of appropriate responses; cognitive overlearning of what was and was not appropriate; alternative strategies to deal with delayed information processing and a TOOTS procedure so reinforcement was not available for inappropriate behaviour. S. K.'s improvement indicates that relatively simple methods can be effective in remediating social interaction deficits in some brain-injured clients.

SUMMARY

The social skills training approach described in this chapter differs from those in many of the published reports of social skills training (Johnson and Newton, 1987; Brotherton *et al.*, 1988). Firstly, the importance of the patient understanding the likely social consequences of his behaviour is emphasized (implied in this, is gaining the individual's active endorsement of the programme, wherever possible). Secondly, the importance of a whole unit approach and 24-hour feedback on behaviour and consequences is stressed (usually, but not always, positive reinforcement). Thirdly, highly concrete criteria for learning and for the tasks used in training needs careful consideration. Programmes for mild to moderately impaired patients can be thought of as a way to direct their attention to habitually ignored aspects of behaviours, and to assist them in replacing the inappropriate behaviour with an appropriate behaviour. This intervention is maintained until the more appropriate behaviours become habitual. In patients with more profound impairments a more orthodox behavioural intervention may be most effective.

13

Facilitating community reintegration

PREPARING FOR COMMUNITY REINTEGRATION

Of particular interest and a central component of community reintegration is the transitional living facility. The most innovative adopted, the therapeutic community model, first developed in the 1950s and early 1960s for psychiatric patients and those with drug and alcohol abuse, has been adapted for use with the traumatically brain-injured. The clients of a therapeutic community for the traumatically brain-injured are medically stable and need to develop to be a more adaptive 'being in the world'. Disruption of cognition, behaviour and mood occur on a background of unrealistic thinking and personality disorganization. Therapists, as well as other clients, can provide persistent gentle confrontation around deficits and foster a global change in lifestyle through multi-dimensional influence and training.

It is the community itself which attempts to set events (discussed in Chapter 7) to aid both the individual's acceptance of his dysfunction and his ability to learn. So, endorsement of deficits within groupwork and the need to spend the day working on specific behavioural goals of recovery is an attempt to manipulate the therapeutic environment which, if successful, is a setting event for later activities. Studies of occupational behaviour show reward and punishment can significantly influence behaviour in a social context. O'Reilly and Puffer (1989) found that the application of a deserved reward or punishment to a group member had positive effects on expressed motivation, satisfaction and perception of equity in observers while failure to use sanctions (for failing to meet required standards) had negative effects. It is possible that a patient's observations of others gaining reward, and failing to gain privileges for poor performance, has a positive effect on their ability to be motivated towards their own rehabilitation goals. The individual's changes in conduct, attitude and emotion are stimulated, monitored and reinforced in the daily regime. Operant conditioning paradigms are used in specific skills building with systematic approaches to achieving two main rehabilitation objectives; reintegration into the community and the development of a 'good enough' position. The entire system is built around the manipulation of motivation and staff must be able to confront clients whose behaviour is not consistent with the group. Privileges are acquired as the individual progresses through treatment.

Treatment fall into a number of stages.

I   Assessment of need and orientation/assimilation of the individual into the community;
II Primary treatment;
III Re-entry autonomous decision making/progress to educational or vocational programmes.

Fussey and Giles (1988) have described the place of this type of model in the overall service system.

Therapy should be pursued towards concrete goals which have relevance outside the treatment facility. Patients need to be actively prepared for discharge in activities of daily living, incorporating the domains of personal, domestic, community, work and leisure skills, social and emotional support and the establishment of a routine daily structure (school/work). Developing the patients' skills in leisure pursuits and teaching them to use their own time constructively can prevent problems from arising in the home situation, where less structure is generally apparent.

Patients often have considerable difficulty in making this change from the hospital or institutional structure to one at home or in a less regimented setting. Community reintegration is facilitated by retraining the individuals in the activities they need to learn in the appropriate settings and the training should be consolidated before treatment is terminated. Activities should be practised in the patient's home environment, if possible, and the relatives and carers trained in the specific methods which could promote the individual's independence in his home environment. Provision of training or management programmes, videos and photograph albums could help the carer (and continuity of care) remember specific information relevant for their relative, when they have returned to their home environment. A gradual transition from the treatment facility to the home environment is ideal.

During the active treatment phase of recovery, the patient develops a rapport with members of the treatment team. Since rehabilitation staff often ask the patient to carry out activities which are unpleasant or frightening, or request them to think about painful issues, the patient needs a high level of trust in them. A period of time usually has to be spent in developing that rapport. As the patient progresses and becomes more independent, therapists have to carefully manage the withdrawal of treatment. This withdrawal from treatment phase is often difficult for patients and staff. The patients' renewed reponsibilities for themselves and feelings of anxiety for the future, could be combined with a sense of mourning for the established relationships with therapists and feelings of rejection. The affective meaning attached to the process of exiting treatment could be considerable. Even if the reason for treatment termination is that the reasonably set goals of treatment have been attained, the patients may none the less feel that the staff are 'giving up on them'. These difficulties can be reduced by a gradual weaning-off process from the rehabilitation establishment, to either home, work or day-care facilities and continuing support to the future placement for a period of time. Also, the adoption of 'rights of passage' such as graduation ceremonies or leaving parties, or associations for patients who have left, could reduce feelings of abandonment. Emotional adjustment is often maintained by family or by a group of friends, once the patient has left active treatment.

Deterioration in the patient's functioning is often the result of a failure to co-ordinate and establish a continuing system of rehabilitation and care for the patient's future. When patients are discharged early from hospital, it is difficult to predict their future needs, therefore, adequate discharge planning and ongoing case management needs to be constructed to reduce the likelihood of this deterioration occurring.

Discharge planning

Before discharge is organized, consideration needs to be given to the home care-givers, the home environment, provision of resources and the availability of social support networks.

When the patient returns home, the family support system assumes great responsibility for the brain-injured relative, often on a 24-hour, 7-day-a-week basis. There are major sources of stress involved in being the constant observers of a relative's discomforts and pain, or his emotional and behavioural demonstrations of distress, apart from the physical pressures of providing care. Family members often have to learn to deal with their own bouts of depression and feelings of hostility towards their loved one. As exhaustion sets in, it is more difficult for them to conceal personal frustrations because of having to put their relative's requests before their own needs.

In many hospitals it is taken for granted that families will automatically care for their relative (even if they were not living with them before the accident). Many care-givers assume this role because they presume that they could adjust to the round-the-clock care-giving, whilst others are unaware of the stresses of care-giving or feel guilty because they have never previously shared in the care and treatment of their loved one. Consideration needs to be given to the suitability of this in discharge planning. Assessment of the family support system needs to include the carers' ages (as well as the patient's); their mental and physical condition; their knowledge of the relative's condition; their understanding of relevant medical or rehabilitation approaches; and their support networks. In order to facilitate decisions, ongoing education about head injury and their relative's difficulties after the brain injury is valuable to help them gain insight and more realistic expectations of their loved one's potential for recovery. Specific information about the options for future care, resources available and financial assistance aid this decision-making process. For the severely injured patient, this process often involves a long-term experiment, with trips home at weekends and for holidays, to help the relatives gain greater understanding of the difficulties and establish methods of coping within the home.

Discharge planning involves establishing the resources required for the patient to return home, to new accommodation or alternative placements. The type of accommodation, access in and around the home, locality and availability of local resources, for example shops, transport, day centres, and the social support networks, all need to be identified to ensure the individual or family can manage. Before patients are discharged, the home environment needs to be assessed and possibly redesigned or adapted to their specific requirements to facilitate further independence or ease the burden of caring. In conjunction with architects and housing authorites, structural alterations require planning and the financial aspects of the work considered. Whilst the physical limitations of a person's home can be adapted, for example, with ramps, lifts, hoists or environmental controls to open doors etc., the application of these have to be carefully considered within the patient's physical and cognitive abilities, their potential progress and social and cultural environment.

Equipment should be provided, if necessary, but only after adequate training has been given to the individual and carer of its use in the relevant functional activities. During rehabilitation, the provision of equipment to overcome physical disabilities in functional activities may be actively discouraged or only given temporarily, as a stage in the rehabilitation process, to ensure the patient does not learn to depend on the equipment if he could potentially manage without. When a patient returns home, a re-evaluation of types of equipment within the home environment will be required. Extra demands on time, an increased or reduced level of independence, greater expectations of their role in the family, further leisure pursuits, could justify the provision of alternative equipment.

Outdoor mobility equipment

Some patients and therapists believe that considering an outdoor mobility aid is equivalent to giving up on the possibility of achieving independent ambulation. Unfortunately this belief leads to some patients not being encouraged to reintegrate into the community. When therapists oppose the purchase of an outdoor mobility aid they may unwittingly support the patient's belief that 'everything will be OK when I can walk' and greatly impede the individual's reintegration into daily life. Careful timing in the provision of mobility aids is essential if patients are to accept them. For patients with cognitive deficits, enough time must be allowed for the considerable training necessary to use an outdoor mobility aid. The therapist's reluctance to 'give up' on the patient can result in the hurried acquisition of an aid (and inadequate training in its use) immediately prior to hospital discharge. Patients who are unlikely to be able to ambulate functionally in the community, in the reasonably foreseeable future, should be encouraged to try appropriate outdoor mobility aids. The type of aid will depend on the severity of the patient's motor and cognitive impairments (electric wheelchair, scooter, etc). Training of the patient in the use of the aid in the community (ideally their own home community) is necessary if the patient is actually going to use the equipment after discharge.

Many patients find their frustration is increased when they return home because of increased reliance on others for transportation in their community. This could be as a result of medical advice not to drive, financial restrictions for alternative transport systems, or an inability to organize themselves to arrange other transport, for example, taxis, buses.

Driving

Patients are frequently very eager to resume or, if adolescents, begin driving. Few guidelines are available for the amount of time people need to wait before returning to driving after injury, but the risks of epilepsy and other psychological concerns need to be fully established before restarting this activity. Driving assessments and lessons from driving schools or specialist centres can recommend relevant care adaptations and aid their return.

Jacobs (1988) found that between one and six years post-injury, 37% of severely brain-injured patients in his study returned to driving as compared with 93.7% who were driving pre-injury. Neither therapists' clinical judgements nor objective (paper and pencil) tests have been shown to predict a person's ability in driving skills on the road (Galski *et al.*, 1990). These results are in line with the difficulty discussed throughout this book in attempting to use non-functional activities to predict functional performance. Van Zomeren *et al.* (1988) examined fitness to drive after severe head injury. Driving was studied in (1) an instrumented car that recorded lateral position control and (2) in driving the subject's own car with a professional observer. The brain-injured subjects were all at least 3 years post-injury (mean 6.5) and all were driving. In comparison with a control group the brain-injured subjects performed worse, with five out of nine drivers being classified as incompetent. The only relationship found between neuropsychological measures and driving involved visuomotor ability and lateral position control. No relationship was found between neurological status and driving skill. Deficits may not compromise an individual's ability to drive provided the individual is able to compensate for them. Hence insight and self-criticism may be a more important determinant for a patient's fitness to drive than degree of cognitive deficits.

Kewman and co-workers (1985) attempted to improve the performance of post-acute traumatically brain-injured patients on behavioural aspects of motor vehicle operation, by providing specific training using a small electrically powered vehicle. The authors' primary interest was whether improvement on these tasks would translate to the functional (and complex) task of on-the-road automobile driving. A matched traumatic brain-injury control group was provided with experience using the electrically powered vehicle but were not provided with training. Experimental subjects showed improvements both on the specific exercises and in performance on a structured test of automobile driving on the road when compared with untrained brain-injured control subjects who did not show improvement. Results suggest a significant therapeutic effect of the specific training programme and also that training in specific tasks is more effective than exposure and unstructured experience.

Many individuals are able to live at home if adequate support services are provided to the family. However, the support services for the brain-injured and their families are often either difficult to find or impossible to finance. The type of care provided needs to take into account all the relevant factors, for instance, the patient's physical, cognitive and behavioural status; the level of stress on the home carer; the resources available in the community; and be flexible according to the fluctuating needs of the carer. These services could include the provision of care ranging from a couple of hours a week (for example, to go shopping) to a full-time carer (or two) living within the home. Training of carers is essential to educate them in the problems after brain injury and provide systems for working with the patient. Planned respite care could regularly give relatives and carers a break.

On returning to the community, individuals often need to have a structured active day in which they can learn specific work or follow their own leisure pursuits, within or outside the home. Resources could include the services of therapists in the home, day care centres or supported employment. Community-based day care and residential units are gradually becoming more available, but are usually limited in the number of people they will accept with any degree of behavioural disorder. Integration of the patient into support groups (for example, those operated by Headway in Great Britain or by the local chapter of the National Head Injury Foundation in the USA), day centres, college or work environments can be begun before full discharge.

The adjustment process for the individual

Following brain injury the individual slowly re-evolves from a dependent patient to a more independent person who has had to slowly adapt to altered circumstances. Tasks that were once easy have often become more effortful, fatiguing and laboured and the individual's ability to cope with the difficulties have been reduced. Many of the cognitive, behavioural and social deficits may not be recognized by the individual but none the less severely hamper his ability to reintegrate into the community.

Emotional changes are common. Fordyce *et al.* (1983) found that relatives thought patients who were over six months post-injury were more emotionally distressed than patients in the acute stage of recovery. The authors ascribe the higher level of emotional distress to increased awareness of impaired functioning. Dikman and Reitan (1977) studied the relationships between impairment of cognitive-intellectual abilities and the resulting emotional problems of adjustment. Neuropsychological tests, including the Minnesota Multiphasic Personality Inventory, were completed soon after injury, at 12 and 18 months. The results indicated that, as a group, there was a decline of emotional stress over time and patients with significant deficits experienced greater emotional distress than those with negligible difficulties.

The adjustment process for the family

Initially the patient's family are grateful that their relative has survived, but gradually over time they begin to realize that the brain-injured individual no longer behaves as he did before his injury. In extreme cases the brain-injured relative may not even seem like the same person.

Some degree of personality change is common after severe brain-injury. It has been recognized since the time of Phineas Gage that significant personality change is compatible with preservation of intellectual abilities. However, severe personality change frequently occurs as part of a constellation of cognitive and behavioural change, which could range from mild intellectual impairment accompanied by a subtle loss of vitality, to significant intellectual blunting and gross behaviour disorder. More severe personality changes are associated with severe damage, and could take the form of apathy, inability to inhibit behaviour, selfishness and altered sexual behaviour.

It is difficult to classify personality change precisely and the best-known studies are based on reports of family members. Relatives interviewed by Thomsen (1984) stated that intellectual deficits, and particularly poor memory, presented difficulties but that changes in personality created the greatest troubles in everyday life. Among the most frequent symptoms were childishness, aspontaneity, emotional lability and irritability and, most seriously disruptive in family life, were aggression and lack of sexual inhibition. Brooks and co-workers (1986) when comparing relative's responses at one and five years, noted an increase from 60% to 70% reporting personality change, an increase from 15% to 54% reporting threats of violence, and an increase from 10% to 20% reporting actual violence. The patients may or may not be aware of the changes in themselves.

Over recent years considerable effort has been devoted to assessing the reaction of family members to severe brain trauma in a loved one. Livingstone (1987) found measures of expressed burden were significantly higher in relatives of the severely brain-injured than of the mildly brain-injured, and this level was relatively stable up to one year. The major factor for predicting relative's distress was the complaints voiced by the patient. The major determinant of the family members' psychosocial adjustment was their previous psychiatric and health history. Families show different coping mechanisms after a member of the family has suffered a brain-injury but clearly many individuals had difficulty in coping with their change of role (Livingstone, 1987). As described by Lees (1988), a long relationship and the presence of a supportive extended family network are likely to increase the chances of a marriage surviving.

Many survivors return to live with their parents, instead of returning to their previous situation, for example living alone or with others. Jacobs found that 47.8% of his sample were living with their parents, compared with 35% who were doing so pre-injury. 22% lived with spouses compared with 30.7% pre-injury and 11.6% lived in therapeutic or professionally supervised environments (Jacobs, 1988). Caring for an individual after brain-injury can be physically demanding, emotionally draining, and socially isolating. Support from people knowledgeable about the consequences of brain injury is frequently lacking, and training for the relatives is often forgotten when the individual is discharged home.

The development of a realistic understanding of the patient's deficits may be difficult for both the patient and family members and they may require extensive counselling and support. Helping the individual and relatives adjust to their new altered circumstances is essential and provision of assistance for the families of an emotionally or behaviourally disordered relative is invaluable for family members, who are understandably emotionally engrossed in their relative's problems.

Family roles

Before the brain-injury, the individual and his family are likely to have had consciously and unconsciously defined roles. These roles may change as a consequence of trauma, but often the relatives, rather than making adjustments, expect the injured individual to return to his original role. A number of role assessment tools have been developed for use by occupational therapists. The Role Change Assessment (RCA) of Jackoway *et al.* (1987) was developed for use with older adults but can also be used with other populations. The RCA considers 48 roles, ten family and social roles, ten vocational roles, eight self-care roles, eight organizational roles, nine leisure roles and three health care roles. The RCA is a semi-structured interview which takes about an hour to administer. Initially information about present role status is elicited. The interview process is then repeated with a focus on past role participation in order to make comparisons. The roles assessed by the Role Checklist are those of the participant in organizations, hobbies/amateur sport, as friend, family member, care-giver, home-maintainer, student, religious participant, worker and volunteer.

Watts and co-workers have described the Assessment of Occupational Functioning. This assessment consists of two parts, a semi-structured interview schedule and a series of five-point rating scale items. The scaled items consist of statements describing a range of functions and these are rated from absent to fully adaptive. A total score may be derived from adding the scores on the six areas assessed: values, personal causation, interest, roles, habits and skills. The total screening takes approximately 25 minutes. It is not clear how reliable the brain-injured group are in completing role asessments, but these measures can be used with family members. It is important to discuss the patient's roles with family members and alert them to possible changes. An understanding of roles may assist in the development of treatment priorities, if properly used. Vauce-Earland (1991) found that standardized role assessment tools are little understood and little used by therapists.

Roles may need to be redefined or new roles established to ensure the individual with injury has a sense of 'worth' following the long process of rehabilitation. Adaptations to the changed situation or altered roles may not be easy to accept. Functioning in the sexual role, caring role, work, income, and domestic roles may be influenced by any of the deficits remaining after the brain-injury.

The individual could be more dependent on the family for achieving functional activities and need physical assistance or instructions to manage, for example, mobility, transferring and bathing. Family members may have to make more decisions about the organization of the daily routine, the management of the household, or maintain some form of work to ensure adequate income is available. The role of organizing may have had to be taken over from the injured person, whilst he/she was in hospital. Uncertainly about the effects of the brain-injury may make it difficult for other family members to withdraw from these roles and return them to the individual. This reinforces the more 'dependent role' and 'helplessness'. After the individual returns to the community, it is important that he has a 'feeling of worth' and the extent of the responsibilities needs to be carefully managed to ensure the individual with brain-injury does not reassume former roles too rapidly and fail as a consequence.

Disputes are likely in 'role re-establishment' after the individual returns to the community and can be constructive. Resolving issues can determine 'role identification' and the results need to be acceptable for all of the family. Counselling for the individual and the family members is helpful in identifying methods of achieving this goal. Zarski *et al.* (1988) suggest that family satisfaction after brain trauma is related to how much families are able to reorganize roles and responsibilities and focus on the brain-injured member's normality rather than his symptomatology. Less satisfied families evolve around the significant losses and limitations of the brain-injured member. Denial in the family may be a road block to further adaptation.

Wiley (1983) has criticized the conceptualization of family members in roles as overly static emphasizing the importance of transactional patterns. Transactional patterns are the repetitive behaviour by which individuals live with others. They are the distillation of a myriad of behaviour options into relatively predictable routines and involve 'family mythology'. The family needs ways of altering its transactional structure. Frequently, the brain-injured adult does not have the resources available to help balance the system and other family members fail to comprehend how the system works. Helping family members understand how responsibilities have been divided, and how each has helped the other, may assist in the development of a new balanced transactional pattern (Wiley, 1983). Empirical methods have rarely been used to assess families of the severely brain injured. A number of interview measures are now widely available and are reviewed by Bishop and Miller (1988). As well as their use in research, most family assessment devices are able to discriminate between normal and distressed families and could be used to help target family support resources.

Sexual dysfunction after brain trauma

Many individuals experience sexual dysfunction after brain-injury. Boller (1982) found that three out of four brain-injured patients experienced decreased frequency of sexual relations. The incidence of sexual dysfunction increases with severity of injury (Lishman, 1973) with reduced sexual drive being seen most often. Damage to the central nervous system may directly interfere with sexual behaviour and performance, for instance damage to the temporal lobes usually decreases libido, and of the frontal lobes influences behaviour, including marked changes in sexual behaviour. Disinhibited behaviour is usually a result of frontal injury or damage to deep limbic structures and changes in sexual activities and preferences may be marked (Miller *et al.*, 1986).

In acute-care settings patients often display themselves, manually stimulate their erogenous zones and masturbate. This behaviour may be perturbing to others and is probably best managed by providing privacy. Patients who are more alert but still confused or in PTA, may make sexual jokes or attempt to sexually touch care staff or therapists. This type of behaviour is best managed by making clear statements as to what is and is not appropriate and removing the patient's hand or moving away for a few seconds. Family members should be informed that this type of behaviour is not uncommon in people emerging from coma and does not necessarily indicate any new facts about their relative.

Inappropriate sexual behaviour where impulses are not controlled may persist into the post-acute stage. Impaired sexual function could continue and include amenorrhoea or orgasmic failure, as well as reduced sexual interest and problems in maintaining arousal. Adolescents could go through a period of regression and sexual confusion.

Treatment depends on the nature of the deficit and the social context, but education and counselling should be initiated early in the recovery process. Treatment could involve the provision of sexual outlets, wherever possible; a behavioural approach to the inappropriate behaviour; or for the brain-injured person with altered sexual reponsiveness, behavioural sex therapy may be indicated.

The impact of sexual changes on the family

Brain injury changes roles in ways which affect sexual relationships. For example, a wife may change role and become a carer or spouses may feel trapped and under pressure to meet the individual's 'needs'. Alternatively, a reduced level of libido in the brain-injured person may leave the non brain-injured partner feeling unfulfilled. Rosenbaum and Najensen (1976) described a crisis in wives of brain-injured servicemen, wounded in the Yom Kippur war, which was far worse for them than for the wives of paraplegics injured in the conflict. There was a drastic reduction in sexual relations and wives reported a tendency to dislike any physical contact with their husbands. For many, this seemed associated with personality change, with increased selfishness and immaturity in the husband.

Table 13.1 Sexual behaviour and problems of couples

Problems of the injured individual
Changes in organic sexual function (e.g. inability to become erect in the male)
Altered (decreased or increased) sexual drive
Changes in preferred sexual behaviour (perceived sexual grossening)
Change in sexual orientation
Sexual talk (public or private)
Interference in sexual activity as a result of changes in other domains (e.g. leg adduction due to spasticity)
Infantile behaviour/dependency
Selfish sexual behaviour

Problems of partners
Partner no longer attracted to injured individual due to physical changes
Partner no longer attracted to injured individual due to personality changes
Partner no longer attracted to injured individual due to changes in role (partner is now care-giver)
Partner submits to injured individual's sexual requests but does not want to
Brain-injured individual not able to fulfil partner's sexual needs

Family members as lay therapists

Dut to the highly labour-intensive nature of working with the brain-injured population, there has been recurrent interest in the family as lay therapists (Giles and Shore, 1989a; LeWinn, 1980). Quine *et al.* (1988) studied the performance of relatives as lay therapists at a university hospital in Sydney, Australia. They found almost all of those relatives approached were willing to participate. Parents were the most frequent lay therapists and the amount of time lay therapists worked with their relatives decreased as time from injury increased. This was partly accounted for by the fact that family members often found it to be an economic necessity to return to work. This study also showed that, particularly as the post-injury interval increased, time that family members could have spent carrying out therapy was spent passively sitting by the bedside. Whilst some positive benefits were found in involving family members, the relatives could not be relied upon to provide intensive regular therapy even when present and able to do so. The reduction of rehabilitation costs was less than had been anticipated. The authors suggested that families as lay therapists would be best thought of as appropriate adjuncts to customary services (Quine *et al.*, 1988).

McKinlay and Hickox (1988) have described the preliminary results of training family members to help their severely brain-injured relatives in the post-acute stage of recovery. Family members were taught to utilize practical behavioural methods to improve memory (diary) and reduce temper outbursts by a variety of coping strategies. Results indicated marked improvement in three of the four clients. The authors suggest that training the family member may reduce the difficulties the client has in generalizing behaviour to real-world settings, since this is primarily where they are learned. McKinlay and Hickox's results support our own in training family members as therapists in the domains of self-care skills and the use of compensatory memory devices (Giles and Shore 1989a, 1989b). They do, however, note the difficulties in managing family dynamics.

LONG-TERM SUPPORT

Family support groups

Model programmes of community support for the brain-injured and their families exist in various parts of the world, but in the vast majority of locations services are inadequate. Headway in Great Britain and the National Head Injury Foundation in the United States organize support groups but these may be geographically thinly spread and difficult for an already overburdened family to attend. Family support groups can offer the relatives a time away from the brain-injured survivor and allow opportunities for family members to voice their concerns and discuss their emotional reaction to caring for their relative. It can also serve as a focus for a referral network.

Client counselling

Counselling the brain-injured client may be difficult and time-consuming. Ongoing counselling, however, can be especially helpful for patients with anxiety and a lack of confidence who are attempting to re-organize their lives in the community. It is important to set appropriate goals to help the clients establish a role for themselves in the family and in their social community. Insight-oriented psychotherapy, for instance, is inappropriate with a client who does not recognize deficits and who is extremely concrete in his or her thinking.

Support groups for the brain-injured

Blanchard (1984) had made a number of suggestions on setting up and running support groups for the brain-injured. The ability of the group leader is likely to be very important in order to

1. stimulate each member's participation and interaction in the group;
2. moderate and interpret for clients, using language they can understand;
3. be stabilizing, organized and calm and prepared to provide a structured approach;

4. work with clients' needs and capitalize on each individual's strength;
5. not deny or minimize the clients' problems;
6. maintain reality boundaries: confront clients with reality in a calm and non-threatening way;
7. introduce role-play of practical situations.

It is important not to impose goals from outside the group. Blanchard noted that interpersonal group behaviour, group cohesion and client's skills should not be devalued because of the client's level of deficit (Blanchard, 1984).

Case management

A case manager is a specialist who is an advocate for the patient and his family, and co-ordinates his rehabilitation and care package from immediately after injury to return to work or long-term care. By maintaining an overall long-term view of the situation, and working closely with the patient and family, referrals can be made to relevant, experienced professionals at the most appropriate time. The role of the case manager also involves not only helping the client and family member organize aspects of life in the early stages, but also in establishing the long-term care and support required when the patient has returned home. The head-injured patient and his relatives need to have a key person to contact especially after the return to the community.

SUMMARY

Early planning for community reintegration is essential if a successful outcome for the brain-injured person is to be achieved. At the earliest opportunity estimates of the patient's likely level of functioning should be made and work directed towards highly concrete goals. Establishing a physically suitable environment which will assist the patient in maintaining his or her level of functioning is an essential component of community reintegration. Long-term supportive services are required by many patients if they are to maintain community living. Support for family members or other carers may also be required to keep the brain-injured individual out of long-term institutionalization. Unfortunately support services are often geographically or financially unattainable.

14

Work skills

INTRODUCTION

Employment brings monetary reward, status, and a sense of personal worth (Brooks *et al.*, 1987). Having a job is very important for most people and many patients believe returning to gainful employment defines 'recovery'. Increasingly therapists are recognizing 'return to work' as a central aspect of the rehabilitation programme following brain trauma.

FACTORS INFLUENCING RETURN TO WORK

Severity of injury

There continues to be considerable dispute in the literature about the likelihood of return to work after brain injury. The populations studied have not been uniform with respect to severity of injury. Definitions of return to work, methods of follow-up and time from treatment to follow-up vary (Giles, 1989). A series of patients followed up from an acute hospital show a higher frequency of vocational return than those from a rehabilitation unit; because the rehabilitation unit only receives a more severely disabled subgroup of patients. Gilchrist and Wilkinson (1979) describe a consecutive series of 84 patients treated on a rehabilitation unit. All patients were unconscious for longer than 24 hours and had a median coma duration of four weeks. Seventy-two patients were followed up nine months to 15 years after injury. Of these patients 28 (38.9%) were working, 17 (23.6%) in the same job as before the injury, and 11 (15.3%) in different work usually of a lower skill level; 27 (37.5%) were at home but not working. Thirteen patients (18%) were in hospital, four in psychiatric units and four patients had died, two of these having commited suicide. Duration of unconsciousness was a major factor affecting outcome. Of those unconscious for between 24 hours and one week, 81% returned to work compared with 46.9% of those unconscious for 2–4 weeks and 18.2% of those unconscious 5–7 weeks. Only 11.1% of those unconscious for eight weeks or longer returned to work (Gilchrist and Wilkinson, 1979). Brooks *et al.* (1987) examined return to work in 98 severely brain-injured patients seven years after injury. Patients and their relatives were asked about the patient's work status in the week before the injury and the week before the interview. Eighty-six percent of patients were employed before injury – 29% after. Within the first four years 27% had returned to work, but five years after injury 70% were still unemployed (Brooks *et al.*, 1987). Jacobs (1988) surveyed individuals with severe brain-injury in Los Angeles and found that 26.7% of patients had their primary source of income from employment compared with 77.9% pre-injury. An additional 13.3% had returned to work post-injury but had been unable to maintain employment.

Age

Brooks *et al.* (1987) found that below the age of 45, there was no effect of age on return to work. However, those individuals aged 45 and over were considerably less likely to return to work than those in the younger age range. Thirty-nine percent of people aged 45 or less returned to work, but only 12% of those aged 45 or older did so. Humphrey and Oddy (1980) suggested that the older patient's lower rate of return to work results both from the patients' reduced power of adaptation and an increasing unwillingness of employers to take on a patient with residual deficits and a reduced working life. Weddell *et al.* (1980) failed to find that age or educational level had an influence on outcome possibly due to the less diverse nature of their sample.

Sex

There is some evidence that women are more likely to return to work than men, but the small numbers of cases makes interpretation difficult (Brooks *et al.*, 1987) and confounding variables (such as type of work) are likely.

Socio-economic factors

Brain-injured unskilled workers are less likely to return to work (21%) then brain-injured managerial workers (50%) (Brooks *et al.*, 1987). Humphrey and Oddy (1980) suggest that the better education and training of those in the higher social classes could result in a higher level of residual skill which allow continued employment. Binder (1986), however, suggests that patients in a higher socio-economic class may find returning to work easier because their jobs offer more flexibility and potential to delegate work to subordinates.

Epilepsy

Miller and Stern (1965) followed up 92 survivors of traumatic brain injury and 18 of these people suffered from epilepsy as a result of the brain injury. Only three patients had changed their jobs because of epilepsy, and only four patients were unemployed solely because of recurrent seizures (Miller and Stern, 1965).

Pre-injury work history

Younger people may have had an irregular work history prior to brain injury and not have established a regular work routine. However, many individuals who suffer brain trauma have problems prior to injury which could hamper them in their work environment. These include learning disability, alcoholism or previous brain injury (Haas *et al.*, 1987). Particularly detrimental for work would be a combination of behavioural and cognitive deficits.

DEFICITS AFFECTING RETURN TO WORK

The majority of studies (Brooks *et al.*, 1987) have found the more severe the injury, the less likely is the patient to return to work (failure to find this relationship may usually be explained as an artifact of a truncated sample where the study was confined to only one end of the spectrum of severity). Within the very severely injured groups of patients, severity *per se* may be of less value in predicting return to work than the precise effects of the injury (Brooks *et al.*, 1987). Cognitive and behavioural/emotional effects of injury have been implicated as important predictors of vocational outcome. A severe injury, resulting in the individual being unable to work for a long period of time, adds to the problem of possible erosion of previously acquired work skills.

Physical impairment

Brooks *et al.* (1987) found no significant differences in return to work between patients with and those without physical deficits. There may however be an effect when physical deficits are considered in conjunction with cognitive or behavioural factors.

Cognitive status

Johnson and Gleave (1987) found that the problems of those who succeed in vocational return were similar to the problems of those who fail. Problems found most frequently are memory impairment, slowness and changes in behaviour and attitude. Amongst the severely injured Brooks and co-workers (1987) found that short-term verbal retention (as measured by the logical memory/immediate of the Wechsler Memory Scale) and attention as measured by the PASAT (rapid presentation) had predictive value. Disorders of cognitive functioning could lead to disorganized behaviour and individuals having problems of retaining their place in day-to-day activities. An employer may not understand the brain-injured workers' difficulties sufficiently to adapt a job appropriately (even when this is possible). For example it may be difficult for an employer to accept that a person is able to perform a familiar task without difficulty but not be able to perform a similar but unfamiliar task. The individual with attention deficits may appear lazy or disinterested to a work supervisor or co-workers. Brain-injured workers may proceed with a task without consideration of how they are going to complete the activity. They may be unable to judge when a task is completed, and the quality of the completed work may be unacceptable. The brain-injured worker may be totally unaware of the inadequacy of his or her efforts. Brain-injured individuals frequently misinterpret social and interpersonal events in their environment and fail to understand why they lose their jobs.

Emotional state

Johnson (1989) has highlighted the importance of having the injured worker experience success during the process of return to work to prevent demoralization. An understanding of the patient's actual deficits is important if appropriate compensatory techniques are to be used but continued experience of failure leads to discouragement and reduced chances of employment. Warr (1983) has shown that unemployment leads to a decline in the chances of employment and Fryer and Warr (1984) showed that unemployment is associated with self-report of poor memory and concentration. One of the goals of therapy must be the maintenance of perceived momentum towards employment and success.

Behaviour

Disinhibition, poor social skills and other disruptive or socially inappropriate behaviours represent severe impediments to vocational functioning. These behaviours may be extreme manifestations of difficulties in adapting to novel environmental demands. Training attempts to assist clients in extinguishing these behaviours. Brooks and co-workers (1987) have pointed out that developing a high level of social interaction/language skills is necessary (though not sufficient) for re-entering competitive employment (Brooks *et al.*, 1987). Central also are higher order self-care skills requiring subtle attention to appearance and grooming (Brooks *et al.*, 1987). The work of Heaton *et al.* (1978) suggests that neuropsychological and personality tests may be useful in predicting employability in individuals with a variety of diagnoses including brain-injury. The MMPI was a particularly powerful predictor with all those in full-time competitive employment scoring within the normal range of all MMPI clinical scales.

Table 14.1 Causes of failure to resume competitive employment after acute rehabilitation

Reduced drive or reduced behavioural control.
Denial of deficits leading to failure to compensate for deficits and unrealistic expectations.
Reduced ability to self-monitor or self-correct errors.
Memory deficits.
Reduced ability to sustain attention.
Poor judgement; inability to weigh factors appropriately; impulsivity.

ESTABLISHING JOB OPTIONS

Jellinek and Harvey (1982) found that active counselling and assistance in pursuing job resources significantly improved the rate of employment in a series of brain-injured patients seen in a medical facility. The patient's pre-morbid functioning, the extent of individual patient's awareness and acceptance of the disability and the family support system all influenced the probability for successful rehabilitation. Appropriate placement and the informed support of employers and co-workers are also vital. Johnson and Gleave (1987) found that both the provision of special work conditions and the maintenance of those conditions over a protracted period were associated with successful return to work. In the Johnson and Gleave (1987) series no one who changed both employer and type of work had a successful return. Johnson and Gleave (1987) noted that the average duration of work trial and altered work conditions was longer than the average total work duration in those who lost their jobs (i.e. those patients who returned to work prematurely were terminated in less time than it took for those who returned more gradually to resume a full workload). Employers of those working in professional occupations were more able to provide moderated work conditions. We have found a trial of work without pay to be of use in persuading employers of workers in more manual employment to re-hire a brain-injured individual. Establishing a relationship with the employer is a prerequisite for a good outcome. It is important to know if the employer is committed to the employee returning to work. Educating the employer and co-workers about the difficulties the brain-injured individual may encounter, and how to help them learn or function more effectively, is a central task in ensuring successful vocational reintegration. The therapist also needs to evaluate the feasibility of adjusting the employment to the employee's needs, e.g. providing extra supervision, more frequent rest periods, daytime work shifts or half days. In our experience the employer's willingness to be flexible often relates more to the interpersonal climate of the job site and the nature of the job than to the employee's particular work history. Some employers are willing to be extremely flexible to accommodate an employee (some of whom may have been marginal workers prior to injury). It is important that employers understand that work reintegration may be a lengthy process and is best accomplished by on-the-job training rather than formalized classroom instruction. An employer must also be informed that for some individuals, change in routine may involve considerable disruption and anxiety until the new routine is learned.

ASSESSMENT OF WORK SKILLS

Vocational assessment considers the abilities and deficits of the brain-injured individual, his relationship with his previous employer, the degree to which a job can be modified, and the different forms of employment or retraining available. Individualized assessment of vocational potential is typically carried out by a physician, a psychologist and an occupational therapist. Additional disciplines may be involved depending on local practice. Industrial therapists (Great Britain) and Certified Vocational Counsellors (United States) have specific skills in vocational rehabilitation. Assessment procedures may be categorized as vocational interest inventories, objective tests relating to sub-skills involved in particular classes of occupation and work trials. The assessment of work skills varies according to the individual's stage of recovery. Vocational interest inventories are typically administered by a psychologist or a vocational specialist. Examples include the Strong Vocational Interest Blank (SVIB) (Hansen, 1985) and the Vocational Preference Inventory (VPI) (Holland, 1985). A language-free vocational interest inventory is available (Becker, 1981) which is made up of 165 pictures of individuals involved in occupations. These are presented in triads and are appropriate for use with the severely impaired.

A number of tests are available which have been used to assess an individual's perceptual-motor ability as this relates to vocational return. The Purdue pegboard measures finger dexterity and has been used to assist in the selection of employees for the industrial (manufacturing) industry. The test-retest reliability is good for the average of three trials. Normative data is available (Mathiowetz *et al.*, 1986). The use of the Purdue pegboard is based on the premise that a small sample of a specialized and complex manual activity will correlate highly with an individual's ability to perform similar tasks. The Minnesota Rate of Manipulations Test and the Minnesota Manual Dexterity Test are both intended to provide samples of arm, hand, eye co-ordination and visuo-perceptual speed which may then be used in an attempt to predict the ability to perform in semi-skilled tasks. Therapists should remember that these tests are intended to correlate with performance of specific types of occupations and not employment *per se*. Another similar test is the Crawford Small Parts Dexterity Test (Crawford and Crawford, 1981). A somewhat more extensive test, referred to as Work Samples, examines in addition to dexterity the subject's ability to integrate performance into a coherent activity. Frequently, however, the reasons for the brain-injured individuals vocational difficulties are not captured by their performance on a 'work sample'. The ability to complete component skills does not mean the individual will be successful in his work environment, as the work setting may need other skills. For example, arriving to work on time and in the right place, working with colleagues and being able to co-ordinate and plan the day's work. In addition the brain-injured worker may have difficulty in self-direction and in adjusting behaviour when problems arise. By systematically defining the needs of the individual's job, retraining can be directed towards the injured worker's specific areas of deficit. An adequate assessment should take into account the demands of the job, analysis of the task requirements, the expectations of the employers, the individual's present skills and his ability to adapt to new situations. As elsewhere 'objective tests' should never be preferred to observations of real samples of behaviour where these are available. Many hospitals have been able to develop volunteer employment sites in various hospital jobs which may be used by therapists to assess the client's work skills. In the 'later stages of recovery from brain injury the hospital-based therapist can work closely with outside agencies for volunteer placement. In Great Britain brain-injured individuals may be assessed by the Employment Rehabilitation Centre (ERC). The ERC may recommend courses of vocational training, special employment schemes or other equipment and aids which may enhance the individual's employment prospects. In the United States assessment and job placement assistance may be available via the Department of Rehabilitation (DR).

Table 14.2 Causes of failure to maintain employment after return to work

Work was not appropriate for the patient's current level of functioning; co-workers/employer ceased 'carrying' the patient (this is often presented to the patient by the employer as a change in job requirements or work rationalization).
Failure to maintain functional compensatory techniques possibly as a result of reinstatement of denial of deficits, social isolation, substance abuse.
Psychiatric illness: e.g. depression, paranoid behaviour, obsessions.
Abortive return to academic pursuits or career change.
Anti-social or disinhibited behaviour; failure to maintain emotional continence, egocentricity.
Disincentives to work.

RETRAINING WORK SKILLS

Hospital-based rehabilitation model

The standard model of vocational rehabilitation for the brain-injured adult is a medical one. Clients are serially assessed, trained and placed (often at separate sites). To be effective this model demands the independent transfer of skills used in one environment to another. Lyons and Morse (1988) have reported the effectiveness of a hospital-based therapeutic work programme (TWP) for brain-injured adults. The programme has eight phases, shown in Table 14.3. As part of a follow-up study an attempt was made to contact by telephone all patients who had been treated in the programme. Of the 32 patients treated one had died and two could not be contacted leaving a total of 29 subjects. Information derived from the interview was confirmed by independent sources in 65% of the cases. Time since discharge range was from 2–39 months (mean 16:2 months). The mean length of time in the TWP was 6.2 months. Length of stay was shorter for subjects who were working at follow-up. Of the 26 patients who were employed pre-injury, 17 were employed at follow-up, four were homemakers, two were students and six were unemployed. Interestingly the authors did not find the expected positive correlation between length of time with a specific employer prior to injury and return to work for the same company. The majority of respondents (80.6%) were working 40 hours per week. 65% of the respondents had 1 or 2 jobs since discharge and 13.8% had three or more. The majority of subjects (78.3) reported that they liked their jobs. Many indicated that they found their jobs challenging and looked forward to going to work. Four respondents said that they did not enjoy their work. Three of the homemakers reported that they would have preferred to be in competitive employment. Fifty-two percent felt that the easiest tasks were those that were repetitious, familiar and made few cognitive demands; 65.2% felt the most difficult aspects of their jobs were those that required memory or new learning and those that had high cognitive demands such as problem-solving and planning or organization. Of the 29 subjects, 22 responded to a self-evaluation of their job performance. Asked to compare their present work skills with their skills prior to injury 19 respondents (82.6%) thought their present work skills were 70–100% or what they had been formerly. Seventeen of this group had been discharged for a year or more. Three respondents who rated themselves 50–65% had been discharged within the past 4 months. The study of Lyons and Morse (1988) suggests the type of outcome which may be expected from work retraining performed during a rehabilitation hospital stay. The report also indicates the difficulties experienced by patients immediately following return to work.

Ben Yishay *et al.* (1987) have reported attempts to assist the post-acute brain-injured person return to work. Time from injury to admission was in the range 4–27 months but all but two patients were 12 months post-injury (possibly indicating

Table 14.3 Eight phases of the Therapeutic Work Program (Lyons and Morse, 1988)

1. Individual assessment and treatment.
2. Group treatment in a variety of skill areas. This includes group treatment in interaction and interpersonal skills, functional retraining, debate and effective communication and family education.
3. Prevocational assessment. Assessment in specific work skills, e.g. constructional tasks, collating, etc. Patient's performance is analysed to assess attention, memory, and organizational and planning skills as well as physical abilities.
4. Therapeutic work groups. Transition from role of patient to role of worker, e.g. time card, seeking assistance, etc. Various forms of work tasks may be used. Emphasis on developing prevocational and work readiness skills (e.g. arriving on time, relating to others, etc.), not on training for specific jobs.
5. Work placements within the hospital. Work placements may occur in a variety of departments. Placements may be varied to suit a patient's functional level by modifying the structure and amount of supervision required, or by modifying the tasks required.
6. Supervised work placements in the community. Placing patients in supervised work situations outside the hospital further integrates them into the worker role and reduces their identification with the patient role.
7. Vocational placement. Competitive or non-competitive employment. DRO provides vocational counselling, conducts work-site evaluations, and meets with former and potential employers to assist with the transition to the actual work setting.
8. Ongoing follow-up. Follow-up to help the individual with any transitional issues and to monitor the patient's status and progress.

Not all patients go through each phase or follow the sequence described.

more severe impairment than the patients in the Lyons and Morse study). Severity of injury varied widely (coma duration was 1–120 days). Although none of those admitted to the programme were working, the population was otherwise highly selected (18–55 years old, IQ of at least 80, ambulatory, only minimally aphasic, no previous brain injury, no history of alcohol or drug abuse or psychiatric history). Patients were treated with cognitive rehabilitation followed by a series of graded occupational trials. Results at discharge showed 64% were competitively employed and 30% non-competitively employed. Of those who were 36 months post-discharge at follow-up, 50% were employed competitively and 22% were non-competitively employed. Patients were able to maintain employment for a period but many patients were unable to remain employed (i.e. the longer post-discharge the lower the percentage of people found to be employed).

The supported employment model

Supported employment involves the provision of on-the-job training and support services to handicapped individuals to allow them to hold competitive employment (which they would otherwise be unable to hold). The major emphasis of the supported employment model is on not excluding even the most handicapped in society from employment. Individual placement, enclave, mobile work crew and small business models are all used. Many centres are now utilizing the supported employment model with various populations so that there is considerable practical experience from which to draw. This 'new' approach is really the application of well-known principles to a new domain. Supported employment takes the best of behavioural methodology and applies it in the naturalistic work setting. Problems of the transfer of skills are therefore avoided. This highly practical approach represents a significant departure from traditional concepts of vocational rehabilitation in which the attainment of independence and productivity is judged in relation to general society norms. The four major components of the supported employment model are job placement, job site training carried out by a job coach, ongoing client assessment and the continuing follow-along component (Kreutzer *et al.*, 1988). On-the-job support may continue for as long as it is required.

Inter-agency co-operation, educational and funding issues are particularly important to the approach. Indeed it could be argued that the truly novel aspects of supported employment are creative funding options. Wehman *et al.* (1988) report a study of the efficacy of supported employment in individuals who have a long history of unemployment or inability to maintain employment. Time in coma averaged 76 days and time since injury five years. Of the 32 clients referred 15 were placed (the reasons for non-placement are not reported). Mean pay levels for this group were $5.52 before injury and $4.43 in supported employment. When followed up 9 months after placement 11 out of the 15 placed were still employed (73.4%). Staff intervention at the job site declined significantly over the time each client was in work. The initial intervention time averaged 90% of the time that the client was in work. By week 28 however this had decreased to 10%. Over the entire course of intervention employment specialists were with the client on the job approximately 50% of the time. Given the size of the sample these results are not significantly different from the results of those of Ben-Yishay and co-workers (1987) who also used a highly selected sample. In addition, since much of the difficulty with this population is not finding, but retaining employment, an adequate assessment of the intervention requires a considerably longer period of follow-up. The low educational attainment and income of this sample prior to injury could lead to an increased level of acceptance on entry level positions than would be found in a sample of brain-injured persons with a higher socio-economic status. Also many of the individuals in this study reportedly had earlier experience of job failure which might affect outcome. While placed and non-placed patients are similar on neuropsychological and MMPI scales, behavioural factors which are central to job placement are not described. The report of Wehman *et al.* (1988) describes an encouraging beginning to research into utilization of the supported employment model with the severely handicapped brain-injured population. The stated objective to work with the most profoundly handicapped makes it of special interest. While of demonstrable efficacy with the mentally retarded, the model is of unproven superiority over other forms of intervention with the brain-injured. Much further research is required to firmly establish supported employment as a general intervention for the severely brain-injured.

RETURNING TO COLLEGE

The central focus of some young people prior to injury was college, and return to college life may therefore be the most appropriate option. The existence of college programmes for brain-injured adults provides special resources in some locations, but evening or day classes that are offered by community groups offer structured settings for return into community and educational environments. Very similar principles however apply to return to college as to work. Return to college should be gradual. Students might begin their return with one class while in the rehabilitation setting to evaluate fatigue, the need to develop compensatory strategies and the ability to follow lectures and other class requirements.

DEVELOPING SPECIFIC COMPONENT SKILLS

Job modification to make daily tasks routine may be the most effective strategy for developing job skills. Visual prompts such as posters illustrating task steps may be helpful for severely impaired clients. 'Place Markers' are physical cues for location: one client with a severe memory impairment would place his backpack in a prominent position where he was working so that after he went to the bathroom or took a break in the lunch room he could find his work station. Organization of materials at the work site and labelling the contents of drawers may dramatically increase the client's productivity. Due to the difficulties experienced by some clients in sustaining attention, several short training periods may be more effective than a small number of lengthy sessions. Directions or check-lists should be kept brief and concise. Tasks may be chained together over several sessions and a task analysis may be used to develop a check-list (a pictorially illustrated check-list if necessary) for the client to follow. This may be the most effective strategy in training a traumatically brain-injured individual. Check-lists should be precise and each step described concretely. A simple step-by-step task analysis helps clients organize their activity. Check-lists may be used to assist the client in monitoring the quality of his/her work. A check-list may instruct a client to check a measurement twice or to go over a step where accuracy is essential. Clients who are resistant to the use of strategies should be encouraged to participate in their creation. For physically handicapped clients careful organization of the work environment may be necessary. Adaptations and equipment, e.g. wheelchair ramps, wheelchair lifts, stair lifts, modified toilets, grab rails, visual alarm systems for telephones, modified lighting, modified machinery and electronic equipment can be utilized. The individual needs to be assessed and the appropriate adaptations and equipment supplied if necessary.

Job performance and the development of new skills will be

impeded by high levels of anxiety. Since return to work may be overburdened with meaning for the client, setting realistic goals and only short work periods may assist him in managing his anxiety. It may take time for a client to habituate to a novel set of distractors. Techniques for developing cognitive skills required for work do not differ from those discussed throughout this text.

STATUTORY SUPPORT SERVICES

In the United States the availability of support services varies considerably from region to region. Unfortunately many of the most innovative services (outside the commercial sector) are supported by special grants or private charity and so are of limited duration. In Great Britain services are less targeted to the brain-injured but are more uniform in character and funding. The British government provides training and incentive schemes to assist its disabled citizens in returning to work. The training schemes are likely to be of limited use to the severely injured. The Job Introduction Scheme exists to encourage employers to take on disabled individuals for a trial period. This allows doubts which the employer may have regarding the client's ability to cope with the proposed job or place of work to be resolved. The usual trial period is six weeks and so does not allow training or time to adapt to disabilities.

In Great Britain, Employment Rehabilitation Centres provide (1) retraining to improve the individual's work capacity within the limits of his residual disabilities (2) reconditioning of basic work behaviours and (3) recommendation of appropriate work replacements. Courses may last 7–8 weeks and may be reduced or extended to meet individual needs. Interests are established and training may be available in commercial or clerical work, bench engineering, machine operating, light work, woodwork, outdoor work, catering, and professional and managerial employment.

Residential training

In Great Britain the Training Division of the Manpower Services Commission sponsors retraining for disabled people in skill centres, colleges of further education, private colleges or with employers. Some individuals may attend residential training colleges. Vocational training in the colleges is intended to prepare disabled people for open employment in industry or commerce. The duration of the courses depends on individual needs; account is taken of learning difficulties and an individual's training may be extended if necessary. As well as technical skills, general instruction about new work situations, for example applying for a job, relationships with work colleagues, trade union membership and what an employer expects of his staff, is provided. Unfortunately the work of Johnson (1989) suggests that the retraining schemes are of limited assistance to brain-injured people (they may be of more assistance to younger people without a work history). Johnson (1989) suggests a number of reasons for their failure including: they are not specifically designed for the brain-injured, they require the transfer of skill (from training site to job) and they are too short.

Travelling to work

In Great Britain grants are available if a disabled individual incurs extra costs in travelling to and from work because of disability. If individuals are severely disabled and cannot travel to work, home-based employment may be possible. Suitable equipment can be loaned to the individual free of charge for as long as it is needed through the Special Aids to Employment scheme. In the United States local government often provides considerable transportation assistance to the disabled. These may include reduced fares, wheelchair accessible buses, special disabled bus services and subsidized taxi fares.

Sheltered work groups

In Great Britain sheltered workgroups provide employment opportunities for individuals with severe disability. Individuals appropriate for sheltered work groups can work, but not at the speed or level which would be acceptable to most employers. The employer provides the work, the work place, tools and training and pays the sponsor for the work done by the disabled person. The sponsor, which is a local authority or a voluntary organization, e.g. Remploy, is the employer and is responsible for paying wages and benefits. The Manpower Services Commission approves the scheme and shares the cost with the sponsor.

Case study 14.1
When admitted to the Transitional Living Centre B.A. was able to wash and dress and perform basic self-care tasks. Once shown his local environment he could find his way around. Areas of deficit included diplopia, poor gait, limited left wrist ROM and decreased wrist and hand strength secondary to a displaced distal radial fracture. All these problems resolved with treatment at the TLC. Continuing problems were a persisting moderate memory impairment, worse for verbally presented information, difficulty in problem solving and a tendency towards mental inflexibility. With training B.A. was able to shop, cook and carry out domestic and community activities of daily living. In work trials conducted with materials provided by his previous employer, he was able to do the tasks requiring transfer of information involving materials handling and shipping. However complex information processing, drawing inferences, and any kind of major decision-making was extremely difficult. He had a tendency to rumination (going over ideas again and again in his mind). Major decisions paralysed B.A. into inactivity. While B.A. was at the treatment facility the patient's wife completed the emotional withdrawal that had begun prior to the injury and which culminated in a divorce; B.A.'s parents lived out of State. Volunteer placement arranged with his employer for two days per week showed B.A. capable of performing the job requirements but he was very tired by a 4-hour work shift. He was capable of going back to his former employer at a lower level of work but left to his own resources was unable to do so. Helping B.A. in his transition to the community involved assisting him to find, organize and move into an apartment, and in arranging routines to help him perform his daily life activities and get to work. From then on the time spent at the TLC was gradually reduced and time at work increased until B.A. returned to full-time employment.

SUMMARY

Vocational evaluation should be integrated into the overall treatment process. A thorough work analysis is essential to assess the likely impact of physical, cognitive and behavioural changes on vocational status and plans. It is important that the client and the therapist have as good an understanding as possible of the client's deficits. Similarly, whilst the employer may understand physical impairments, cognitive problems may be ignored or misinterpreted if appropriate education has not been carried out at the work site. If the client can no longer perform his or her previous job then the possibility of transfer to a similar but less demanding post may be explored. This type of re-entry at a lower level of responsibility allows the employee to use already overlearned skills. Where return to work for the same employer is not possible employment in a related field is advised. In some cases retraining to a new occupation may be indicated. When progress to competitive employment is not possible, volunteer work establishes work experience and various work components skills, e.g. time-keeping, and improves the client's feelings of usefulness and purpose. New models of vocational rehabilitation are becoming available to assist the most handicapped clients. There is increasing recognition for those involved in vocational rehabilitation that the brain-injured represent a population requiring specialized rehabilitation services. The relative efficacy of the various models of rehabilitation is unclear. For many mildly to moderately impaired individuals success at work appears to be heavily influenced by the conditions of work (e.g. availability of part-time or reduced work load). The work of the rehabilitationist should therefore place heavy emphasis on developing the preconditions for successful return to work at the job site and acceptance of the prerequisites of successful return in the prospective worker. The supported employment model may offer a maintenance programme for severely impaired people who would not otherwise be employable.

15

Future directions

INTRODUCTION

In this brief chapter, the prevention of primary and secondary injury and the organization of cost-effective rehabilitation services are discussed. Changes in the law and in public attitudes could have a considerable impact on primary prevention efforts and research is providing new avenues in the prevention of secondary injury. Pressure from organizations of the families of brain-injury survivors, as well as the increasing number of survivors, are helping professionals and policy makers re-evaluate the structure of service provision.

PREVENTION

Haddon (1972) described a logical framework for categorizing highway safety phenomena. An accident can be divided into the pre-event phase, the event phase and the post-event phase. In the pre-event phase, various factors operate which determine if accidents are likely to happen. For example, in driving these would include the types of driving behaviour (e.g. slow reaction times due to the influence of alcohol). The event phase describes the actual incident and safety measures in this phase are directed towards protecting the people and property involved. Measures include seat belts, energy absorbing steering assemblies and impact air bags. Design of both the motor vehicle itself and impactable objects at the roadside, for example lampposts, should attempt to minimize damage. The post-event phase includes attempts to minimize the final effects of the damage after the incident, and therefore includes rescue services and emergency medical systems. It was noted in Chapter one how the introduction of air rescue services decreased mortality in San Diego County (Klauber et al., 1985). Air rescue and transportation (of severely injured individuals to tertiary care centres) is now widely available in the United States. Here, the alteration

of pre-event behaviour (highway safety campaigns and legis-
lations) and event stage interventions is discussed.

The pre-event stage

Job (1988) describes the use of fear in health promotion campaigns. A major disadvantage of fear (or punishment) is that
it does not necessarily direct the person towards the desired
behaviour. The introduction of a competing adaptive behaviour,
which is rewarded, is likely to be more effective.

The anxiety produced by the campaign should not be so
extreme that it leads to denial. Concentration on short-term
effects, such as prosecution for drinking and driving, may be
more effective than highlighting the lethal or maiming consequences of drinking and driving. A mild to moderate anxiety-
producing event, for example being stopped by a police officer,
followed by realistic options, for instance, one sober member
of a group driving people home, is more likely to be effective
(with the relevant prosecutions). Health promotion campaigns
should attempt to shape healthy, sensible behaviour, whereas
high fear evoking campaigns are likely to reduce the effectiveness of subsequent campaigns.

Individuals responsible for fatal or near-fatal accidents are not
representatives of the general population of drivers. Drivers
who cause accidents are usually male between 20 and 35; have
a high school education or less; a previous alcohol-related arrest
or two or more speeding arrests; a suspended or revoked
license; single, separated or divorced; and prefer to drink beer
(Fell, 1977). This information can be used to target individuals
at risk, once they are in the justiciary system (see Fell, 1977 for
a discussion). Decker *et al.* (1988) examined attempts to reduce
mortality from motor vehicle accidents in Tennessee. Raising
the legal drinking age resulted in a 38% decline in alcohol-
related deaths in 19–20-year-olds. The introduction of a legal
measure to stiffen penalties and increase enforcement was
associated with a 33% reduction of alcohol-related deaths in
15–18-year-olds. Decker and co-workers (1988) note, however,
that the reduced mortality is also likely to be due to increased
anti-drink driving publicity and the wave of social disapproval,
which usually precedes and stimulates legislation. The effect in
Tennessee appeared to last at least four years. The pressures
causing changes in behaviour could be particularly effective
with high school students. As noted by Decker and associates
(1988), sustained effort to maintain awareness among high-
school students about the risks of drinking and driving could

address an open-minded, but potentially at risk, population, and have a more significant effect than when attempting to produce significant effects within society as a whole.

The event phase

Seat-belt

Orsay and co-workers (1988) provided further evidence for the efficacy of seat-belt use in reducing the effects of accidents in the USA. The authors evaluated 1364 patients prospectively at Chicago area hospitals and found that those wearing seat-belts were much less severely injured than those not wearing a seat-belt. Only 6.8% of seat-belt wearers required hospital admission, whereas 19.2% of those not wearing seat-belts required hospital admission. Average hospital charges for those with seat-belts were approximately one-third of the charges for the unrestrained driver.

Latimer and Lave (1987) studied the introduction of a seat-belt law in New York state and found the introduction of the law and publicity surrounding it led to a significant reduction in mortality and severe, moderate and mild injury. Williams *et al.* (1987) found reminders, in conjunction with enforcement campaigns, could also be effective. Chorba *et al.* (1988) discovered that a mandatory seat-belt law was effective in reducing the severity of injury in drivers and front seat passengers, when it was introduced in North Carolina. This study did not control for the severity of the crash but alcohol use was still associated with more severe injury. The use of rear seat restraints significantly reduces injury and the severity of injury in rear seat passengers (Christian and Bullimore, 1989). In addition, emphasis should be placed on the use of child restraints and elimination of the practice of children riding unrestrained in open vehicles (for example, pick-up trucks) (Agran *et al.*, 1990).

Helmets

Worrell (1987) studied whether helmets worn by pedal cyclists prevented injury. He examined one hundred consecutively injured patients, of whom eleven were admitted to hospital, eight had loss of consciousness and one died. The author concluded that in all cases, where there was loss of consciousness, severity of injury would have been reduced and, in the case of the fatality, death would have been averted if a helmet had been worn. Dorsh *et al.* (1984) found a statistically significant association between helmet use and reduced severity of head injury in a study of South Australian cycling enthusiasts. Dorsh and associates (1984) estimate that the risk of death from head injury is 3–10 times greater for those cyclists not wearing helmets.

Air bags

The most effective protection in a severe head-on crash is a combination of seat-belt (with shoulder harness) and air bags. Air bags are often considered supplementary restraint systems meaning the air bag is best used in conjunction with a seat-belt. The United States department of transportation issued a ruling in 1984 stating that all new automobiles must be equipped with passive restraints (automatic seat-belts and/or air bags) from 1990 onwards. The air bag inflates automatically at an impact of a certain velocity (usually of 12 miles per hour or faster) following the initial impact, but prior to the 'human collision' where the moving occupants slams into the hard interior surface. The air bag, which inflates in 1/25 seconds, diffuses the harmful forces of the collision by acting as a cushion between the occupants and the vehicle interior.

Post-event phase

Biochemical interventions

Some neurones are destroyed or damaged at the time of the initial injury and intrinsic neurophysiological processes occur which cause neurones to die hours or days later. Recently, a good deal of effort has focused on attempts to interrupt these intrinsic destructive processes. Various research groups have studied the possible efficacy of anticholinergic agents (Lyeth *et al.*, 1985; Dixon *et al.*, 1985; Hayes *et al.*, 1985) catecholaminergic agents (Feeney *et al.*, 1982), opiate antagonists (McIntosh *et al.*, 1986), free radical scavengers (Suzuki *et al.*, 1987) and other agents (Karpiak, 1983). It is hoped that the introduction of one of these (or an undiscovered compound) can interrupt the chain of events which currently result in late neuronal death. Although currently largely limited to animal models, the introduction of this type of treatment could have beneficial results. Research continues into the transplantation of neuronal material with controversial results (Lipton, 1989) and other neurochemical and structural methods of promoting cell process regeneration also continues (Lipton, 1989).

UNIFIED TREATMENT SERVICES

From a rehabilitation management perspective, provision of services must be balanced in some way with the cost of service. Services must retain their client-centred orientation but, at the same time, relate to clinical effort and outcome. Programmes are needed which increase the patient's level of functioning in the community (however defined) and reduce emotional distress. This requires careful documentation and ways of evaluating clinical efforts.

The aim is to develop interventions which require the minimum in financial resources and provide the greatest return in helping individuals become well-functioning and self-respecting in the community. One of the key elements here is to provide the required services in a way that movement towards reducing service demand is maintained. It is important to have a range of services allowing for flexibility of approach and to have appropriate entry and discharge criteria. At possible entry, it must be determined if the client is an appropriate referral. Planning the rehabilitation/care must involve an evaluation of the issues, the goals and the likely discharge placement (wherever possible). Ongoing review is essential as goals are met and the situation changes.

In order to prepare for discharge, placement and follow-up services should include

1. treatment to raise an individual's level of functioning by influencing the individual's behaviour or life situation;
2. intervention to prevent deterioration to a lower level of function;
3. support to maintain an individual in a community setting, the level of support relating to the level of dysfunction.

Case management would provide the individual with a person who traces progress, consults about transfer between services and designs the optimum service package.

SUMMARY

Progress continues to be made in the spheres of brain injury prevention and early and late treatment approaches. Therapists have a duty to advocate for effective preventative measures to be introduced.

Conclusion

The reader of the this book will have noted that many of the same theoretical issues recur in many domains. For example, similar considerations apply to motor skills acquisition as to the learning of other functional tasks. The neurofunctional approach provides a preliminary formulation of a way to manipulate the learning environment to maximize the reacquisition of functional skills and the development of emotional well-being in brain-injured individuals. Goals of rehabilitation must take into account the constraints on human learning established by the neurological disruption as well as the individual's social and environment context. Only by developing an understanding of how and why performance breaks down can therapists develop rational interventions. The key variables to be manipulated by the therapist are attention and practice in a certain class of action, for instance, attending and practicing what needs to be learned and not something else.

Central to an understanding of many of the problems experienced by patients is an appreciation of the role of the frontal lobes in the development of novel action plans. The highest level of complex human function requires the ability to plan and use those plans to execute novel behaviours. Plans can also be used as referents for interrupting 'stimulus generated' or automatic behaviours. Although the relationship appears very complex the regulative function of the frontal lobes is undoubtedly involved in these activities. There is evidence that as behaviours become overlearned, participation of the frontal lobes is required less and less, thus explaining the reason why practiced behaviours are less cognitively demanding. Patients whose frontal lobe functioning is impaired have difficulty in planning and using these plans to govern action. Even patients with mild deficits can have difficulty in initiating highly novel behaviours. Moderately impaired patients have difficulty in generating plans of action over time and in forseeing the consequences of their actions. In addition, these individuals may be unable to suppress powerful response tendencies and engage in impulsive or poorly thought out behaviours. For some patients planning of novel behaviours and complex problem solving may be impossible. Patients can achieve many functional activities with practice and by establishing appropriately selected routine procedures. Patients with the most profound impairments could have difficulty in initiating any action. Rehabilitation involves an attempt to create overlearnt behaviours so they become activated even when patients have profound difficulties in initiation. Much of the change in behaviour resulting from treatment is probably subserved by a combination of procedural and semantic learning. The role of procedural acquisition of skills in humans has been underestimated, but can be very effective. Social skills retraining, for example, could be designed to make use of procedural learning via specific training programmes and more non-specific manipulation of the environment by setting events. The development of the neurofunctional approach has been an attempt to describe a rational approach to therapy for the brain-injured individual, the goal being to assist in the redevelopment of functional behaviours.

References and further reading

Abreu, B. C. and Toglia, J. P. (1987) Cognitive rehabilitation – a model for occupational therapy. *The American Journal of Occupational Therapy*, **41**, 439–48.

Achte, K. A., Hillbom, E. and Aalberg, V. (1969) Psychoses following war brain injuries. *Acta Psychiatrica Scandinavica*, **45**, 1–8.

Acker, C., Jacobson, R. R. and Lishman, W. A. (1987) Memory and ventricular size in alcoholics. *Psychological Medicine*, **17**, 343–8.

Acton, N. (1982) The world's response to disability: evolution of a philosophy. *Archives of Physical Medicine and Rehabilitation*, **63**, 145–9.

Adams, A. L. (1978) Theoretical issues for knowledge of results, in *Information Processing in Motor Control and Learning*, (ed G. E. Stelmach), Academic Press, New York, pp. 229–40.

Adams, J. A. (1971) A closed-loop theory of motor learning. *Journal of Motor Behaviour*, **3**, 111–49.

Adams, J. A. (1976) Issues for a closed-loop theory of motor learning, in *Motor Control: Issues and Trends*, (ed G. E. Stelmach), Academic Press, New York, pp. 87–107.

Adams, J. A., Goetz, E. T., and Marshall, P. H. (1972) Response feedback and motor learning. *Journal of Experimental Psychology*, **92**, 391–7.

Adams, J. H., Graham, D. I. and Gennarelli, T. A. (1983) Contemporary neuropathological considerations regarding brain damage in head injury. Central Nervous System Trauma Status Report. National Institute of Neurological and Communicative Disorders and Stroke.

Adams, J. H., Graham, D. I., Scott, G. *et al.* (1980a) Brain damage in fatal non-missile head injury. *Journal of Clinical Pathology*, **33**, 1132–45.

Adams, J. H., Scott, G., Parker, L. S. *et al.* (1980b). The contusion index: a quantitative approach to cerebral contusions in head injury. *Neuropathology and Applied Neurobiology*, **2**, 323–32.

Agran, P. F., Winn, D. G. and Castillo, D. N. (1990) Pediatric injuries in the back of pickup trucks. *Journal of the American Medical Association*, **264**, 712–16.

Aiken, L. R. (1987) *The Assessment of Intellectual Functioning*. Allyn and Bacon Inc., Boston.

Alberico, A. M., Ward, J. D., Choi, S. C. *et al.* (1987) Outcome after severe head injury: Relationship to mass lesion, diffuse injury and ICP course in pediatric and adult patients. *Journal of Neurosurgery*, **67**, 648–56.

Alberti, R. E. and Emmons, M. L. (1982) *Your Perfect Right: A guide to assertive living* (4th edn.) Impact Publishers, San Luis Obispo, California.

Alexander, J. L. and Fuhrer, M. J. (1984) Functional assessment of individuals with physical handicaps, in *Functional Assessment in Rehabilitation* (eds A. S. Halpern and M. J. Fuhrer), Paul H. Brookes, pp. 45–59.

Alexander, J. L. and Willems, E. (1981) Quality of life: Some measures requirements. *Archives of Physical Medicine and Rehabilitation*, **62**, 261–6.

Alexander, M. P., Stuss, D. T. and Benson, D. F. (1979) Capgras syndrome and reduplication phenomenon. *Neurology*, **29**, 334–9.

Alexandre, A., Colombo, F., Nertempi, P. and Benedetti, A. (1983) Cognitive outcome and early indices of severity of head injury. *Journal of Neurosurgery*, **59**, 751–61.

Allen, C. K. (1982) Independence through activity: The practice of occupational therapy (psychiatry). *American Journal of Occupational Therapy*, **36**, 731–9.

Allport, D. A., Antonis, B. and Reynolds, P. (1972) On the division of attentions: a disproof of the single channel hypotheses. *Quarterly Journal of Experimental Psychology*, **24**, 225–35.

American Psychiatric Association (1987) *The Diagnostic and Statistical Manual of Mental Disorders*, 3rd edn, American Psychiatric Association, Washington.

Anastasi, A. (1988) *Psychological Testing*, 6th edn, Macmillan Publishing Company, New York.

Anderson, D. W. and McLaurin, R. L. (eds) (1980) The national head and spinal cord injury survey. *Journal of Neurosurgery* (Supplement) S21.

Anderson, J. R. and Bower, G. H. (1973) *Human Associative Memory*, Winston, Washington D.C.

Anderson, T. P. (1989) Rehabilitation 'Treatment' (versus training) for 'recovery'. *Archives of Physical Medicine and Rehabilitation*, **70**, 647.

Annegers, J. F., Grabow, J. D., Kurland, L. T. and Laws, E. R. (1980) The incidence, causes and secular trends in head trauma in Olmstead county, Minnesota, 1935–1974. *Neurology*, **30**, 912–19.

Anokhin, P. K. (1969) Cybernetics and the integrative activity of the brain, in *A Handbook of Contemporary Soviet Psychology*, (eds M. Cole and I. Maltzman), Basic Books, New York, pp. 830–56.

Argyle, M. (1981) *Social Skills and Health*, Methuen, London.

Armstrong, K. K., Sahgal, V., Block, R. *et al.* (1990) Rehabilitation outcomes in patients with post-traumatic epilepsy. *Archives of Physical Medicine and Rehabilitation*, **71**, 156–60.

Arts, W. F. M., Van Dongen, H. R., Van Hof-Van Duin, J. V. and Lammens, E. (1985) Unexpected improvement after prolonged post-traumatic vegetative state. *Journal of Neurology, Neurosurgery and Psychiatry*, **48**, 1300–3.

Atkinson, R. C. and Shiffrin, R. M. (1968) Human memory: a proposed system and its control processes, In *The Psychology of learning and motivation: Advances in Research and Theory*, vol 2, (eds K. W. Spence and J. T. Spence), Academic Press, New York, pp. 89–195.

Bach-Y-Rita, P. (ed) (1980) *Recovery of Function: Theoretical considerations for Brain Injury Rehabilitation*, University Park Press, Baltimore.

Bach-Y-Rita, G., Lion, J., Climent, C. and Ervin, F. (1978) Episodic dyscontrol: A study of 130 violent patients. *American Journal of Psychiatry*, **127**, 1473–8.

Baddeley, A. D. and Warrington, E. K. (1973) Memory coding and amnesia. *Neuropsychologia*, **11**, 159–65.

Baddeley, A. D., and Hitch, G. (1974) Working Memory, in *The Psychology of Learning and Motivation*, vol 8, (ed G. H. Bower), Academic Press, New York, pp. 47–89.

Baethmann, A. (1987) Multidisciplinary international symposium: Mechanisms of secondary brain damage. February 23–26, 1986. Mauls/Vipitino, Italy. *Neurosurgery*, **20**, 343–4.

Baker, L. L., Parker, K. and Sanderson, D. (1983) Neuromuscular electrical stimulation of the head-injured patient. *Physical Therapy*, **63**, 1967–74.

Balliet, R., Blood, K. M. T. and Bach-Y-Rita, P. (1985) Visual Rehabilitation in the cortically blind? *Journal of Neurology, Neurosurgery and Psychiatry*, **48**, 1113–24.

Balliet, R., Harbst, K. B., Kim, D. and Stewart, R. V. (1987) Retraining of functional gait through the reduction of upper extremity weight-bearing in chronic cerebellar ataxia. *International Rehabilitation Medicine*, **8**, 148–53.

Banaji, M. R. and Crowder, R. G. (1989) The bankruptcy of everyday memory. *American Psychologist*, **44**, 1185–93.

Bandura, A. (1977) *Social Learning Theory*, Prentice-Hall, Englewood Cliffs, NJ.

Barnard, P., Dill, H., Edgredge, P. *et al.* (1984) Reduction of hypertonicity by early casting in a comatose head-injured individual, *Physical Therapy*, **64**, 1540–2.

Baron, J. C., Bousser, M. G., Comar, D. and Castaigne, P. (1980) Crossed cerebellar diaschisis in human supratentorial brain infarction. *Annals of Neurology*, **8**, 128.

Barrer, A. E. and Girard, D. (1987) A systems approach to working with families. Paper presented at Head Injury Frontiers: Sixth Annual National Head Injury Symposium, San Diego, California.

Barry, P., Clark, D. E., Yaguda, M. *et al.* (1989) Rehabilitation inpatient screening of early cognitive recovery. *Archives of Physical Medicine and Rehabilitation*, **70**, 902–6.

Basmajian, J. V., Gowland, C. A., Finlayson, M. A. J. *et al.* (1987) Stroke treatment: Comparison of integrated behavioural-physical therapy vs traditional physical therapy programs. *Archives of Physical Medicine and Rehabilitation,* **68**, 267–72.

Bates, D., Caronna, J. J., Cartlidge, N. E. F. *et al.* (1977) A prospective study of nontraumatic coma: Methods and results in 310 patients. *Annals of Neurology,* **2**, 211–20.

Battig, W. F., (1979) The flexibility of human memory, in *Levels of Processing in Human Memory,* (eds L. S. Cermak and F. I. M. Craik), Erlbaum, Hillsdale. NJ. pp. 23–44.

Bauer, R. M. and Rubens, A. B. (1985) Agnosia, in *Clinical Neuropsychology,* 2nd edn, (eds K. M. Heilman and E. Valenstein), Oxford University Press, New York, pp. 187–241.

Baum, B. and Hal, K. M. (1981) Relationship between constructional praxis and dressing in the head-injured adult. *American Journal of Occupational Therapy,* **35**, 438–42.

Baxt, W. G. and Moody, P. (1987a) The differential survival of trauma patients. *The Journal of Trauma,* **27**, 602–6.

Baxt, W. G. and Moody, P. (1987b) The impact of advanced prehospital emergency care on the mortality of severely brain injured patients. *The Journal of Trauma,* **27**, 365–9.

Baxter, D. M. and Warrington, E. K. (1986) Ideational agraphia: a single case study. *Journal of Neurology, Neurosurgery and Psychiatry,* **49**, 369–74.

Baxter, R., Cohen, S. B. and Ylvisaker, M. (1985) Comprehensive cognitive assessment, in *Head Injury Rehabilitation: Children and Adolescents,* (ed M. Ylvisaker) College Hill Press, San Diego, pp. 247–74.

Beatty, W. W., Salmon, D. P. Bernstein, N. *et al.* (1987) Procedural learning in a patient with amnesia due to hypoxia. *Brain and Cognition,* **6**, 386–402.

Beck, A. T., Rush, A. J., Shaw, B. F. and Emory, G. (1979) *Cognitive Therapy of Depression: A Treatment Manual,* Guilford, New York.

Beck, A. T., Ward, C. H., Mendelson, M. *et al.* (1961) An inventory for measuring depression. *Archives of General Psychology,* **4**, 561–71.

Becker, D. P., Miller, D., Ward, J. D. *et al.* (1977) The outcome from severe head injury with early diagnosis and intensive management. *Journal of Neurosurgery,* **47**, 491–502.

Becker, G. M. and McClintock, C. G. (1967) Value: behaviour decision theory. *Annual Review of Psychology,* **18**, 239–86.

Becker, R. L. (1981) *Reading-Free Vocational Interest Inventory,* Edmark Corporation, Bellevue, Washington.

Bellack, A. S. (1979) A critical appraisal of strategies for assessing social skills. *Behavioural Assessment,* **1**, 157–76.

Bellack, A. S. and Hersen, M. (1978) Chronic psychiatric patients: Social skills training, in *Behaviour Therapy in the Psychiatric Setting,* (eds M. Hersen and A. S. Bellack), Williams and Wilkins, Baltimore, pp. 169–95.

Bellack, A. S., Hersen, M. and Lamparski, D. (1979) Role-play tests for assessing social skills: are they valid? are they useful? *Journal of Consulting and Clinical Psychology,* **47**, 335–42.

Ben-Yishay, Y., Diller, L. and Rattok, J. (1978) A modular approach to optimizing orientation, psychomotor alertness and purposive behaviour in severe head trauma patients, in *Working Approaches to Remediation of Cognitive Deficits in Brain Damaged Persons*, Rehabilitation Monographs No. 50, Institute of Rehabilitation Medicine, New York University Medical Center, New York, pp. 63–7.

Ben-Yishay, Y., Silver, S. M., Piasetsky, E. *et al.* (1987) Relationship between employability and vocational outcome after intensive holistic cognitive rehabilitation. *Journal of Head Trauma Rehabilitation*, **2**, 35–48.

Bender, M. B. (1952) *Disorders of Perception*, C. C. Thomas, Springfield, Illinois.

Bennett-Levy, J. and Powell, G. E. (1980) The Subjective Memory Questionnaire (SMQ). An investigation into the self-reporting of real-life memory skills. *British journal of Social and Clinical Psychology*, **19**, 177–88.

Benson, D. F., Gardner, H. and Meadows, J. C. (1976) Reduplication Paramnesia. *Neurology*, **26**, 147–51.

Benton, A. L. (1969) Disorders of spacial orientation, in *Handbook of Clinical Neurology*, Vol 3, (eds P. J. Vinken and G. W. Bruyn), North-Holland Publishing Company, pp. 212–28.

Benton, A. (1979) Behaviourial consequences of closed head injury. Central nervous system trauma status report. National Institutes of Health, Washington D. C.

Benyakar, M., Tadir, M., Groswasser, Z. and Stern, M. J. (1988) Dreams in head-injured patients. *Brain Injury*, **2**, 351–6.

Berlyne, D. E. (1951) Attention to change. *British Journal of Psychology*, **42**, 269–79.

Bernstein, N., (1967) *The Co-ordination and Regulation of Movement*, Pergammon Press, London.

Berrol, S. (1986a) Evolution and the persistent vegatative state. *Journal of Head Trauma Rehabilitation*, **1**, 7–13.

Berrol, S. (1986b) Considerations of management of the persistent vegetative state. *Archives of Physical Medicine and Rehabilitation*, **67**, 283–5.

Berrol, S. (1988) Risk of restraint in head injury. *Archives of Physical Medicine and Rehabilitation*, **69**, 537–8.

Beukelman, D. R., Yorkston, K. M. and Losing, C. A (1984) Functional communication assessment of adults with neurogenic disorders, in *Functional Assessment in Rehabilitation*, (eds A. S. Halpern and M. J. Fuhrer), Paul H. Brookes, Baltimore and London,

Bilodeau, E. A., and Bilodeau, I. M. (1958) Variable frequency of knowledge of results and the learning of a simple skill. *Journal of Experimental Psychology*, **55**, 379–83.

Bilodeau, E. A. and Ryan F. J. (1960) A test for interaction of delay of knowledge of results and two types of interpolated activity. *Journal of Experimental Psychology*, **59**, 414–9.

Binder, L. M. (1986) Persisting symptoms after mild head injury: a review of the post-concussive syndrome. *Journal of Clinical and Experimental Neurosychology*, **8**, 323–46.

Binder, L. M., and Schreiber, J., (1980) Visual Imagary and verbal mediation as memory aids in recovering alcoholics. *Journal of Clinical Psychology*, **2**, 71–4.

Bird, A. M. and Riki, R. (1983) Observational learning and practice variability. *Research Quarterly for Exercise and Sport*, **54**, 1–4.

Birdwhistell, R. L. (1970) *Kinesics and Context: Essays on Body Motion Communication*, University of Pennsylvania Press, Philadelphia.

Bishop, B. (1982) Neural plasticity 4. *Physical Therapy*, **62**, 1442–51.

Bishop, D., Baldwin, L., Epstein, N and Keitner, G. (1984) Assessment of family functioning, in *Functional Assessment in Rehabilitation Medicine*, (eds C. V. Granger and C. E. Gresham), Williams and Wilkins, Baltimore and London, pp. 305–23.

Bishop, D. S. and Miller, I. W. (1988) Traumatic brain injury: Empirical family assessment techniques. *Journal of Head Trauma Rehabilitation*, **3**, 16–30.

Bisiach, E., Capitani, E. Luzzatti, C. and Perani, D. (1981) Brain and conscious representation of outside reality. *Neuropsychologia*, **19**, 543–51.

Bjork, R. A. and Allen, T. W. (1970) The spacing effect: Consolidation or differential encoding. *Journal of Verbal Learning and Verbal Behaviour*, **9**, 567–72.

Black, B., Adler, J. E., Dreyfus, C. F. *et al.* (1988) Experience and the biochemistry of information storage in the nervous system, in *Perspectives in Memory Research*, (ed. M. S. Gazzaniga), The MIT Press, Cambridge, Massachusetts, pp 3–22.

Black, P., Markowitz, R. S. and Cianci, S. N. (1975) Recovery of motor function after lesions in the motor cortex of monkey. In CIBA Foundation Symposium 34. New Series. Outcome of Severe Damage to the Central Nervous System. Elsevier, Amsterdam.

Blanchard, M. K. (1984) *Counselling Head Injured Patients: Guidelines for Community Mental Health Workers*, New York State Head Injury Association, New York.

Bloom, B. S. and Broder. L. J. (1950) *Problem-Solving Processes of College Students*, University of Chicago Press, Chicago.

Bobath, B. (1978) *Adult Hemiplegia: Evaluation and Treatment*, Heinemann, London

Boller, F. (1982) *Sexual Dysfunction in Neurological Disorders: Diagnosis Management and Rehabilitation*, Raven Press, New York, p. 141.

Bond, M. R. (1975) Assessment of the psychosocial outcome after severe head injury, in CIBA Foundation Symposium 34. New Series. Outcome of Severe Damage to the Central Nervous System, Elsevier, Amsterdam, pp 141–57.

Bond, M. R. (1976) Assessment of the psychosocial outcome of severe brain injury. *Acta Neurochirgica*, **34**, 57–70.

Booth, B. J., Doyle, M. and Montgomery, J. (1983) Serial casting for the management of spasticity in the head-injured adult. *Physical Therapy*, **63**, 1961–6.

Bornstein, B., Sroka, H., and Munitz, H. (1969) Prosopagnosia with animal face agnosia, *Cortex*, **5**, 164–9.

Bornstein, R. A., Miller, H. and Schoor, J. T. (1989) Neuropsychological deficit and emotional disturbance in head-injured patients. *Journal of Neurosurgery*, **70**, 509–13.

Borod, J. C., Koff, E. and White, B. (1983) Facial asymmetry in posed and spontaneous expression of emotion. *Brain and Cognition*, **2**, 165–75.

Botte, M. J. and Moore, T. J. (1987) The orthopedic management of extremity injuries in head trauma. *The Journal of Head Trauma Rehabilitation*, **2**, 13–27.

Boughton, A. and Ciesla, N. (1986) Physical therapy management of the head-injured patient in the intensive care unit. *Topics in Acute Care and Trauma Rehabilitation*, **1**, 1–18.

Bowe F. G. (1979) Transportation: A key to independent living. *Archives of Physical Medicine and Rehabilitation*, **60**, 483–6.

Bowman, B. R. and Baker, L. L. (1985) Effects of waveform parameters on comfort during transcutaneous neuromuscular electrical stimulation. *Annals of Biomedical Engineering*, **13**, 59–74.

Bradley, K. P. (1982) The effectiveness of constructional praxis tests in predicting upper extremity dressing abilities. *Occupational Therapy Journal of Research*, **2**, 184–5.

Bransford, J. D. and McCarrell, N. S. (1977) A sketch of a cognitive approach to comprehension, in *Thinking: Readings in Cognitive Science*, (eds P. N. Johnson-Laird and P. C. Wason), Cambridge University Press, Cambridge,

Braun, C. M. J., Baribeau, J. M. C. and Ethier, M. (1988) A prospective investigation compairing patients' and relatives' symptom reports before and after a rehabilitation program for severe closed head injury. *Journal of Neurological Rehabilitation*, **2**, 109–15.

Braun, C. M. J., Lussier, F., Baribeau, J. M. C. and Ethier, M. (1989) Does severe traumatic closed head-injury impair sense of humor. *Brain-Injury*, **3**, 345–54.

Braunling-McMorrow, D., Lloyd, K. and Fralish, K. (1986) Teaching social skills to brain injured adults. *Journal of Rehabilitation*, Jan/Feb/March, 39–44.

Bricolo. A., Turrazzi, S. and Feriotti, G. (1980) Prolonged post-traumatic unconsciousness: Therapeutic assets and liabilities. *Journal of Neurosurgery*, **52**, 625–34.

Brink, J. D., Imbus, C. and Woo-Sam, J. (1980) Physical recovery after severe closed head trauma in children and adolescents. *Journal of Pediatrics*, **97**, 721–7.

Brismar, B., Engstrom, A. and Rydberg, U. (1983) Head injury and intoxication: a diagnostic and therapeutic dilemma. *Acta Chirugica Scandinavica*, **149**, 11–14.

Broadbent, D. (1958) *Perception and Communication*, Pergamon Press, Oxford.

Brooks, D. N. (1984) *Closed Head Injury: Psychosocial, Social and Family Consequences*, Oxford University Press, Oxford.

Brooks, D. N., Campsie, L., Symington, C. *et al.* (1986) The five year outcome of severe blunt head injury: A relative's view. *Journal of Neurology, Neurosurgery and Psychiatry*, **49**, 764–70.

Brooks, D. N., Symington, C., Beattie, A. *et al.* (1989) Alcohol and other predictors of cognitive recovery after severe head injury. *Brain Injury*, **3**, 235–46.

Brooks, D. N. (1972) Memory and head injury. *The Journal of Nervous and Mental Disease*, **155**, 350–5.

Brooks, D. N. (1975) Long and short-term memory in head injury patients. *Cortex*, **11**, 329–40.

Brooks, D. N. and Baddeley, A. D. (1976) What can amnesics learn? *Neuropsychologia*, **14**, 111–22.

Brooks, D. N., and McKinlay, W. W. (1983) Personality and behavioural change after severe blunt head injury. *Journal of Neurology, Neurosurgery and Psychiatry*, **46**, 336–44.

Brooks, D. N., Hosie, J., Bond, M. R. *et al.* (1986) Cognitive sequelae of severe head injury in relation to the Glasgow outcome scale. *Journal of Neurology, Neurosurgery and Psychiatry*, **49**, 549–53.

Brooks, N., McKinlay, W., Symington, C. *et al.* (1987) Return to work within the first seven years of head injury. *Brain Injury*, **1**, 5–19.

Brotherton, F. A., Thomas, L. L., Wisotzek, I. E. and Milan, M. A. (1988) Social skills training in the rehabilitation of patients with traumatic head injury. *Archives of Physical Medicine and Rehabilitation*, **69**, 827–32.

Brown, M., Diller, L., and Gordon, W. A. (1982) Functional assessment and outcome measurement: an integrative review. *Annual Review of Rehabilitation*, **3**, 93–120.

Bruce, D. (1983) Head trauma management, in *Handbook of Neuroanesthesis*, (eds P. Newfield and J. E. Cottrell), Little Brown, Boston, pp. 282–301.

Brudney, J. B. Korein, J., Grynbaum, B. B. *et al.* (1976) EMG Feedback Therapy: Review of Treatment of 114 Patients. *Archives of Physical Medicine and Rehabilitation*, **57**, 55–61.

Bruett, T. L. and Overs, R. P. (1968) A critical review of 12 ADL scales. *Physical Therapy*, **49**, 859–61.

Brunstromm, S. (1970) *Movement Therapy in Hemiplegia: A Neurophysiological Approach*, Harper Row, New York.

Bryant, E.T., Scott, M.L., Golden, C.J. and Tori, C.D. (1984) Neuropsychological deficits, learning disability and violent behavior. *Journal of Consulting and Clinical Psychology*, **52**, 323–4.

Burke, D. (1980) A reassessment of the muscle spindle contribution to muscle tone in normal and spastic man, in *Spasticity: Disordered Motor Control*, (eds. R.G. Feldman, R.R. Young and W.P. Koella), Year Book Medical Publications, Chicago, pp. 261–78.

Burke, W.H. Wesolowski, M.D. and Lane, I.M. (1988) A positive approach to the treatment of aggressive brain-injured clients. *International Journal of Rehabilitation Research*, **11**, 235–41.

Buschke, H., and Fuld, P. (1974) Evaluating storage, retention and retrieval in disordered memory and learning. *Neurology*, **24**: 1019–25.

Canavan, Y.M., O'Flaherty, M.J., Archer, D.B. and Elwood, J.H. (1980) A 10-year survey of eye injuries in Northern Ireland 1967–1976. *British Journal of Ophthalmology*, **64**, 618–25.

Cannon, W.B. and Rosenblueth, A. (1949) *The Supersensitivity of Denervated Structures*, Macmillan, New York.

Caplan, A.L., Callahan, D. and Haas, J. (1987) Ethics and policy issues in rehabilitation medicine. A Hastings Center Report: Special Supplement.

Carberry, H. and Burd, B. (1985) The use of psychological theory and content as a media in the cognitive and social training of brain injured patients. *Cognitive Rehabilitation*, July/August, 8–10.

Caresia, L., Pugnetti, L., Besana, R. *et al.* (1984) EEG and clinical findings during pemoline treatment in children and adults with attention deficits disorder. *Neuropsychobiology*, **11**, 158–67.

Carr, J.H., and Shepherd, R. (1980) *Physiotherapy in Disorders of the Brain*, Heinmann Medical Books Limited.

Carter, L.T., Howard, B.E. and O'Neil, W.A. (1983) Effectiveness of cognitive skill remediation in acute stroke patients. *Americal Journal of Occupational Therapy*, **37**, 320–6.

Cartlidge, N.E. and Shaw, D.A. (1981) *Head Injury*, WB Saunders, London.

Cassidy, J.W. (1990a) Neurochemical substrates of aggression: towards a model for improved intervention, part 1. *Journal of Head Trauma Rehabilitation*, **5**, 83–6.

Cassidy, J.W. (1990b) Neurochemical substracts of aggression towards a model for improved intervention, part 2. *Journal of Head Trauma Rehabilitation*, **5**, 70–3.

Casson. J.R., Siegel, O., Sham, R. *et al.* (1984) Brain damage in modern boxers. *JAMA*, **251**, 2663–7.

Catalano, J.F. and Kleiner, B. M. (1984) Distant transfer in coincident timing as a function of variability in practice. *Perceptual and Motor Skills*, **58**, 851–6.

Catania, A.C., Mathews, B.A. and Shimoff, E. (1982) Instructed versus shaped human verbal behavior: Interactions with nonverbal responding. *Journal of the Experimental Analysis of Behavior*, **38**; 233–48.

Cermak, L.S. (1976) The encoding capacity of a patient with amnesia due to encephalitis. *Neuropsychologia*, **14**, 311–26.

Chan, C.W.Y. (1986) Motor and Sensory deficits following a stroke: Relevance to a comprehensive evaluation. *Physiotherapy Canada*, **38**, 29–34.

Cherry, D.B. (1980) Review of physical therapy alternatives for reducing muscle contracture. *Physical Therapy*, **60**; 877–81.

Cherry, D.B. and Weigand, G.M. (1981) Plaster drop out splints as a dynamic means to reduce muscle contracture. *Physical Therapy*, **61**, 1601–3.

Childs, A. (1987) Naltrexone in organic bulimia: a preliminary report. *Brain Injury*, **1**, 49–55.

Chorba, T.L., Reinfurt, D. and Hulka, B.S. (1988) Efficacy of mandatory seatbelt use legislation: The North Carolina experience from 1983 through 1987, *JAMA*, **260**, 3593–7.

Christian, M.S. and Bullimore, D.W. (1989) Reduction in accident injury severity in rear seat passengers using restraints. *Injury*, **20**, 262–4.

Cicerone, K.D., Lawar, R.M. and Shapiro, W.R. (1983) Effects of frontal lobe lesions on hypothesis sampling during concept formation. *Neuropsychologia*, **21**, 513–24.

Ciminero, A.R., Calhoun, K.S., and Adams, H.E. (eds) (1977). *Handbook of Behavioural Assessment*, Wiley, New York.

Clark-Wilson (1988) The use of a computer in aiding functional skills training: a single case study. *Clinical Rehabilitation*, **2**, 199–206.

Clark-Wilson, J. and Gent. A. (1989) A conductive education approach to individuals with motor disorders. *British Journal of Occupational Therapy*, **52**, 271–2.

Clarke, J.M. (1974) Distribution of microglial scars in the brain after head injury. *Journal of Neurology, Neurosurgery and Psychiatry*, **34**, 463–74.

Coates, H. and King, A. (1982) *The Patient Assessment. A Handbook for Therapists*, Churchill Livingstone, Edinburgh.

Cohen, B.F. and Anthony, W.A. (1984) Functional Assessment in Psychiatric Rehabilitation, in *Functional Assessment in Rehabilitation*, (eds A.S. Halpern and M. J. Fuhrer), Paul H. Brooks, Bathmore and London.

Cohen, M., Groswasser, Z., Barchadski, R. and Appel, A. (1989) Convergence insufficiency in brain-injured patients. *Brain Injury*, **3**, 187–91.

Cohen, R.E. (1986) Behavioural treatment of incontinence in a profoundly neurologically impaired adult. *Archives of Physical Medicine and Rehabilitation*, **67**, 833–4.

Cohn, K.C., Wright, R.J. and DeVaul, R. (1977) Post head trauma syndrome in an adolescent treated with lithium carbonate – case report. *Disorders of the Nervous System*, **38**, 630–1.

Cole, J.R., Cope, N. and Cervelli, L. (1985) Rehabilitation of the severely brain injured patient: A community based, low cost model program. *Archives of Physical Medicine and Rehabilitation*, **66**, 38–40.

Collins, K., Oswald, P., Burger, G. and Nolden, J. (1985) Customized adjustable orthoses: Their use in spasticity. *Archives of Physical Medicine and Rehabilitation*, **66**, 397–9.

Conine, T.A., Sullivan, T., Mackie, T. and Goodman, M. (1990) Effects of serial casting for the prevention of equinus in patients with acute head injury. *Archives of Physical Medicine and Rehabilitation*, **71**, 310–12.

Cook, M. (1969) Experiments on orientation and proxemics. *Human Relations*, **23**, 61–76.

Cope, D.N. (1985) Traumatic closed head injury; status of rehabilitation treatment. *Seminars in Neurology*, **5**, 212–20.

Cope, D.N. and Hall, K. (1982) Head injury rehabilitation: Benefits of early intervention. *Archives of Physical Medicine and Rehabilitation*, **63**, 433–7.

Cope, D.N., Date, E.S. and Mar. E.Y. (1988) Serial computerized tomographic evaluations in traumatic head injury. *Archives of Physical Medicine and Rehabilitation*, **68**, 483–6.

Corkin, S. (1968) Acquisition of motor skills after bilateral medial temporal lobe excision. *Neuropsychologia*, **6**, 255–65.

Cornes, P. (1987) Vocational rehabilitation. *International Rehabilitation Medicine*, **8**; 38–141.

Corrigan, J.D. and Mysiw, W.J. (1988) Agitation following traumatic head injury: Equivocal evidence for a discrete stage of cognitive recovery. *Archives of Physical Medicine and Rehabilitation*, **69**, 487–92.

Corrigan, J.D., Arnett, J.A., Houck, L.J. and Jackson, R.D. (1985) Reality orientation for brain injured patients: Group treatment and monitoring of recovery. *Archives of Physical Medicine and Rehabilitation*, **66**, 626–30.

Cosgrove, J.L., Vargo, M. and Reidy, M. (1989) A prospective study of peripheral nerve lesions occurring in traumatic brain-injured patients. *American Journal of Physical Medicine and Rehabilitation*, **68**, 15–17.

Cotton, E., and Kinsman, R. (1983) *Conductive Education for Adult Hemiplegia*, Croom Helm, London.

Craik, F.I.M. and Lockhart, R.S. (1972) Levels of Processing: a framework for memory research. *Journal of Verbal Learning and Verbal Behaviour*, **11**, 671–84.

Crawford, J.E. and Crawford, D.M. (1981) *Crawford Small Parts Dexterity Test*, Psychological Corporation, New York.

Crewe, N. and Athlestan, G (1981) Functional assessment in vocational rehabilitation: A systematic approach to diagnosis and goal setting. *Archives of Physical Medicine and Rehabilitation*, **62**, 299–305.

Crewe, N. and Turner, R. (1984) A functional assessment system for vocational rehabilitation, in *Functional Assessment in Rehabilitation*, (eds A.S. Harper and M.J. Fuhrer), Paul H. Brookes, Baltimore and London, pp. 223–38.

Crosson, B. and Buenning, W. (1984) An individualized memory retraining program after closed head-injury: a single case study. *Journal of Clinical Neuropsychology*, **6**, 287–301.

Crovitz, H.F. (1979) Memory rehabilitation in brain damaged patients: The airoplane list. *Cortex*, **15**, 131–4.

Crovitz, H.F., Harvey, M.T., and Horn, R.W. (1979) Problems in the acquisition of imagery mnemonics: Three brain-damaged cases. *Cortex*, **15**, 225–34.

Crow, T.J. (1980) Molecular pathology of schizophrenia. More than one dimension of pathology. *British Medical Journal*, **280**, 66–8.

Cummings, J.L. (1985) Organic delusions: Phenomenology, anatomical correlations, and review. *British Journal of Psychiatry*, **146**, 184–97.

Cummings, J.L., Landis, T., and Bensom, F. (1983) Environment disorientation: Clinical and radiological findings. *Neurology*, **33** (Supplement 2), 103.

D'Zurilla, T.J., and Goldfried, M.R. (1971) Problem solving and behaviour modification. *Journal of Abnormal Psychology*, **78**, 107–26.

Damsio, A.R. and Hoesen, G.W.V. (1985) The limbic system and localization of herpes simplex encephalitis. *Journal of Neurology, Neurosurgery and Psychiatry*, **48**, 297–301.

Dannenbaum, R.M. and Dykes, R.W. (1990) Evaluating sustained touch-pressure in severe sensory deficits: Meeting an unanswered need. *Archives of Physical Medicine and Rehabilitation*, **71**, 455–9.

Davidoff, G., Doljanac. R., Berent, S. *et al.*, (1988) Galveston orientation and amnesia test: Its utility in the determination of closed head injury in acute spinal cord injury patients. *Archives of Physical Medicine and Rehabilitation*, **69**, 432–3.

Davidoff, G., Morris, J., Roth E. and Bleiberg, J. (1985) Closed head injury in spinal cord injured patients: Retrospective study of loss of consciousness and post-traumatic amnesia. *Archives of Physical Medicine and Rehabilitation*, **66**, 41–3.

Davis, G.A. and Manske, M.E. (1966) An instructional method of increasing originality. *Psychonomic Science*, **6**, 73–4.

Davison, K. and Bagley, C.R. (1969) Schizophrenia-like psychosis associated with organic disorders of the central nervous system: a review of the literature, in *Current Problems in Neuropsychiatry*, (ed. R.N. Herrington), British Journal of Psychiatry Special Publication, Vol 4, pp. 113–84.

De Renzi, and Spinnler, H. (1966) Facial recognition in brain-damaged patients. *Neurology*, **16**, 145–52.

De Renzi, E., Motti F., and Nichelli P. (1980) Imitating gestures: A quantitative approach to ideomotor apraxia. *Archives of Neurology*, **37**, 6–10.

Decker, M.D., Graiter, P.L. and Schaffner, W. (1988) Reduction in motor vehicle fatalities associated with an increase in the minimum drinking age. *JAMA*, **260**, 3604–10.

Delamater, R.J. and Mcnamara, J.R. (1986) The social impact of assertiveness; Research findings and clinical implications. *Behaviour Modification*, **10**, 139–58.

Delay, J. (1935) Les astereognosies. Pathologie due toucher. *Clinique, Physiologie, Topographie*, Mason, Paris.

Delgado-Escueta, A.V., Mattson, R.H., King, L. et. al. (1981) The nature of aggression during epileptic seizures. *New England Journal of Medicine*, **30**, 711–6.

Deutsch, J.A. and Deutsch, D. (1963) Attention: some theoretical considerations. *Psychological Review*, **80**, 80–90.

Dickstein. R., Hocherman, S., Pillar, T., and Shaham R. (1986) Stroke rehabilitation. Three exercise therapy approaches. *Physical Therapy*, **66**, 1233–8.

Dietz, V. and Berger, W. (1983) Normal and impaired regulation of muscle stiffness in gait: a new hypothesis about music hypertonia. *Experimental Neurology*, **79**, 680–7.

Dikman, S. and Reitan, R.M. (1977) MMPI correlates of adaptive ability: Deficits in patients with brain lesions. *Journal of Nervous and Mental Diseases*, **165**, 247–54.

Dikman, S., McLean, A. and Temkin, N. (1986) Neuropsychological and psychosocial consequences of minor head injury. *Journal of Neurology, Neurosurgery, and Psychiatry*, **49**, 1227–32.

Dikman. S., Temkin, N., Mclean, A. *et al.* (1987) Memory and head injury severity. *Journal of Neurology, Neurosurgery and Psychiatry*, **50**, 1613–8.

Diller, L. (1976) A model for cognitive retraining in rehabilitation. *The Clinical Psychologist*, **29**, 13–15.

Diller, L. and Weinberg, J. (1972) Differential aspects of attention in brain damaged persons. *Perceptual and Motor Skills*, **35**, 71–81.

Diller, L., Ben-Yishay, Y., Gerstman, L.J. *et al.* (1974) *Studies in Cognitive Rehabilitation in Hemiplegia*. Rehabilitation Monographs No. 50. Institute of Rehabilitation Medicine, New York University Medical Center, New York.

Dixon, C.E., Lyeth, B.G., Giebel, M.L. *et al.* (1985) Pre-treatment with scopolamine accelerates recovery of locomotor functioning following cerebral concussion in the rat. *Society for Neuroscience Abstracts*, **11**, 432.

Dolan, M.P. (1979) The use of contingent reinforcement for improving the personal appearance and hygiene of chronic psychiatric inpatients. *Journal of Clinical Psychology*, **35**, 140–4.

Dolan, M.P. and Norton, J.C. (1977) A programmed training technique that uses reinforcement to facilitate acquisition and retention in brain damaged patients. *Journal of Clinical Psychology*, **33**, 496–501.

Donaldson, S.W., Wagner, C.C. and Gresham, G.E. (1973) A unified ADL evaluation form. *Archives of Physical Medicine*.

Dorsch, M.M., Woodward, A.J. and Somers, R.L. (1984) Effect of helmet use on reducing head injury in bicycle accidents. *Proceedings of the American Association for Automotive Medicine*, **28**, 247–57.

Dougherty, P. and Radomski, M.V. (1987) *The Cognitive Rehabilitation Workbook: A Systematic Approach to Improve Independent Living Skills in Brain Injured Adults*, Aspen.

Drake, M.E., Jackson, R.D. and Miller, C.A. (1986) Paroxymal choeoathetosis after head injury. *Journal of Neurology, Neurosurgery and Psychiatry*, **49**, 837–8.

Drummond, L.M. (1988) Delayed emergence of obsessive-compulsive neurosis following head injury. *British Journal of Psychiatry*, **153**, 839–42.

Dube, A.H. and Mitchell, E.K. (1986) Accidental strangulation from vest restraints. *Journal of the American Medical Association*, **256**, 2725–6.

Duda, P.D. and Brown, J. (1984) Lateral asymmetry of positive and negative emotions. *Cortex*, **20**, 253–61.

Duncan, G.W., Shahani, B.T., and Young R.R., (1976) An evaluation of baclofen treatment for certain symptoms in patients with spinal cord lesions. *Neurology* (Minneap), **26**, 441–6.

Duncan, P.W. (1990) Physical therapy assessment, in *Rehabitation of the Child with Traumatic Brain Injury*, (eds M. Rosenthal *et al.*), F.A. Davis, Philadelphia,

Duncan, S. (1972) Some signals and rules for taking speaking turns in conversations. *Journal of Personality and Social Psychology*, **23**, 283–92.

Eames, P. and Wood, R. (1985a) Rehabilitation after severe brain injury: a follow-up study of a behaviour modification approach. *Journal of Neurology, Neurosurgery, and Psychiatry*, **48**, 613–19.

Eames, P. and Wood, R. (1985b) Rehabilitation after severe brain injury: a special-unit approach to behaviour disorders. *International Rehabitation Medicine*, **7**, 130–3.

Edna, T-H. and Cappelen, J. (1987) Late post concussion symptoms in traumatic head injury. An analysis of frequency and risk factors. *Acta Neurochirgica* (Wien), **86**, 12–17.

Edney, J. (1988) Education for the severely impaired brain-injured adult, in *Rehabilitation for the Severely Brain-Injured Adult: A Practical Apparoach*, (eds I. Fussey and G.M. Giles), Croom Helm, London,

Ehrlich, J. and Barry, P. (1989) Rating communication behaviours in the head-injured adult. *Brain Injury*, **3**, 193.

Ehrlich, J.S. (1988) Selective characteristics of narrative discourse in head-injured and normal adults. *Journal of Communication Disorders*, **21**, 1–9.

Eisler, R.M., Hersen, M., Miller, P.M. and Blanchard, E.G. (1975) Situational determinants of assertive behavior. *Journal of Consulting and Clinical Psychology*, **43**, 330–40.

Ekman, P., and Oster, H. (1979) Facial expressions of emotion. *Annual Review of Psychology*, **30**, 527–55.

Elliot, F.A. (1977) Propranolol for the control of belligerent behaviour following acute brain damage. *Annals of Neurology*, **1**, 489–91.

Ellsworth, R.B., Foster, L., Childers, B. *et al.* (1968) Hospital and community adjustment as perceived by psychiatric patients, their families, and staff. *Journal of Consulting and Clinical Psychology*, (monograph supplement), **32**, 1–41.

Elsass, L., and Kinsella, G. (1987) Social interaction following severe closed brain injury. *Psychological Medicine*, **17**, 67–78.

Elstein, A.S., Shulman, L.S. and Sprafka, S.A. (1978) *Medical Problem Solving: An Analysis of Clinical Reasoning*, Harvard University Press, Cambridge.

Elwell, J.L. and Grindley, G.C. (1938) The effect of knowledge of results on learning and performance. *British Journal of Psychiatry*, **29**, 39–54.

Epstein, N. (1980) Social consequences of assertion, aggression, passive aggression and submission: Situational and dispositional determinants. *Behaviour Therapy*, **11**, 662–9.

Eriksson, A. and Bjornstig, V. (1982) Fatal snowmobile accidents in northern Sweden. *The Journal of Trauma*, **22**, 977–82.

Evans, G.W., Palsane, M.N. and Carrere, S. (1987a) Type A behaviour and occupational stress: A cross cultural study of blue-collar workers. *Journal of Personality and Social Psychology*, **36**, 1213–20.

Evans, R.W., Gualtieri, C.T. and Patterson, D. (1987b) Treatment of chronic closed head injury with psychostimulant drugs: A controlled study and an appropriate evaluation procedure. *Journal of Nervous and Mental Disease*, **175**, 106–10.

Ewing, R. McCarthy, D., Gronwall, D. and Wrightson, P. (1980) Persisting effects of minor head injury observable during hypoxic stress. *Journal of Clinical Neuropsychiatry*, **2**, 147–55.

Fahy, T.J., Irving, M.H. and Millac, P. (1967) Severe head injuries. *Lancet*, **i**, 475–9.

Farver, P.F. and Farver, T.B. (1982) Performance of normal older adults on tests designed to measure parietal lobe functions. *The American Journal of Occupational Therapy*, **36**, 444–9.

Feeney, D.M., Gonzales, A. and Law, W.A. (1982) Amphetamine, haloperidol and experience interact to affect rate of recovery after motor cortex injury. *Science*, **217**, 855–7.

Fell, J.C. (1977) A profile of fatal accidents involving alcohol, in *Proceedings of the 21st Conference of the American Association for Automotive Medicine*, American Association for Automotive Medicine, Chicago, pp. 197–218.

Fenwick, P. (1989) The nature and management of aggression in epilepsy. *Journal of Neuropsychiatry*, **1**, 418–25.

Fife, D. (1987) Head injury with and without hospital admission: Comparison of incidence and short term disability. *American Journal of Public Health*, **77**, 810–12.

Fife, D., Faich, G., Hollingshead, W. and Boynton, W. (1986) Incidence and outcome of hospital treated head injury in Rhode Island. *American Journal of Public Health*, **76**, 773–8.

Finger, S. and Stein, D.G. (1982) *Brain Damage and Recovery*, Academic Press, New York.

Fishbone, H. (1976) Irreversable injury of the last four cranial nerves, in *Handbook of Clinical Neurology*, Vol 24, (eds P.J. Vinken and G.W. Bruyn), North–Holland, Amsterdam, pp. 179–81.

Fisk, A.D. and Schneider, W. (1984) Memory as a function of attention, levels of processing and automatisation. *Journal of Experimental Psychology: Learning, Memory anmd Cognition*, **10**, 181–97.

Fitts, P.M. (1964) Perceptual-motor skill learning, in *Categories of Human Learning*, (ed A.M. Melton), Academic Press, New York.

Fitts, P.M. and Posner, M.I. (1967) *Human Performance*, Brooks/Cole, Belmont, California.

Flamm, E.S., Demopoulos, H.B., Seligman, M.L. *et al.* (1977) Ethanol potentiation of central nervous system trauma. *Journal of Neurosurgery*, **46**, 328–35.

Flor-Henry, P. (1983) *Cerebral Basis of Psychopathology*, John Wright, Boston MA.

Folstein, M.F., Folstein, S.E. and McHugh, P.R. (1975) Mini-mental state: a practical method for grading cognitive state of patients for the clinician. *Journal of Psychiatric Research*, **12**, 189–98.

Ford, C.V., King, B.H. and Hollander, M.H. (1988) Lies and liars: Psychiatric aspects of prevarication. *American Journal of Psychiatry*, **145**, 554–62.

Fordyce, D.J., Roueche, J.R. and Prigatano, G.P. (1983) Enhanced emotional reactions in chronic head trauma patients. *Journal of Neurology, Neurosurgery and Psychiatry*, **46**, 620–4.

Fox, J. and Harlowe, D. (1984) Construct validation of occupational therapy measures used in CVA evaluation: A beginning. *American Journal of Occupational Therapy*, **38**, 101–6.

Franz, S.I. (1923) *Nervous and Mental Re-education*, New York, Macmillan.

Freedman, P.E., Bleiberg, J. and Freedland K. (1987) Anticipatory behaviour deficits in closed head injury. *Journal of Neurology, Neurosurgery and Psychiatry*, **50**, 398–401.

French, L.R., Schuman, L.M., Mortimer, J.A. *et al.* (1985) A case control study of dementia of the Alzheimer type. *American Journal of Epidemiology*, **121**, 414–21.

Frey, W.D. (1984) Functional assessment in the 80's: A conceptual enigma, a technical challenge, in *Functional Assessment in Rehabilitation*, (eds A.S. Halpern and M.S. Fuhrer) Paul H. Brookes, Baltimore and London, pp. 11–43.

Frisch, M.B. and Froberg, W. (1987) Social validation of assertion strageties for handling aggressive criticism. Evidence for consistency across situations. *Behaviour Therapy*, **2**, 181–91.

Frith, C.D. (1987) The positive and negative symptoms of schizophrenia reflect impairments in the perception and initiation of action. *Psychological Medicine*, **17**, 631–48.

Fryer, D. and Warr, P. (1984) Unemployment and cognitive difficulties. *British Journal of Clinical Psychology*, **23**, 67–71.

Fukuyama, H., Kameyama, M. and Harada, K. (1986) Thalmic tumours invading the brain stem produce crossed cerebellar diaschisis demonstrated by PET. *Journal of Neurology, Neurosurgery and Psychiatry*, **49**, 524–28.

Fuld, P.A. and Fisher, P. (1977) Recovery of intellectual ability after closed head injury. *Developmental Medicine and Child Neurology*, **19**, 495–502.

Fussey, I. and Giles, G.M. (1988) *Rehabilitation of the Severely Brain Injured Adult: A Practical Approach*, Croom Helm, London.

Fussey, I. and Tyerman, D. (1985) An exploration of memory retraining in rehabilitation following closed head injury. *International Journal of Rehabilitation Research*, **8**, 465–7.

Gaines, A.T. (1986) Trauma: cross cultural issues. *Advances in Psychosomatic Medicine*, **16**, 1–16.

Gajar, A., Schloss, P.I., Schloss, C. and Thompson, C.K. (1984) Effects of feedback and self-monitoring on brain trauma youth's conversational skills. *Journal of Applied Behavior Analysis*, **17**, 353–8.

Galski, T., Ehle, H.T. and Bruno, R.L. (1990) An assessment of measures to predict the outcome of driving evaluations in patients with cerebral damage. *The American Journal of Occupational Therapy*, **44**, 709–13.

Gans, J.S. (1983) Hate in the rehabitation setting. *Archives of Physical Medicine and Rehabilitation*, **64**, 176–9.

Gardner, W.I., Karan, O.C. and Cole, C.L. (1984) Assessment of setting events influencing functional capacities of mentally retarded adults with behaviour difficulties, in *Functional assessment in Rehabilitation*, (eds A.S. Halpern and M.S. Fuhrer), Paul H. Brookes, Baltimore and London,

Garland, D.E. and Baily, S. (1981) Undetected injuries in head injured adults. *Clinical Orthopedics*, **155**, 162–265.

Garland, D.E., Glogova, S.V. and Waters, R.L. (1979) Orthopedic aspects of pedestrian victims of automobile accidents. *Orthopedics*, **2**, 242.

Gennarelli, T.A. (1988) Heterotopic Ossification. *Brain Injury*, **2**, 175–8.

Gennarelli, T.A., Adams, J.H. and Graham, D.I. (1986) Diffuse axonal Injury – a new conceptual approach to an old problem, in *Mechanisms of Secondary Brain damage*, (eds A. Baethman, K.G. G. and A. Unterberg), Plenum Publishing, New York, pp. 15–28.

Gennarelli, T. A., Thibault, L.E., Adams, J.H. *et al* (1982) Diffuse axonal injury and traumatic coma in the primate. *Annals of Neurology*, **12**, 564–74.

Gentilini, M., Nichelli, P., Schoenhuber, R. *et al*, (1985) Neuropsychological evaluation of mild head injury. *Journal of Neurology, Neurosurgery and Psychiatry*, **48**, 137–40.

Geschwind, N. (1975) The apraxias: neuronal mechanisms of disorders of learned movement. *American Scientist*, **63**, 188–95.

Gianutsos, R. (1980) What is cognitive rehabilitation? *Journal of Rehabilitation*, **46**, 36–40.

Gianutsos, R. (1981) Training the short- and long-term verbal recall of a post encephalitic amnesia. *Journal of Clinical Neuropsychology*, **3**, 143–53.

Gianutsos, R., Ramsey, G. and Perlin, R.R. (1988) Rehabilitative optometric services for survivors of acquired brain injury. *Archives of Physical Medicine and Rehabilitation*, **69**, 573–8.

Gibb, W.R.G. and Lee, A.J. (1986) The clinical phenomenon of akathisia. *Journal of Neurology, Neurosurgery and Psychiatry*, **49**, 861–6.

Gibson, E.J. (1969) *Principles of Perceptual Learning and Development*, Appleton Century Crofts, New York.

Gilchrist, M. and Wilkinson, M. (1979) Some factors determining prognosis in young people with severe head injuries. *Archives of Neurology*, **36**, 355–8.

Giles, G.M. (1989) Demonstrating the effectiveness of occupational therapy after severe brain trauma. *The American Journal of Occupational Therapy*, **43**, 613–15

Giles, G. M. and Clark-Wilson, J. (1988a) The use of behavioural techniques in functional skills training after severe brain injury. *The American Journal of Occupational Therapy*, **42**, 658–65.

Giles, G. M. and Clark-Wilson, J. (1988b) Functional skills training after severe brain injury, in *Rehabilitation of the Severely Brain-Injured Adult: A Practical Approach*, (eds I. Fussey and G. M. Giles), Croom Helm, London, pp. 69–101.

Giles, G. M. and Fussey, I. (1988) Models of brain-injury rehabilitation: From theory to practice, in *Rehabilitation of the Severely Brain-Injured Adult: A Practical Approach*, (eds I. Fussey and G. M. Giles), Croom Helm, London, pp. 1–29.

Giles, G. M. and Morgan, J. H. (1989) Training functional skills following herpes simplex encephalitis: A single case study. *Journal of Clinical and Experimental Neuropsychology*, **11**, 311–18.

Giles, G. M. and Shore, M. (1989a) A rapid method for teaching severely brain injured adults to wash and dress. *Archives of Physical Medicine and Rehabilitation*, **70**, 156–8.

Giles, G. M. and Shore, M. (1989b) The effectiveness of an electronic memory aid for a memory-impaired adult of normal intelligence. *The American Journal of Occupational Therapy*, **43**, 409–11.

Giles, G. M., and Gent, A. (1988) Conductive Education and Motor Learning, in *Rehabilitation of the Severely Brain Injured Adult: A Practical Approach*, (eds I. Fussey and G. M. Giles), Croom Helm, London, pp. 130–48.

Giles, G. M., Fussey, I. and Burgess, P. (1988) The behavioral treatment of verbal interaction skills following severe head injury: a single case study. *Brain Injury*, **2**, 75–9.

Gjerris, F. (1976) Traumatic lesions of the visual pathways, in *Handbook of Clinical Neurology*, Vol. 24, Elsevier, Oxford and New York, pp. 27–58.

Glasgow, R. E., Zeiss, R. A., Barrera, M., and Lewinsohn, P. (1977) Case Studies on remediating memory deficits in brain-damaged individuals. *Journal of Clinical Psychology*, **33**, 1049–54.

Glick, S. D. and Greenstein, S. (1973) Possible modulatory influences of frontal cortex on nigro-striatal function. *British Journal of Pharmacology*, **49**, 316–21.

Glisky, E. L. and Schacter, D. A. (1988) Long-term retention of computer learning by patients with memory disorders. *Neuropsychologia*, **26**, 173–8.

Glisky, E. L., Schacter, D. L. and Tulving, E. (1986) Computer learning by memory impaired patients: acquisition and retention of complex knowledge. *Neuropsychologia*, **24**, 313–28.

Gloag, D. (1985a) Rehabilitation after head injury: 1: Cognitive problems. *British Medical Journal*, **290**, 834–7.

Gloag, D. (1985b) Rehabilitation after head injury: 11: Behaviour and emotional problems, long term needs and the requirements for services. *British Medical Journal*, **291**, 557–8.

Godfrey, H. P. D. and Knight, R. G. (1987) Intervention for amnesics: a review. *British Journal of Clinical Psychology*, **26**, 83–91.

Godfrey, H. P. D., Knight, R. G., Marsh, N. V. *et al.* (1989) Social interaction and speed of information processing following very severe head-injury. *Psychological Medicine*, **19**, 175–82.

Goff, B. (1969) Appropriate afferent stimulation. *Physiotherapy*, **55**, 9–17.

Goffman, E. (1961) *Asylums. Essays on the Social Status of Mental Patients and Inmates*, Penguin, Harmondsworth.

Gold, R. L. (1958) Roles in sociological field observations. *Social Forces*, **36**, 217–23.

Goldberg, E. and Bilder, R. M. (1987) The frontal lobes and hierarchical organization of cognitive control, in *The Frontal Lobes Revisited*, (ed. E. Perecman), The IRBN Press, New York, New York.

Goldspink, D. F. (1977) The influence of activity on muscle size and protein turnover. *Journal of Physiology,* **264**, 283–96.

Goldstein, G., Ryan, C., Turner, S. M. *et al.* (1985) Three methods of memory training for severely amnesic patients. *Behaviour Modification,* **9**, 357–74.

Goldstein, L. H. and Oakley, D. A. (1986) Colour versus orientation discrimination in severely brain-damaged and normal adults. *Cortex,* **22**, 261–6.

Goldstein, L. H. and Oakley, D. A. (1983) Expected and actual behavioral capacity after diffuse reduction in cerebral cortex: A review and suggestions for rehabilitative techniques with the mentally handicapped and head injured. *British Journal of Clinical Psychology,* **24**, 13–24.

Goodglass, H., and Kaplan, E. (1963) Disturbances of gesture and pantomime in aphasia. *Brain,* **86**, 703–20.

Gordon, W. A., Hibbard, M. R., Egelko, S. *et al.* (1985) Perceptual remediation in patients with right brain damage: A comprehensive programme. *Archives of Physical Medicine and Rehabilitation,* **66**, 353–9.

Grafman, J., Vance, S. C., Weingartner, H. *et al.* (1986) The effect of lateralized frontal lesions on mood regulation. *Brain,* **109**, 1127–48.

Graham, D. I. (1977) Pathology of hypoxic brain damage in man, in Hypoxia and Ischemia, (ed. B. C. Morson), *Journal of Clinical Pathology,* Supplement 30, **11**, 170–80.

Graham, D. I., McLellan, D. R., Adams, J. H., *et al.* (1983) The neuropathology of severe disability after non-missile head injury. *Acta Neurochirurgica,* (Suppl.) (Wien), **32** : 65–67.

Granger, C. V. and Barret, J. E. (1979) Stroke Rehabilitation: Analysis of repeated Barthel Index measures. *Archives of Physician Medicine and Rehabilitation,* **60**, 14–17.

Granger, C. V. and Gresham, G. E. (1984) *Functional Assessment in Rehabilitation Medicine,* Williams and Wilkins, Baltimore and London.

Granger, C. V., Albrecht, G. L., and Hamilton, B. B. (1979) Outcome of comprehensive medical rehabilitation: measurement by PULSES profile and the Barthel Index. *Archives of Physical Medicine and Rehabilitation,* **60**, 145–54.

Granger, C. V., Dewis, L. S., Peters, N. C. *et al.* (1982) *The Neuropsychology of Anxiety: An Enquiry into the Functioning of the Septohippocampal System,* Oxford University Press, New York.

Gray, J. A. (1982) *The Neuropsychology of Anxiety: An Enquiry into the Functions of the Septo-Hippocampal System,* Clarendon Press, Oxford.

Gray, J. A. and Wedderburn, A. A. (1960) Grouping strategies with simultaneous stimuli. *Quarterly Journal of Experimental Psychology,* **12**, 180–4.

Green, H. J., Miskimins, R. W. and Keil, E. C. (1968) Selection of psychiatric patients for vocational rehabilitation. *Rehabilitation Counseling Bulletin,* **11**, 297–302.

Green, C. W., Reid, D. H., White, L. K. *et al.* (1988) Identifying reinforcers for persons with profound handicaps: Staff opinion versus systematic assessment of preferences. *Journal of Applied Behavioral Analysis*, **21**, 31–43.

Greendyke, R. M., Kanter, D. R., Schuster, D. B. *et al.* (1986) Propranolol treatment of assaultive patients with organic brain disease. A double blind crossover placebo-controlled study. *Journal of Nervous and Mental Diseases*, **174**, 290–4.

Greenwood, R., Bhalla, A., Gordon, A. and Roberts, J. (1983) Behaviour disturbance during recovery from herpes simplex encephalitis. *Journal of Neurology, Neurosurgery and Psychiatry*, **46**, 809–17.

Gresham, G. E., Phillips, T. A. and Labi, M. L. C. (1980) ADL status in stroke: Relative merits of three standard indexes. *Archives of Physical Medicine and Rehabilitation*, **61**, 355–58.

Grillner, S., and Rossignol, S., (1978) Contralateral reflex reversal controlled by limb position in the acute spinal cat injected with clonidine iv. *Brain Research*, **144**, 411–14.

Groher, M. (1977) Language and memory disorders following closed brain trauma. *Journal of Speech and Hearing Research*, **20**, 212–24.

Gronwall, D. (1977) Paced auditory serial addition task: A measure of recovery from concussion. *Perceptual and Motor Skills*, **44**, 367–73.

Gronwall, D. and Wrightson, P. (1981) Memory and information processing capacity after closed head injury. *Journal of Neurology, Neurosurgery, and Psychiatry*, **44**, 889–95.

Grossman, M. R., Sahrmann, S. A. and Rose, S. J. (1982) Review of length associated change in muscle: Experimental evidence and clinical implications. *Physical Therapy*, **62**, 1799–807.

Grosswasser, Z., Cohen, M., Reider-Grosswasser, I. and Stern, M. J. (1988) Incidence, CT findings and rehabilitation outcome of patients with communicating hydrocephalus following severe brain injury. *Brain Injury*, **2**, 167–272.

Gualtieri, C. T. (1988) Pharmacotherapy and the neurobehavioural sequelae of traumatic brain injury. *Brain Injury*, **2**, 101–29.

Gualtieri, C. T. and Evans, R. W. (1988) Stimulant treatment for the neurobehavioural sequelae of traumatic brain injury. *Brain Injury*, **2**, 273–90.

Guidice, M. A., LeWitt, P. A. and Berchou, R. C. (1986) Improvement of motor functioning with Levodopa and Bromocriptine following closed head injury. *Neurology*, Supplement 1, (Abstract) **36**, 198–9.

Haas, J., Cope, D. N. and Hall, K. (1987) Premorbid prevalence of poor academic performance in severe head injury. *Journal of Neurology, Neurosurgery, and Psychiatry*, **50**, 52–6.

Habib, M. and Sirigu, A. (1987) Pure topographical disorientation: A definition and anatomical basis. *Cortex*, **23**, 73–85.

Haddon, W. (1972) A logical framework for categorizing highway safety phenomena and activity. *Journal of Trauma*, **12**, 193–207.

Hagen, C., Malkmus, D. and Durham, P. (1972) *Levels of Cognitive Functioning*, Rancho Los Amigos Hospital, Downey California.

Haig, A. J., Katz, R. T. and Sahgal, V. (1987) Mortality and complications of the locked-in syndrome. *Archives of Physical Medicine and Rehabilitation*, **68**, 24–7.

Hall, E. T. (1959) *The Silent Language*, Doubleday and Co., New York.

Halligan, P. W. and Marshall, J. C. (1990) Two techniques for the assessment of line bisection in visuo-spatial neglect: a single case study. *The Journal of Neurology, Neurosurgery and Psychiatry*, **52**, 1300–2.

Halpern, A. S. (1984) Functional assessment and mental retardation, in *Functional Assessment in Rehabilitation*, (eds A. S. Halpern and M. J. Fuhrer), Paul H. Brookes, Baltimore and London,

Hamilton, D. W. (1979) A cognitive-attribution analysis of stereotyping, in *Advances in Experimental Social Psychology*, vol. 12, (ed L. Berkowitz), Academic Press, New York,

Hansen, J. I. C. (1985) *Manual for the Strong Vocational Interest Blank – Strong-Campbell Interest Inventory*, Stanford University Press, Stanford, California.

Hargie, O. (ed.) (1986) *Handbook of Communication Skills*, New York University Press, New York.

Harrigan, J. A. (1985) Listeners body movements and speaking turns. *Communication Research*, **12**, 233–50.

Harris, J. E. (1984a) Remembering to do things: a forgotten topic, in *Everyday Memory, Actions and Absent-Mindedness*, (eds J. E. Harris and P. E. Morris), Academic Press, London, pp. 71–92.

Harris, J. E. (1980) Memory aids people use: Two interview studies. *Memory and Cognition*, **8**, 31–8.

Harris, J. E. (1984b) Methods of improving memory, in *Clinical Management of Memory Problems*, (eds. B. A. Wilson and N. Moffat), Croom Helm, London, pp. 46–62.

Harris, J. E. and Morris, P. E. (1984) (eds) *Everyday Memory, Actions and Absent-Mindedness*, Academic Press, London.

Harris, J. E. and Sunderland, A. (1981) A brief survey of the management of memory disorders in rehabilitation units in Britain. *International Rehabilitation Medicine*, **3**, 206–9.

Harris, L. J. and Gitterman, S. R. (1978) University professors' self-descriptions of left-right confusability: sex and handedness differences. *Perceptual and Motor Skills*, **47**, 819–23.

Hartlage, L. C., and Telzrow, C. F. (1983) The neuropsychological basis of educational intervention. *Journal of Learning Difficulties*, **16**, 521–28.

Hasselkus, B. R. and Safrit, M. J. (1976) Measurements in occupational therapy. *American Journal of Occupational Therapy*, **30**, 429–36.

Haviland, S. E. H. and Clark, H. H. (1974) What's new? Acquiring new information as a process of comprehension. *Journal of Verbal Learning and Verbal Behaviour*, **13**, 512–21.

Hayes, R. L., Lyeth, B. G., Dixon, C. E. *et al.* (1985) Cholinergic antagonist reduces neurological deficits following cerebral concussion in the rat. *Journal of Cerebral Blood Flow and Metabolism*, **5** (Suppl. 1), 395–6.

Heacock, L., McNeny, R. and Zasler, N. D. (1989) Training the brain injured (Letter). *Archives of Physical Medicine and Rehabilitation*, **70**, 720.

Heaton, R. K. and Pendleton, M. T. (1981) Use of neuropsychological tests to predict adult patients everyday functioning. *Journal of Consulting and Clinical Psychology*, **49**, 807–21.

Heaton, R. K., Baade, L. E. and Johnson, K. L. (1978) Neuropsychological test results associated with psychiatric disorders in adults. *Psychological Bulletin*, **85**, 141–62.

Hecaen, A. (1968) Suggestions for a typology of the apraxia, in *The Reach of Mind*, (ed. M. L. Simmel) Springer, New York,

Hedley, D. W., Maroun, J. A. and Espir M. L. E. (1975) Evaluation of baclofen (Lioresal) for spasticity in multiple sclerosis. *Postgraduate Medical Journal*, **51**, 615–18.

Heilman, K. M. and Valenstien, E. (1972) Frontal lobe neglect in man. *Neurology*, **22**, 660–4.

Heilman, K. M. and Valenstien, E. (1979) Mechanisms underlying hemispatial neglect. *Annals of Neurology*, **5**, 166–70.

Heilman, K. M., Watson, R. T. and Valenstein, E. (1985) Neglect and related disorders, in *Clinical Neuropsychology*, 2nd ed. (eds K. M. Heilman and E. Valenstein), Oxford University Press, New York, pp. 378–402.

Heilman, K. M. and Rothi, L. J. G. (1985) Apraxia, in *Clinical Neuropsychology*, (eds K. M. Heilman and E. Valenstein), Oxford University Press, New York, pp. 131–50.

Heilman, K. M., Schwartz, H. D. and Geschwind, N. (1975) Defective motor learning in ideomotor apraxia. *Neurology*, **25**, 1018–20.

Heiskanen, O. and Sipponen, P. (1970) Prognosis of severe brain injury. *Acta Neurologica Scandinavica*, **46**, 343–8.

Heit, G., Smith, M. E. and Halgren, E. (1988) Neural encoding of individual words and faces by the human hippocampus and amygdala. *Nature*, **333**, 773–5.

Helffestein, D. and Weschler, F. (1982) The use of interpersonal process recall (IPR) in the remediation of interpersonal and communication skill deficits in the newly brain-injured. *Clinical Neuropsychiatry*, **4**, 139–43.

Henderson, S., Duncan-Jones, P., McAuley, H., and Ritchie, K. (1978). The Patients Primary Group. *British Journal of Psychiatry*, **132**, 74–86.

Herrstein, R. J. (1970) On the law of effect. *Journal of the Experimental Analysis of Behavior*, **13**, 243–66.

Hersen, M. and Barlow, D. H. (eds) (1976) *Single-Case Experimental Design: Strategies for Studying Behavior Change*, Pergamon, Elmsford, New York.

Hersen, M. and Turner, M. (1978) Role-play tests for assessing social skills: Are they valid? *Behavior Therapy*, **9**, 448–61.

Hick W. E. (1952) On the rate of gain of information. *Quarterly Journal of Experimental Psychology*. **4**, 11–26.

Hillbom, E. (1951) Schizophrenia-like psychosis after brain trauma. *Acta Psychiatrica Scandanavica*, (Suppl.), **60**, 30–47.

Hillbom, E. (1960) After effects of brain-injuries. *Acta Psychiatrica and Neurologica Scandinavica*, (Suppl.), **142**, 1–135.

Hillbom, M. and Holm, L. (1986) Contribution of traumatic head injury to neurosychological deficits in alcoholics. *Journal of Neurology, Neurosurgery and Psychiatry*, **49**, 1348–53.

Hinkeldey, N. S. and Corrigan, J. D. (1990) The structure of head-injured patients' neurobehavioral complaints: A preliminary study. *Brain Injury*, **4**, 115–33.

Ho, L. and Shea, J. B., (1978) Levels of processing and the coding of position cues in motor short-term memory. *Journal of Motor Behaviour*, **10**, 113–21.

Hoberman, M., Cicenia, E. F. and Stephenson, G. R. (1952) Daily activity testing in physical therapy and rehabilitation. *Archives of Physical Medicine*, **33**, 99–108.

Hogarty, G. E. and Katz, M. M. (1971) Norms of adjustment and social behaviour. *Archives of General Psychiatry*, **25**, 470–80.

Hogue, R. E. and McCandless, S. (1983) Genu recurvatum: Auditory biofeedback treatment for adult patients with stroke or head injuries. *Archives of Physical Medicine and Rehabilitation*, **64**, 368–70.

Holland, J. L. (1985) *Vocational Preference Inventory (VPI) Manual*, Psychological Assessment Resources, Odessa, Florida.

Hooper, H. E. (1958) *The Hooper Visual Organization Test*, (Manual), Western Psychological Services, Los Angeles.

Hooper-Row, J. (1988) Rehabilitation of physical deficits in the post acute brain-injured: Four case studies, in *Rehabilitation of the Severely Brain-Injury Adult: A Practical Approach*, (eds I. Fussey and G. M. Giles), Croom Helm, London, pp. 102–16.

Horton, A. M. and Howe, N. R. (1981) Behavioral treatment of the traumatically brain injured: a case study. *Perceptual and Motor Skills*, **53**, 349–50.

Houten, R. V., Axelrod, S., Baily, J. S. *et al.* (1988) The right to effective behavioral treatment. *Journal of Applied Behavioral Analysis*, **21**, 381–4.

Howes, J. L. (1983) Effects of experimenter and self-generated imagery on the Korsakoff patients memory performance. *Neuropsychologia*, **21**, 341–9.

Hubel, D. H., and Wiesel, T. N., (1962) Receptive fields, binocular interaction and functional architecture in the cat's visual cortex. *Journal of Physiology*, **160**, 106–54.

Hufschmidt, A. and Mauritz, K-H. (1985) Chronic transformation of muscle in spasticity: A peripheral contribution to increased tone. *Journal of Neurology, Neurosurgery and Psychiatry*, **48**, 676–85.

Hull, D. B. and Schroeder, H. E. (1979) Some interpersonal effects of assertion, nonassertion and aggression. *Behaviour Therapy*, **10**, 20–8.

Humphrey, M. and Oddy, M. (1980) Return to work after head injury: a review of post-war studies. *Injury*, **12**, 107–14.

Husak, W. S. and Reeve, T. G. (1979) Novel response production as a function of variability and amount of practice. *Research Quarterly*, **50**, 215–21.

Imle, P. C., Eppinghaus, C. E. and Boughton, A. C. (1986) Efficacy of non-bivalved and bivalved serial casting on head injured patients in intensive care. (Abstract) *Physical Therapy*, **66**, 784.

Inaba, M., Edberg, E., Montgomery, M., and Gillis, M. K. (1973) Effectiveness of functional training, active exercise and resistive exercise for patients with hemiplegia. *Physical Therapy*, **53**, 28–35.

Ivan, L. P., Choo, S. H. and Ventureyera, E. C. (1983) Head injuries in childhood: a 2-year survey. *Canadian Medical Association Journal*, **128**, 281–4.

Jackoway, I. S. Rogers, J. C. and Snow, T. (1987) The role change assessment: An interview tool for evaluating older adults. *Occupational Therapy in Mental Health*, **1**, 17–37.

Jackson, H. F. (1980) Impaired emotional recognition following severe brain injury. *Cortex*, **23**, 293–300.

Jackson, H. F. and Moffit, N. J. (1987) Impaired emotional recognition following severe head injury. *Cortex*, **23**, 293–300.

Jackson, R. D., Corrigan, J. D. and Arnett, J. A. (1984) Amytriptyline for agitation in head injury. *Archives of Physical Medicine and Rehabilitation*, **66**, 180–1.

Jackson, R. D., Mysiw, W. J. and Corrigan, J. D. (1989) Orientation group monitoring system: An indicator for reversible impairments in cognition during posttraumatic Amnesia. *Archives of Physical Medicine and Rehabilitation*, **70**, 33–6.

Jacobs, H. E. (1988) The Los Angeles head injury survey: Procedures and initial findings. *Archives of Physical Medicine and Rehabilitation*, **69**, 425–31.

Jaffe, D. T. (1985) Self renewal: personal transformations following extreme trauma. *Journal of Humanistic Psychology*, **25**, 99–124.

Jaffe, M. B., Mastrilli, J. P., Molitor, C. B. and Valko, A. S. (1985) Intervention for motor disorders, in *Head Injury Rehabilitation: Children and Adolescents*, (ed. M. Ylvisaker), College Hill Press, San Diego, pp. 167–94.

Jagger, J., Fife, D., Vernberg, K. and Jane, J. A. (1984) Effect of alcohol intoxication on the diagnosis and apparent severity of brain injury. *Neurosurgery*, **15**, 303–6.

James, J. (1890) *Principles of psychology*, Vols 1 and 2, Holt, New York.

Jane, J. A., Rimel, R. W., Pobereskin, L. H. *et al.* (1982) Outcome and pathology of head injury, in *Head Injury: Basic and Clinical Aspects*, (eds R. G. Granman and P. L. Gildenberg), Raven Press, New York, pp. 229–37.

Jankowski, L. and Sullivan, S. J. (1990) Aerobic and neuromuscular training: effects on the capacity, efficiency and fatigability of patients with traumatic brain-injuries. *Archives of Physical Medicine and Rehabilitation*, **71**, 500–4.

Jebsen, R. H., Taylor, N., Trieschmann, R. B. *et al.* (1969) An objective and standardized test of hand function. *Archives of Physical Medicine and Rehabilitation*, **50**, 311–9.

Jellineck, H. M., Torkelson, R. M. and Harvey, R. F. (1982) Functional abilities and distress levels in brain injured patients at long-term follow up. *Archives of Physical Medicine and Rehabilitation*, **63**, 160–2.

Jellinek, H. M. and Harvey, R. F. (1982) Vocational/educational services in a medical rehabilitation facility: outcomes in spinal cord and brain injured patients. *Archives of Physical Medicine and Rehabilitation*, **63**, 87–8.

Jennett, B. and Plum, F. (1979) Persistent vegetative state after brain damage. A syndrome in search of a name. *Lancet*, i, 734–7.

Jennett, B. (1990) Post traumatic epilepsy, in *Rehabilitation of the Head Injured Adult*, (eds M. Rosenthal *et al.*), F. A. Davis Company, Philadelphia, pp. 89–93.

Jennett, B. and Bond, M. (1975) Assessment of outcome after severe brain damage: A practical scale. *Lancet* **1**, 480–4.

Jennett, B. and Plum, F. (1972) Persistent vegetative state after brain damage. *Lancet*, **1**, 734–7.

Jennett, B. and Teasdale, G. (1981) *Management of Head Injuries*, F. A. Davis, Philadelphia.

Jennett, B., Teasdale, G., Galbraith, S. *et al.* (1977) Severe head injuries in three countries. *Journal of Neurology, Neurosurgery and Psychiatry*, **40**, 291–8.

Jette, A. M. (1980) Functional capacity evaluation: an empirical approach. *Archives of Physical Medicine and Rehabilitation*, **61**, 85–9.

Joannette, Y., Brouchon, M. and Samson, M. (1986) Pointing with left vs right hand in left visual field neglect. *Neuropsychologia*, **24**, 391–6.

Job, R. F. S. (1988) Effective and ineffective use of fear in health promotion campaigns. *American Journal of Public Health*, **78**, 163–7.

Johnson, D. A. and Newton, A. (1987a) Brain injured persons social interaction group: A basis for social adjustment after brain injury. *British Journal of Occupational Therapy*, **50**, 47–52.

Johnson, D. A. and Newton, A. (1987b) Social adjustment and interaction after severe brain injury: 2. Rationale and bases for intervention. *British Journal of Clinical Psychology*, **26**, 289–98.

Johnson, R. (1989) Employment after severe head injury: Do the manpower services commission schemes help? *Injury*, **20**, 5–9.

Johnson, R. and Gleave, J. (1987) Counting the people disabled by head injury. *Injury*, **18**, 7–9.

Johnson, R. and McCabe, J. (1982) Schema theory: A test of the hypothesis, variation in practice. *Perceptual and Motor Skills*, **55**, 231–4.

Johnston, P. B. and Armstrong, M. F. (1986) Eye injuries in Northern Ireland two years after seat belt legislation. *British Journal of Opthalmology*, **70**, 460–2.

Jolles, J. (1983) Vasopressin-like peptides and the treatment of memory disorders in man, in the neurohypophysis: Structure, function and control, (eds B. A. Cross and G. Leng), *Progress in Brain Research*, **60**, 169–82.

Jones, W. H., Hobbs, S. A. and Hockenbury, D. (1982) Loneliness and social skills deficits. *Journal of Personality and Social Psychology*, **42**, 682–9.

Jones, W. H., Freemon, J. E. and Goswick, R. A. (1981) The persistence of loneliness: Self and other determinants. *Journal of Personality*, **49**, 27–48.

Kahn, R. L. and Cannell, C. F. (1957) *The Dynamics of Interviewing, Theory Techniques and Cases,* John Wiley and Sons, New York.

Kahneman, D. (1973) *Attention and Effort,* Prentice-Hall, Englewood Cliffs, NJ.

Kalisky, Z., Morrison, D. P., Meyer, C. A. and Von Laufen, A. (1985) Medical problems encountered during rehabilitation of patients with head injury. *Archives of Physical Medicine and Rehabilitation,* 66, 25–9.

Karlson, T. A. (1982) The incidence of hospital treated facial injuries from vehicles. *Journal of Trauma,* 22, 303–10.

Karpiak, S. E. (1983) Ganglioside treatment improves recovery of alternation behavior after unilateral entorhinal cortex lesions. *Experimental Neurology,* 81, 330–9.

Katz, M. M. and Lyerly, S. B. (1963) Methods of measuring adjustment and social behaviour in the community: Rationale, description, discrimination validity and scale development. *Psychological Reports,* 13, 503–35.

Katz, S., Ford, A. B., Mosowitz, R. W. *et al.* (1963) Studies of illness in the aged. The index of A. D. L. in a standard measure of biological and psychosocial function. *JAMA,* 185, 914–19.

Kaufert, J. (1983) Functional ability indices: measurement problems in assessing their validity. *Archives of Physical Medicine and Rehabilitation,* 64, 260–7.

Kazdin, A. E. (1976) Statistical analysis for single case experimental designs, in *Single-Case Experimental Design: Strategies for Studying Behavior Change,* (eds M. Hersen and D. H. Barlow), Pergamon, Elmsford, New York, pp. 265–316.

Kazdin, A. E. (1978) Methodology of applied behavior analysis, in *Handbook of Applied Behavior Analysis,* (eds A. C. Catinia and T. A. Brigham), Irvington Publishers, New York, pp. 61–104.

Kazdin, A. E. (1982) *Single Case Research Designs.* Oxford University Press, New York.

Kendon, A. (1967) Some functions of gaze direction in social interaction. *Acta Psychologia,* 26, 1–47.

Kendon, A. and Ferber, A. (1973) A description of some human greetings, in *Comparative ecology and behaviour of primates* (eds R. Michael and J. Crook), Academic Press, London.

Kent, B. E. (1965) Sensory-motor testing: The upper limb of adult patients with hemiplegia. *Journal of the American Physical Therapy Association,* 45, 550–61.

Kern, J. M. (1982) Predicting the impact of assertive, empathetic-assertive and non-assertive behaviour: The assertiveness of the assertee. *Behaviour Therapy,* 13, 486–98.

Kewman, D. G., Seigerman, C., Kinter, H. *et al.* (1985) Simulation training of psychomotor skills: Teaching the brain-injured to drive. *Rehabilitation Psychology,* 30, 11–26.

Kewman, D. G., Yanus, B. and Kirsch, N. (1988) Assessment of distractibility in auditory comprehension after traumatic brain injury. *Brain Injury,* 2, 131–7.

King, G. (1972) *Open and closed questions; the reference interview*, RQ – Reference and Adult Sciences Division, **12**, 157–60.

King, T. I. (1982) Plaster splinting as a means of reducing elbow flexor spasticity: A case study. *American Journal of Occupational Therapy*, **36**, 671–3.

Kinsbourne, M. and Warrington, E. K., (1962) A disorder of simultaneous form perception. *Brain*, **85**, 461–86.

Kintsch, W., (1970) Models for free recall and recognition, in *Models of Human Memory*, (ed. D. A. Norman) Academic Press, New York, pp. 333–73.

Klauber, M. R., Barrett-Conner, E., Marshall, L. F. and Bowers, S. A. (1981) The epidemiology of head trauma: A prospective study of an entire community – San Diego County California, 1978. *American Journal of Epidemiology*, **113**, 500–9.

Klauber, M. R., Marshall, L. F., Toole, B. M. *et al.* (1985) Cause of decline in head-injury mortality rate in San Diego Country, California. *Journal of Neurosurgery*, **62**, 528–31.

Klein, R. M. and Bell, B. (1982) Self-care skills: Behavioural measurement with Klein-Bell scale. *Archives of Physical Medicine and Rehabilitation*, **63**, 335–8.

Kleinman, A. (1980) *Patients and Healers in the Context of Culture*, University of California Press, Berkeley.

Kleinmuntz, B. (1984) The scientific study of clinical judgment in psychology and medicine. *Clinical Psychology Review*, **4**, 111–6.

Klingbell, G. E. G. (1988) Airway problems in patients with traumatic brain injury. *Archives of Physical Medicine and Rehabilitation*, **69**, 493–5.

Klonoff, P. S., Costa, L. D. and Snow, W. D. (1986) Predictors and indicators of quality of life in patients with closed head injury. *Journal of Clinical and Experimental Neuropsychology*, **8**, 469–85.

Kluver, H. and Bucy, P. C. (1939) Preliminary analysis of functions of the temporal lobes in monkeys. *Archives of Neurology and Psychiatry*, **42**, 979–1000.

Knott, M., and Voss, D. E. (1968) *Proprioceptive Neuromuscular Facilitation, Patterns and Techniques*, 2nd ed., Hoeber, New York.

Kolpan, K. I. (1987) Functional outcome evaluation of the head injured: its effect of legal rights. *Journal of Head Trauma Rehabilitation*, **2**, 93.

Kopelman, M. D. (1987) Two types of confabulation. *Journal of Neurology, Neurosurgery and Psychiatry*, **50**, 1482–7.

Kosljanetz, M. (1981) Sexual and hypothalamic dysfunction in the post-concussional syndrome. *Acta Neurologica Scandinavica*, **63**, 163–80.

Kottke, F. J. (1982) Therapeutic exercise to develop neuromuscular coordination, in *Krusen's Handbook of Physical Medicine and Rehabilitation*, (eds F. J. Kottke *et al.*), W. B. Saunders, Philadelphia, pp. 403–26.

Kottke, F. J., Halpern, D., Easton, J. K. M. *et al.* (1978) The training of coordination. *Archives of Physical Medicine and Rehabilitation*, **59**, 567–72.

Kraus, J. F., Black, M. A., Hessol, N. *et al.* (1984) The incidence of acute brain injury and serious impairment in a defined population. *American Journal of Epidemiology*, **119**, 186–201.

Kraus, J. F., Fife, D. and Conroy, C. (1987) Incidence, severity and outcomes of brain injury involving bicycles. *American Journal of Public Health*, **77**, 76–8.

Krauthammer, C. and Klerman, G. L. (1978) Secondary mania: Manic syndromes associated with antecedent physical illness or drugs. *Archives of General Psychiatry*, **35**, 1333–9.

Kreutzer, J. S., Wehman, P., Morton, M. V. and Stonnington, H. H. (1988) Supported employment and compensatory strategies for enhancing vocational outcome following traumatic brain injury. *Brain Injury*, **2**, 205–23.

Kupke, T. E., Calhoun, K. S., and Hobbs, S. A. (1979) Selection of heterosexual skills. *Behaviour Therapy*, **10**, 336–46.

Kwentus, J. A., Hart, R. P., Peck, E. T. and Kornstein, S. (1985) Psychiatric complications of closed head trauma. *Psychosomatics*, **26**, 8–17.

Lal, S., Merbtiz, C. P. and Grip, J. C. (1988) Modification of function in head-injury patients with sinemet. *Brain Injury*, **2**, 225–33.

Lamm-Warburg, C. (1988). Assessment and treatment planning strategies for perceptual deficits, in *Physical Rehabilitation: Assessment and Treatment*, 2nd edn, (eds S. O'Sullivan and T. Schmitz), F. A. Davis, Philadelphia, pp. 93–117.

Lance, J. W. (1980) Pathophysiology of spasticity and clinical experience with baclofen, in *Spasticity Disordered Motor Control*, (Eds. R. G. Feldman *et al.*) Year Book Medical Publications, Chicago, pp. 185–202.

Langer, E., Rodin J., Beck, *et al.* (1979) Environmental determinants of memory improvement in late adulthood. *Journal of Personality and Social Psychology*, **37**, 2003–13.

Langfitt, W. (1981) Measuring the outcome for head injuries. *Journal of Neurosurgery*, **48**, 637–78.

Lashley, B. and Drabman, R. (1974) Facilitation of the acquisition and retention of sight-word vocabulary through token reinforcement. *Journal of Applied Behavioral Analysis*, **7**, 307–312.

Laszlo, J. I. (1967) Training of fast tapping with reduction of kinesthetic, tactile, visual and auditory sensations. *Quarterly Journal of Experimental Psychology*, **19**, 344–9.

Latimer, M. S. and Lave, L. B. (1987) Initial effects of the New York State auto safety belt law. *American Journal of Public Health*, **77**, 183–6.

Laurence, S. and Stein, D. G. (1978) Recovery after brain damage and the concept of localization of function, in *Recovery from Brain Damage*, (ed. S. Finger), Plenum Press, New York, pp. 369–407.

Lavond, D. G., McCormick, D. A. and Thompson, R. F. (1984) A non-recoverable learning deficit. *Physiological Psychology*, **12**, 103–10.

Lawes, N. (1989) Course on Neural Plasticity and the Neural Control of Movement. Cardiff 11–13th May 1989.

Lazarus, A. A. (1971) *Behavior Therapy and Beyond*. McGraw-Hill, New York.

Lazarus, R. S. and Folkman, S. (1984) *Stress, Appraisal, and Coping*, Springer, New York.

Leahy, P. (1988) Precasting worksheet – an assessment tool: a clinical report. *Physical Therapy*, **66**, 748.

Lee, T. D., Magill, R. A., and Weeks, D. J. (1985) Influence of practice schedule on testing schema theory predictions in adults. *Journal of Motor Behavior*, **17**, 283–99.

Lees, M. (1988) The social and emotional consequences of severe brain injury: The social work perspective, in *Rehabilitation of the Severely Brain-Injury Adult: A Practical Approach*. (eds I. Fussey and G. M. Giles), Croom Helm, London, pp. 166–82.

Levin, H. S. and Goldstein, F. (1986) Organisation of verbal memory after severe closed-head injury, *Journal of Clinical and Experimental Neuropsychology*, **8**, 643–56.

Levin, H. S. and Grossman, R. G. (1978) Behavioral sequelae of closed head injury. A quantitative study. *Archives of Neurology*, **35**, 720–7.

Levin, H. S., Goldstein, F. C., High. W. M., and Williams, D. (1988a) Automatic and effortful processing after severe closed head injury. *Brain and Cognition*, **7**, 283–97.

Levin, H. S., Grossman, R. G. and Kelly, P. J. (1977) Assessment of long term memory in brain damaged patients. *Journal of Consulting and Clinical Psychology*, **45**, 484–88.

Levin, H. S., High, W. M. and Eisenberg, H. M. (1988b) Learning and forgetting during post traumatic amnesia in head injured patients. *Journal of Neurology, Neurosurgery and Psychiatry*, **51**, 14–20.

Levin, H. S., High, W. M., Goethe, K. E. *et al.* (1987a) The neurobehavioural rating scale: assessment of the behavioural sequelae of head injury by the clinician. *Journal of Neurology, Neurosurgery and Psychiatry*, **50**, 183–193.

Levin, H. S. High, W. M., Meyers, C. A. *et al.* (1985) Impairment of remote memory after closed head injury. *Journal of Neurology, Neurosurgery and Psychiatry*, **48**, 556–63.

Levin, H. S., Lippold, S. C., Goldman, A. *et al.* (1987b) Neurobehavioral functioning and magnetic resonance imaging finding in young boxers. *Journal of Neurosurgery*, **67**, 657–67.

Levin, H. S., O'Donnell, V. M. and Grossman, R. G. (1979) The Galveston orientation and amnesia test: A practical scale to assess cognition after head injury. *The Journal of Nervous and Mental Diseases*, **167**, 675–84.

Levine, A. M. (1988) Buspirone and agitation in head injury. *Brain Injury*, **2**, 165–7.

Levin, D. N. and Grek, A. (1984) The anatomical basis of delusions after right cerebral infarction. *Neurology* (Cleveland), **34**, 577–82.

Lewicki, P., Czyzenska, M. and Hoffman, H. (1987) Unconscious acquisition of complex procedural knowledge. *Journal of Experimental Psychology; Learning, Memory and Cognition*, **13**, 523–30.

Lewicki, P., Hill, T. and Bizot, E. (1988) Acquisition of procedural knowledge about a pattern of stimuli that cannot be articulated. *Cognitive Psychology*, **20**, 24–37.

LeWinn, E. B. (1980) The coma arousal team. Procedures for the patient's professional attendants and for his family. *Royal Society of Health Journal*, **100**, 19–21.

LeWinn, E. B. and Dimancescu, M. M. (1978) Environmental deprivation and enrichment in coma. *Lancet*, i, 156–7.

Lewinsohn, P. M., Danaher, B. G., and Kikel, S. (1977) Visual imagery as a mnemonic aid for brain injured persons. *Journal of Consulting and Clinical Psychology*, **45**, 717–23.

Lewis, J. L. (1970) Semantic processing of unattended messages using dichotic listening. *Journal of Experimental Psychology*, **85**, 225–8.

Lewis, D. O. and Pincus, J. H. (1989) Epilepsy and violence: Evidence for a neuropsychotic-aggressive syndrome. *Journal of Neuropsychiatry*, **1**, 413–8.

Lewis, D. O., Pincus, J. H. Bard, *et al.* (1988) Neuropsychiatric, psychoeducational, and family characteristics of 14 juveniles condemned to death in the United States. *American Journal of Psychiatry*, **145**, 584–9.

Lewis, D. O., Pincus, J. H., Feldman, M. *et al.* (1986) Psychiatric, neurological, and psychoeducational characteristics of 15 death row inmates in the United States. *American Journal of Psychiatry*, **143**, 838–45.

Lewis, F. D., Nelson, J., Nelson, C. and Reusink, P. (1988) Effects of three feedback contingencies on the socially innappropriate talk of a brain-injured adult. *Behavior Therapy*, **19**, 203–11.

Lewis, J. L. (1970) Semantic processing of unattended messages using dichotic listening. *Journal of Experimental Psychology*, **85**, 225–8.

Lezak, M. D. (1976) *Neurological Assessment*, Oxford University Press, New York.

Lezak, M. D. (1983) *Neurological Assessment*, 2nd edn, Oxford University Press, New York.

Lezak, M. (1978) Living with the characterologically altered brain injured patient. *Journal of Clinical Psychiatry*, **39**, 592–8.

Lezak, M. (1979) Recovery of memory and learning functions following traumatic brain injury. *Cortex*, **15**, 63–72.

Lezak, M. D. (1987) Relationship between personality disorders, social disturbances and physical disability following traumatic brain injury. *Journal of Head Trauma Rehabilitation*, **2**, 57–69.

Lhermitte, F. and Pillon, B. (1975) La prosopagnosie: Role de l'heisphere droit dans la perception visuelle. *Revue de Neurology*, **131**, 791–812.

Lincoln, N. B., Whiting, S. E., Cockburn, J. and Bhavnani, G. (1985) An evaluation of perceptual retraining. *International Rehabilitation Medicine*, **7**, 99–101.

Lipton, S. A.(1989) Growth factors for neuronal survival and process regeneration: Implications in the mammalian central nervous system. *Archives of Neurology*, **46**, 1241–8.

Lishman, W. A. (1968) Brain damage in relation to psychiatric disability after head injury. *British Journal of Psychiatry*, **114**, 373–410.

Lishman, W. A. (1972) Selective factors in memory: I. Age sex and personality attributes. *Psychological Medicine*, **2**, 121–38.

Lishman, W. A. (1973) The psychiatric sequelae of head injury: A review. *Psychological Medicine*, **3**, 304–18.

Lishman, W. A. (1978) *Organic Psychiatry*, Blackwell Scientific Publications, Oxford.

Lishman, W. A., Ron, M. and Acker, W. (1980) Computed tomography of the brain and psychometric assessment of alcoholic patients – a British study, in *Addiction and Brain Damage*, (ed. D. Richters), Croom Helm, London, pp. 215–27.

Lissauer, H. (1889) Ein fall von seelenblindheit nebst conem beitrage zur theorie derselben. *Archive Psychiatrie*, **21**, 222–70.

Livingston, M. G. and Livingston, H. M. (1985) The Glasgow assessment schedual: Clinical and research assessment of head injury outcome. *International Rehabilitation Medicine*, **7**, 145–9.

Livingstone, M. G. (1986) Assessment of need for coordinated approach in families with victims of head injury. *British Medical Journal*, **293**, 742–4.

Livingstone, M. G. (1987) Head injury: The relatives' response. *Brain Injury*, **1**, 33–9.

Livingstone, M. G., Brooks, D. N. and Bond, M. R. (1985a) Three months after severe head injury: Psychiatric and social impact on relatives. *Journal of Neurology, Neurosurgery and Psychiatry*, **48**, 870–5.

Livingstone, M. G., Brooks, D. N. and Bond, M. R. (1985b) Patient outcome in the year following severe head injury and relatives' psychiatric and social functioning. *Journal of Neurology, Neurosurgery and Psychiatry*, **48**, 876–81.

Logigian, M., Samuels, M. A., Falconer, J., and Zagar R. (1983) Clinical exercise trial for stroke patients. *Archives of Physical Medicine and Rehabilitation*, **64**, 364–7.

Lorayne, H., and Lucas, J. (1974) *The Memory Book*, Stern and Day, Briarcliffe Manor, New York.

Lorch, E. P., Anderson, D. R. and Well, A. D. (1984) Effects of irrelevant information on speeded classification tasks: Interference is reduced by habituation. *Journal of Experimental Psychology: Human Perception and Performance*, **10**, 850–64.

Luna, G. K., Maier, R. V. Sowder, L. *et al.* (1984) The influence of ethanol intoxication on outcome of injured motorcyclists. *The Journal of Trauma*, **24**, 695–9.

Lungren, C. C. and Persechino, E. L. (1986) Cognitive group: A treatment program for head-injured adults. *The American Journal of Occupational Therapy*, **40**, 397–401.

Luria, A. R. (1965) Two kinds of motor perseveration in massive injuries of the frontal lobes. *Brain*, **88**, 1–10.

Luria, A. R. (1968) *The Mind of a Mnemonist*, Basic Books, New York.

Luria, A. R. (1959) Disorders of 'simultaneous perception' in a case of bilateral occipitoparietal brain injury. *Brain*, **83**, 437–49.

Luria, A. R. (1961) *The Role of Speech in Regulation of Normal and Abnormal Behaviour*, Pergamon Press, Oxford.

Luria, A. R. (1966) *Higher Cortical Functions in Man*, Basic Books, New York.

Luria, A. R. (1973) *The Working Brain*, Penguin, Harmondsworth.

Lyeth, B. G., Dixon, C. E., Hamm, R. J. *et al.* (1985) Neurological deficits following experimental cerebral concussion in the rat attenuated by scopolamine pre-treatment. *Society for Neuroscience Abstracts*, **11**, 432.

Lynch, G., and Baudry, M. (1984) The biochemistry of memory: a new and specific hypothesis. *Science*, **224**, 1057–63.

Lynch, W. J. and Mauss N. K. (1981) Brain Injury rehabilitation: Standard problem lists. *Archives of Physical Medicine and Rehabilitation*, **62**, 223–7.

Lyons, J. L. and Morse, A. R. (1988) A therapeutic work program for head injured adults. *The American Journal of Occupational Therapy*, **42**, 364–70.

Mace, C. F., Hock, M. L., Lalli, J. S. *et al.* (1988) Behavioral momentum in the treatment of non-compliance. *Journal of Applied Behavioral Analysis*, **21**, 123–141.

Mace, F. C., Kratochwill, T. R. and Fiello, R. A. (1983) Positive treatment of aggressive behavior in a mentally retarded adult: A case study. *Behavior Therapy*, **14**, 689–96.

Mackworth, N., Mackworth, J. and Cope, D. N. (1982) Towards an interpretation of head injury recovery trends, in Santa Clara Valley Medical Center Institute for Medical Research. Head Injury Rehabilitation Project: Final Report. Santa Clara Valley Medical Center, San Jose California, pp. 1–66.

Macpherson, P., Teasdale, E., Dhaker, S. *et al.* (1986) The significance of traumatic haematoma in the region of the basal ganglia. *Journal of Neurology, Neurosurgery and Psychiatry*, **49**, 29–34.

Magill, R. A., (1985) *Motor Learning: Concepts and Applications*, 2nd Edn., Brown, Duberquer, Iowa.

Magill, R. A., and Lee, T. D., (1987) Verbal label effects on response accuracy and organisation for learning limb positioning movements. *Journal of Human Movement Studies*, **13**, 285–308.

Mahoney, F. I. and Barthel, D. W. (1965) Functional Evaluation: The Barthel Index. *Maryland State Medical Journal*, **14**, 61–65.

Maier, N. R. F. (1960) Screening solutions to upgrade quality: A new approach to problem solving under conditions of uncertainty. *Journal of Psychology*, **49**, 217–31.

Maier, N. R. F. and Hoffman, L. R. (1964) Financial incentives and group decision in motivating change. *Journal of Social Psychology*, **64**, 369–78.

Malec, J., Jones, R., Rao, M., and Stubbs, K. (1984) Video-game practice and sustained attention in patients with craniocerebral trauma. *Cognitive Rehabilitation*, **2**, 18–23.

Malloy, P. (1987) Frontal lobe dysfunction in obsessive-compulsive disorder, in *The Frontal Lobes Revisited*, (ed. E. Perecman), The IRBN Press, New York, New York.

Maltzman, I. (1960) On the training of originality. *Psychological Review*, **67**, 229–42.

Mammucari, A., Caltagirone, C., Ekman, P. *et al.* (1988) Spontaneous facial expressions of emotions in brain-damaged patients. *Cortex*, **24**, 521–33.

Martinelli, P.(1986) Tremor: A clinical and pharmacological survey. *Journal of Neural Transmission*, (Suppl) **22**, 141–8.

Mathiowetz, V., Rogers, S. L., Dowe-Keval, *et al.* (1986) The purdue pegboard: Norms of 14- to 19-year olds. *The American Journal of Occupational Therapy*, **40**, 174–9.

McClain, L. and Todd, C. (1990) Food store accessibility. *The American Journal of Occupational Therapy*, **44**, 487–91.

McDowell, J. J. (1982) The importance of Hernsteins' mathematical statement of the law of effect for behavior therapy. *American Psychologist*, **37**, 771–9.

McFall, R. M. (1982) A review and reformulation of the concept of social skills. *Behaviour Assessment*, **4**, 1–33.

McFarlane, A. C. (1989) The aetiology of post-traumatic morbidity: predisposing, precipitating and perpetuating factors. *British Journal of Psychiatry*, **154**, 221–8.

McHugh, S. and Vallis, T. M. (1986) Illness behavior: Operationalization of the biopsychosocial model, in *Illness Behavior*, (eds S. McHugh and T. M. Vallis), Plenum Press, New York, pp. 1–32.

McIntosh, T. K., Andrews, B., Agura, V. *et al.* (1986) Sterospecific efficacy of the opiate antagonist WIN44, 441–3 in the treatment of head injury in the cat. *Proceedings of the American Association of Neurological Surgeons*, 116–118.

McKeon, J., McGuffin, P. and Robinson, P. (1984) Obsessive-compulsive neurosis following head injury: a report of four cases. *British Journal of Psychiatry*, **144**, 190–2.

McKinlay, W. W. and Brooks, D. N. (1984) Methodological problems in assessing psychosocial recovery following severe brain injury. *Journal of Clinical Neuropsychology*, **6**, 87–99.

McKinlay, W. W. and Hickox, A. (1988) How can families help in the rehabilitation of the head injured? *Journal of Head Trauma Rehabilitation*, **3**, 64–72.

McKinlay, W. W., Brooks, D. N., Bond, M. R. *et al.* (1981) The short-term outcome of severe blunt brain injury as reported by relatives of the injured persons. *Journal of Neurology, Neurosurgery and Psychiatry*, **44**, 727–33.

Mclatchie, G., Brooks, No., Galbraith, S. *et al.* (1987) Clinical neurological examination, neuropsychology, electroencephalography and computer tomographic head scanning in active amateur boxers. *Journal of Neurology, Neurosurgery and Psychiatry*, **50**, 96–9.

McLellan, D. L. (1977) Co-contraction and stretch reflexes in spasticity during treatment with baclofen. *Journal of Neurology, Neurosurgery and Psychiatry*, **40**, 30–8.

McLelland, R. J. (1985) A neurophysiological investigation of minor head injury, in *Clinical and Experimental Neurophysiology*, (eds D. Papakostopoulos et al.), Croom Helm, London, pp. – .

McMillan, T. M. and Gluckman, E. E. (1987) The neuropsychology of moderate head injury. *Journal of Neurology, Neurosurgery and Psychiatry*, **50**, 393–7.

McMordie, W. R. and Barker, S. L. (1988) The financial trauma of head Injury. *Brain Injury*, **2**, 357–64.

McSweeny, A. J., Grant, I., Heaton, R. K. *et al.* (1982) Life quality of patients with chronic obstructive pulmonary disease. *Archives of Internal Medicine*, **142**, 473–8.

Mechanic, D. (1986) Illness behavior an overview, in *Illness Behavior*, (eds S. McHugh and T. M. Vallis), Plenum Press, New York, pp. 101–10.

Mehrabian, A. (1972) *Non-Verbal Communication*, Aldine-Atherton Chicago, Illinois.

Mehrabian, A. and Ferris, S. R. (1967) Inference of attitude from non-verbal communication in two channels. *Journal of Consulting Psychology*, **31**, 248–52.

Meichenbaum, D. (1977) *Cognitive-Behavior Modification: Integrative Approach*, Plenum, New York.

Meissner, W. W. (1978) *The Paranoid Process*, Jason Aronson, Dunmore, Penn.

Mentis, M. and Prutting, C. A. (1987) Cohesion in the discourse of normal and head injured adults. *Journal of Speech and Hearing Research*, **30**, 88–98.

Millar, K., Jeffcoate, W., and Walder, C. (1987) Vasopressin and memory: Improvement in normal short-term recall and reduction of alcohol-induced amnesia. *Psychological Medicine*, **17**, 335–41.

Miller, G. A. (1956) The magical number seven plus or minus two: Some limits on our capacity for processing information. *Psychological Review*, **63**, 81–97.

Miller, B. L., Cummings, J. L., McIntyre, H. *et al.* (1986) Hypersexuality or altered sexual preference following brain injury. *Journal of Neurology, Neurosurgery and Psychiatry*, **49**, 867–73.

Miller, E. (1970) Simple and choice reaction time following head injury. *Cortex*, **6**, 121–7.

Miller, E. (1980) The training characteristics of severely head injured patients: A preliminary study. *Journal of Neurology, Neurosurgery and Psychiatry*, **43**, 525–8.

Miller, E. (1985) Cognitive retraining of neurological patients, in *New Developments in Clinical Psychology* (ed. F. N. Watts), John Wiley, Chichester,

Miller, E. (1987) Hysteria: Its nature and explanation. *British Journal of Clinical Psychology*, **26**, 163–73.

Miller, G. A., Galanter, E. and Pribram, K. H. (1960) *Plans and the Structure of Behaviour*, Holt, Rinehart and Winston, New York.

Miller, H. and Stern, G. (1965) The long-term prognosis of severe head injury. *Lancet*, **ii**, 225–9.

Miller, J. D., Tocher, J. L. and Jones, P. A. (1988) Editorial: Extradural haematoma-earlier detection, better results. *Brain Injury*, **2**, 83–6.

Miller, E. and Cruzat, A. (1981) A note on the effects of relevant information on task performance after mild and severe brain injury. *British Journal of Social and Clinical Psychology*, **20**, 69–70.

Milner, B. (1962) Les troubles de la memoire accompagnant des lesions hippocampiques bilaterales, in *Physiology de l'Hippocampe*, (ed P. Passouant), Centre National de la Recherche Scientifique, Paris. English translation in P. M. Milner and S. Glickman (eds.) (1985) *Cognitive Processes and the Brain*, Van Nostrand, New York,

Milner, B. (1963) Effects of different brain lesions on card sorting. *Archives of Neurology*, **9**, 90–100.

Milner, B., Corkin, S. and Teuber, H.-L. (1968) Further analysis of the Hippocampalamnesic syndrome: 14-year follow up study of H.M. *Neuropsychologia*, **6**, 215–34.

Minnesota Manual Dexterity Test Manual. Lafayette Instrument Co., Indiana.

Minnesota Rate of Manipulations Test. Examiners Manual. (1969) American Guidance Service Inc., Circle Pines, MN.

Mishkin, M. and Petri, H. L. (1984) Memories and habits: Some implications for the analysis of learning and retention, in *Neuropsychology of Memory*, (eds. L. R. Squire and N. Butters), The Guilford Press, New York.

Moffat, N. (1984) Strategies of memory therapy, in Wilson, B. A. and Moffat, N. (eds.) *Clinical Management of Memory Problems*, (eds B. A. Wilson and N. Moffat), Croom Helm, London.

Monakow, C. Von. (1914) *Das Grosshirn und die Abbbavfunktion durch Kortikale*. Bergmann, Herde Weisbaden.

Monroe, R. R. (1970) *Episodic Behavioural Disorders*, Harvard University Press, Cambridge, MA.

Montgomery, A., Fenton, G. W. and McLelland, R. J. (1984) Delayed brain stem conduction time in post-concussional syndrome. *Lancet*, i, 1011.

Monti, P. M., Corneau, D. P. and Curran J. P. (1982) Social skills for psychiatric patients: Treatment and outcome, in *Social Skills Training: A Practical Handbook for Assessment and Treatment*, (eds J. P. Curran and P. M. Monti), Guilford, New York.

Moore, J. W. (1977) The initial interview and interactional analysis. *American Journal of Occupational Therapy*, **31**, 29.

Moore, T. J., Barron, J., Modlin, P. and Bean, S. (1989) The use of tone-reducing casts to prevent joint contractures following severe closed head injury. *Journal of Head Trauma Rehabilitation*, **4**, 63–5.

Moos, R. H. (1988a) *Ward Attitude Scale*, Consulting Psychologists Press, Palo Alto, CA.

Moos, R. H. (1988b) *Community-Oriented Programs Environment Scale*, Consulting Psychologists Press, Palo Alto, CA.

Moos, R. H., Cronkite, R. C., Billing, A. G. and Finney, J. W. (1988) *Health and Daily Living Form Manual*. Social Ecology Laboratory, Veterans Administration Hospital, Palo Alto.

Mroczec, M., Halpern, D. and McHugh, R., (1978) Electromyographic feedback and physical therapy for neuromuscular retraining in hemiplegia. *Archives of Physical Medicine and Rehabilitation*, **59**, 592–6.

Mueller-Jensen, A., Neunzig, H-P. and Emskotter, Th. (1987) Outcome prediction in comatose patients: significance of reflex eye movement analysis. *Journal of Neurology, Neurosurgery and Psychiatry*, **50**, 389–92

Mulder, T. (1985) *Learning of Motor Control Following Brain Damage: Experimental and Clinical Studies*, Swets Publishing Service,

Musa, I. (1986) The role of afferent input in the reduction of spasticity: An hypothesis. *Physiotherapy*, **72**, 179–82.

Mysiw, W. J., Corrigan, J. D., Carpenter, D. and Chock, S. K. L. (1990) Prospective assessment of posttraumatic amnesia: A comparison of the GOAT and the OGMS, *Journal of Head Trauma Rehabilitation*, **5**, 65–72.

Nagi, S. Z. (1976) The disabled and rehabilitation services: A national overview. *American Rehabilitation*, **2**, 26–33.

Najenson, T., Mendelson, L., Schechter, I. *et al.* (1974) Rehabilitation after severe head injury. *Scandinavian Journal of Rehabilitation Medicine*, **6**, 5–14.

Narayan, R. K., Greenberg, R. P., Miller, J. D. *et al.* (1981) Improved confidence in outcome prediction in severe head injury. *Journal of Neurosurgery*, **54**, 751–62.

Nasrallah, H. A., Fowler, R. C. and Judd, L. L. (1981) Schizophrenialike illness following head injury. *Psychosomatics*, **22**, 359–61.

Nation, J. R. and Woods, D. J. (1980) Persistence: The role of partial reinforcement in psychotherapy. *Journal of Experimental Psychology: General*, **109**, 175–207.

National Head Injury Foundation (1989) *Directory of Head Injury Rehabilitation Services*, Southborough MA, NHIF.

Neisser, U. (1967) *Cognitive Psychology*, Appleton Century Crofts, New York.

Neisser, U. (1988) New vistas in the study of memory, in *Remembering Reconsidered: Ecological and Traditional Approaches to the Study of Memory*, (eds U. Neisser and E. Winograd), Cambridge University Press, Cambridge, pp. 1–10.

Neistadt, M. E. (1988) Occupational therapy for adults with perceptual deficits. *The American Journal of Occupational Therapy*, **42**, 434–40.

Neistadt, M. E. (1990) A critical analysis of occupational therapy approaches for perceptual deficits in adults with brain injury. *The American Journal of Occupational Therapy*, **44**, 299–304.

Nelson, R. D. and Hayes, S. C. (1979) The nature of behavioural assessment: A commentary. *Journal of Applied Behaviour Analysis*, **12**, 491–500.

Newcombe, F. (1982) The psychological consequences of closed brain injury; assessment and rehabilitation. *Injury*, **14**, 111–36.

Newman, F. L. and Sorensen, J. E. *Integrated Clinical and Fiscal Management in Mental Health: A Handbook*, Ablex publishing Corporation, Norwood, New Jersey.

Newton, A. and Johnson, D. (1985) Social adjustment and interaction after brain injury. *British Journal of Clinical Psychology*, **24**, 225–34.

Newton, A., Kindness, K. and Mcfadyen, M. (1983) Patients and social skills groups: Do they lack social skills? *Behavioural Psychotherapy*, **11**, 116–26.

Nichols, P. J. R. (1974) Functional assessment. *Proceedings of the Royal Society of Medicine*, **67**, 406–9.

Nihira, K., Foster, R., Shellhaas, M. and Leland, H. (1975) *Adaptive Behavior Scale*, Manual, American Association on Mental Deficiency, Washington.

Nissen, M. J. and Bullemer, P. (1987) Attentional requirements of learning: Evidence from performance measures. *Cognitive Psychology*, **19**, 1–32.

Nolan, M. F. (1982) Two-point discrimination assessment in the upper limb in young adult men and women. *Physical Therapy*, **62**, 965–9.

Nolan, M. F. (1985) Quantitative measures of cutaneous sensation: Two-point discrimination values for the face and trunk. *Physical Therapy*, **65**, 181–5.

Norman, D. A. (1968) Toward a theory of memory and attention. *Psychological Review*, **75**, 522–36.

Nouri, F. M., Tinson, D. J. and Lincoln, N. B. (1987) Cognitive ability and driving after stroke. *International Disability Studies*, **9**, 110–15

O'Keefe, J. and Nadel, L. (1978) *The Hippocampus as a Cognitive Map*, Oxford University Press, London.

O'Reilly, C. A. and Puffer, S. M. (1989) The impact of rewards and punishments in a social context: A laboratory and field experiment. *Journal of Occupational Behavior*, **62**, 41–53.

O'Rourke, N. A., Costello, F., Yelland, J. D. N. and Stuart, G. G. (1987) Head injuries to children riding bicycles. *The Medical Journal of Australia*, **146**, 619–21.

O'Reilly, M. F. and Cuvo, A. J. (1989) Teaching self-treatment of cold symptoms to an anoxic brain injured adult. *Behavioral Residential Treatment*, **4**, 359–75.

Oakley, D. A. (1983) Learning capacity outside the neocortex in animals and man: Implications for therapy after brain injury, in *Animal Models of Human Behavior: Conceptual Evolutionary and Neurobiological Perspectives*. (ed. G. Davey), Wiley, Chichester,

Oakley, F., Kielhofner, G., Barris, R. and Reichler, R. K. (1986) The role checklist: Development and empirical assessment of reliability. *Occupational Therapy Journal of Research*, **6**, 157–70.

Ochipa, C., Rothi, L. J. G. and Heilman, K. M. (1989) Ideational apraxia: a deficit in tool selection and use. *Annals of Neurology*, **25**, 191–3.

Oddy, M. (1985) Seven years after: a follow-up study of severe brain injury in young adults. *Journal of Clinical Experimental Neuropsychology*, **7**, 165.

Oddy, M., Humphrey, M. and Uttley, D. (1978) Stresses upon the relatives of brain-injured patients. *British Journal of Psychiatry*, **41**, 611–16

Ogden, J. A. (1985) Autopagnosia, occurrence in a patient without nominal aphasia and with an intact ability to point to parts of animals and objects. *Brain*, **108**, 1009–22.

Oppenheimer, D. R. (1968) Microscopic lesions in the brain following head injury. *Journal of Neurology, Neurosurgery and Psychiatry*, **31**, 299–306.

Ornato, J. P., Craren, E. J., Nelson, N. M. and Kimball, K. F. (1985) Impact of improved emergency medical services and emergency trauma care on reduction of mortality from trauma. *Journal of Trauma*, **25**, 575–9.

Orsay, E. M., Turnbull, T. L., Dunne, M. *et al*. (1988) Prospective study of the effect of safety belts on morbidity and health care costs in motor-vehicle accidents. *JAMA*, **260**, 3598–603.

Osborn, A. F. (1963) Applied imagination: *Principles and procedures of Creative Problem-solving*, 3rd edn, Scribners, New York.

Overall, J. E. and Gorman, D. R. (1962) The brief psychiatric rating scale. *Psychological Report*, **10**, 799–812.

Overguaard, J. (1973) Prognosis after brain injury based on early clinical examination. *Lancet*, **ii**, 631–5.

Palmer, M. and Wyness, M. A. (1988) Positioning and handling: Important considerations in the care of the severely head-injured patient. *Journal of Neuroscience Nursing*, **20**, 42–9.

Panikoff. L. B. (1983) Recovery trends in functional skills in head injured adults. *AJOT: The American Journal of Occupational Therapy*, **37**, 735–43.

Pantano, J. C., Baron, J. C., Samson, Y. *et al*. (1968) Crossed cerebellar diaschisis: further studies. *Brain*, **109**, 677–694.

Parasuraman, R. (1984) The psychobiology of sustained attention, in *Sustained Attention in Human Performance*, (ed. J. S. Warm), John Wiley, Chichester.

Parente, R. and Anderson-Parente, J. K. (1989) Vocational Memory Training. In *Community Integration Following Traumatic Brain Injury*, (Eds J. S. Kreutzer and P. Wehman), Paul H. Brookes, Baltimore, USA.

Parkin, A. L. (1984) Amnesic syndrome: a lesion-specific disorder? *Cortex*, **20**, 479–80.

Parmelee, D. X. and O'Shanick, G. J. (1988) Neuropsychiatric interventions with head injured children and adolescents. *Brain Injury*, **1**, 41–7.

Parnes, S. J. and Meadow, A. (1960) Evaluation of persistence of effect produced by a creative problem-solving course. *Psychological Reports*, **7**, 357–61.

Pask, G. and Scott, B. C. E. (1972) Learning strategies and individual competence. *International Journal of Man-Machine Studies*, **4**, 217–53.

Pask, G. and Scott, B. C. E.(1973) CASTE: a system for exhibiting learning strategies and regulating uncertainties. *International Journal of Man-Machine Studies*, **5**, 5–52.

Paterson, A. and Zangwill, O. L. (1944) Recovery of spatial orientation in the post-traumatic confusional state. *Brain*, **67**, 54–68.

Pattern, B. M. (1972) The ancient art of memory: Usefulness in treatment. Archives of Neurology, **26**, 25–31.

Patterson, C. H. (1983) *Non-verbal behaviour: a functional perspective*, Springer-Verlag, New York.

Patterson, M. L. (1983) *Non-Verbal Behavior*, Springer-Verlag, New York.

Pavlov, I. P. (1927) *Conditioned Reflexes*, Oxford University Press, London.

Pedretti, L. W. (1981) *Occupational Therapy Practice Skills for Physical Dysfunction*, The C.V. Mosby Company, St. Louis, Missouri.

Pellock, J. M. (1989) Editorial: Who should receive prophylactic antiepileptic drugs following head injury? *Brain Injury*, **3**, 107–8.

Peters, B. H. and Levin, H. S. (1977) Memory enhancement after Physostigmine treatment in the amnesic syndrome. *Archives of Neurology*, **34**, 215–9.

Petito, C. K., Feldmann, E., Pulsinelli, W. A. and Plum, F.(1987) Delayed hippocampal damage in humans following cardiorespiratory arrest. *Neurology*, **37**, 1281–6.

Petrides, M. (1985) Deficits on conditional and associative-learning tasks after frontal and temporal-lobe lesions in man. *Neuropsychologia*, **23**,601–14.

Pilz, P. (1983) Axonal injury in head injury. *Acta Neurochir* (Suppl 32), 119–23.

Pizzamiglio, L., Caltagirone, C., Mammucari, A. *et al.* (1987) Imitation of facial movements in brain damaged patients. *Cortex*, **23**,207–21.

Plienis, A. J., Hansen, D. J., Ford, F. *et al.* (1987) Behavioral small group training to improve the social skills of emotionally disordered adolescents. *Behaviour Therapy*, **18**, 17–32

Plum, F. and Posner, J. B. (1980) *The Diagnosis of Stupor and Coma*, F. A. Davis Company, Philadelphia.

Poeck, K., and Lehmkuhl G. (1980) Ideatory apraxia in a left-handed patient with right-sided brain lesion. *Cortex*, **16**,273–84.

Ponsford, J. L. and Kinsella, G. (1988) Evaluation of a remedial program for attentional deficits following closed-head injury. *Journal of Clinical and Experimental Neuropsychology*, **10**,693–708.

Posner, M. I. (1975) Abstraction and the process of recognition. *Psychology of Learning and Motivation*, **3**, 43–100.

Post, R. M., Uhde, T. W., Putnam, F. W. *et al.* (1982) Kindling and carbamazepine in affective illness. *Journal of Nervous and Mental Disease*, **170**,717–31.

Powell, G. E. (1981) *Brain Function Therapy*, Gower, Aldershot, Hants.

Powell-Proctor, L., and Miller, E., (1982) Reality orientation: A critical appraisal. *British Journal of Psychiatry*, **140**,457–63.

Power, C. (1979) The time sample checklist: Observational assessment of patient functioning. *Journal of Behaviour Assessment*, **1**,199–210.

Priddy, D. A., Mattes, D. and Lam, C. S. (1988) Reliability of self report among non-oriented head-injured adults. *Brain Injury*, **2**,249–53.

Prigatano, G. P. (ed. 1986) *Neuropsychological Rehabilitation After Brain Injury*, Johns Hopkins University Press, Baltimore.

Prigatano, G. P., O'Brien, K. P. and Klonoff, P. S. (1988) The clinical management of paranoid delusions in postacute traumatic brain-injured patients. *Journal of Head Trauma Rehabilitation*, **3**,23–332.

Prigatano, G., Monte, L., William C. *et al* (1982) Sleep and dreaming disturbance in closed head injury patients. *Journal of Neurology, Neurosurgery and Psychiatry*, **45**, 78–80.

Prutting, C. A. and Kirchner, D. M. (1987) A clinical appraisal of the pragmatic aspects of language. *Journal of Speech and Hearing Disorders*, **52**,105–119.

Quine, S., Pierce, J. P. and Lyle, D. M. (1988) Relatives as lay-therapists for the severely head-injured. *Brain Injury*, **2**, 139–49.

Rader, M. A., Alston, J. B. and Ellis, D. W. (1989) Sensory stimulation of severely brain injured patients. *Brain Injury*, **3**,141–7.

Rao, N., Jellinke, H. M. and Woolston, D. C. (1985) Agitation in closed head injury: Haloperidol effects on rehabilitation outcome. *Archives of Physical Medicine and Rehabilitation*, **66**,30–4.

Rao, N., Jellinek, H. M., Harberg, J. K. and Fryback, D. G. (1988) The art of medicine: subjective measures as predictors of outcome in stroke and traumatic brain injury. *Archives of Physical Medicine and Rehabilitation*, **69**,179–182.

Rappaport, M., Hall, K. M., Hopkins, K. *et al.* (1982) Disability rating scale for severe brain trauma; coma to community. *Archives of Physical Medicine and Rehabilitation*, **63**,118–23.

Rapport, M. D., Sonis, W. A., Fialkov, M. J. *et al* (1983) Carbamazepine and behaviour therapy for aggressive behaviour. *Behaviour Modification*, **7**,255–65.

Ratcliff, G. (1982) Disturbances in spacial orientation associated with cerebral lesions, in *Spatial Abilities*, New York academic press, New York,

Reason, J. (1979) Actions not as planned, in *Aspects of Consciousness Vol 1*. (eds G. Underwood and R. Stevens), Academic Press, London and New York. pp 67–89.

Reed, E. S. (1982) An outline of a theory of action systems. *Journal of Motor Behaviour*, **14**, 98–134.

Reilly, E. L., Kelley, J. T. and Fallace, L. A. (1986) Role of alcohol use and abuse in trauma, *Advances in Psychosomatic Medicine*, **16**, 17–30.

Riddoch, M. J. and Humphreys, G. W. (1983) The effect of cueing on unilateral neglect. *Neuropsychologia*, **21**,589–99.

Rimel, R., Giordani, M., Barth, J. *et al.* (1981) Disability caused by minor head injury. *Neurosurgery*, **9**,221–8.

Rinehart, M. A. (1983) Considerations for functional training in adults after brain injury. *Physical Therapy*, **63**, 1975–82.

Roberts, J. (1945) *Pennsylvania Bi-Manual Work Sample*, American Guidance Service Inc., Circle Pines, Minnesota.

Robbertson, I., Gray, J. and McKenzie, S. (1988) Microcomputer based cognitive rehabilitation of visual neglect: 3 multiple baseline single case studies. *Brain Injury*, **2**;151–63.

Robin, J. J. (1977) Paroxymal choeoathetosis following head injury. *Annals of Neurology*, **2**,447–8.

Robinett, C. S. and Vondran, M. A. (1988) Functional ambulation velocity and distance requirements in rural and urban communities. *Physical Therapy*, **68**,1371–3.

Robinson, R. G., Boston, J. D., Starkstein, S. E. and Price, T. R. (1988) Comparison of mania and depression after brain injury: causal factors. *American Journal of Psychiatry*, **145**,172–8.

Robson, P. (1989) Development of a new self report questionnaire to measure self esteem. *Psychological Medicine*, **19**,513–8.

Romano, J. M. and Bellack, A. S. (1980) Social validation of a component model of assertive behaviour. *Journal of Consulting and Clinical Psychology*, **48**,478–90.

Ron, S. (1981) Plastic changes in eye movements in patients with traumatic brain injury. *Progress in Oculomotor Research*, (eds A. F. Fuchs and W. Becker), Elsevier, North Holland, Amsterdam, pp. 223–40.

Rood, M. (1962) The use of sensory receptors to activate and inhibit motor response, autonomic and somatic in developmental sequence, *Approaches to Treatment of Patients with Neuromuscular Dysfunction*, (ed. C Sattely), Brown and Co., Dubuque,

Rose M. (1988) Medical considerations in brain injury rehabilitation, in *Rehabilitation of the Severely Brain-Injured Adult: A Practical Approach*, (eds I. Fussey and G. M. Giles), Croom Helm, London, pp. 1–29.

Rose Y. and Tryon, W. (1979) Judgements of assertive behaviour as a function of speech loudness, latency, content, gestures, inflection and sex. *Behaviour Modification*, **3**, 112–23.

Rosenbaum, A. and Najensen, R. (1976) Sexual dysfunction due to interpersonal changes in life patterns and symptoms of low mood as reported by wives of severely brain-injured soldiers. *Journal of Consulting and Clinical Psychology*, **44**,881–8.

Ross, R. J., Cole, M., Thompson, J. S. *et al* (1983) Boxers – computed tomography, EEG and neurological evaluation. *JAMA*, **249**,211–3.

Rotter, J. B. (1966) Generalised expectancies for internal versus external control of reinforcement. *Psychological Monographs* (no. 609), **80**.

Russell, E. W. (1975) A multiple scoring method for the assessment of complex memory functions. *Journal of Consulting and Clinical Psychology*, **43**,800–9.

Russell, W. R. (1960) Injury to cranial nerves and optic chiasm, in *Injuries on the Brain and Spinal Cord and their Coverings*, 4th edn. (ed. S. Brock), Springer-Verlag, New York, pp. 118–26.

Russell, W. R. and Smith, A. (1961) Post-traumatic amnesia in closed head injuries. *Archives of Neurology*, **5**,16–29.

Russell, W. R. (1971) *The Traumatic Amnesias*, Oxford University Press, Oxford.

Rutherford, W. H. (1977) Diagnosis of alcohol ingestion on mild head injuries. *The Lancet*, **i**,1021–3.

Sage, G. H. (1984) *Motor Learning and Control: A Neuropsychological Approach*, W. C. Brown, Dubuque, Iowa.

Sahrmann, S. A. and Norton, B. J. (1977) The relationship of voluntary movement to spasticity in the upper motor neuron syndrome. *Annals of Neurology*, **2**,460–5.

Sakai, C. S. and Mateer, C. A. (1984) Otological and audiological sequelae of closed head trauma. *Seminars in Hearing*, **5**,157–73.

Santa Clara Valley Medical Center Institute for Medical Research (1988) Head Injury Rehabilitation Project: Final Report. Santa Clara Valley Medical Center, San Jose, California.

Sarno, M. T. (1984) Verbal impairment after closed head injury: Report of a replication study. *Journal of Nervous and Mental Diseases*, **172**,475–9.

Schechter, P. J. and Henkin, R. I. (1974) Abnormalities of taste and smell after head trauma. Journal of Neurology, Neurosurgery and Psychiatry, **37**,802–10.

Schegloff, E. A. and Sacks, H. (1973) Opening-up closings, *Semiotica*, **8**, 289–329.

Schmitt, R. A. (1975) A schema theory of discrete motor skill learning. *Psychological Review*, **82**,225–60.

Schmitt, R. A. (1980) On the theoretical status of time in motor program representation. *Tutorials in Motor Behavior*, (eds. G. E. Steimach and J. Requin) North Holland Publishing Company, Amsterdam,

Schmitt, R. A. (1982) *Motor Learning and Control: A Behavioral Emphasis*, Human Kinetics, Champaign, Illinois.

Schneider, W., Dumais, S. T. and Shiffrin, R. M. (1984) Automatic and control processing and attention. *Varieties of Attention* (eds R. Parasuraman and D. R. Davis), Academic Press, London, pp 1–27.

Scholten, D. J. and Glover, J. L. (1984) Increased mortality following repeal of manditory motorcycle helmet law. *Indiana Med*, **77**,252–5.

Schoenfeld, T. A. and Hamilton, L. W. (1977) Secondary brain changes following lesions: A new paradigm for lesion experimentation. *Physiology and Behavior*, **18**,951–67.

Scott, W. O. and Edelstein, B. A. (1981) The social competence of two interaction strategies: An analog evaluation. *Behaviour Therapy*, **12**,482–92.

Scranton, J., Fogel, M. L. and Erdman, W. J. (1970) Evaluation of functional levels of patients during and following rehabilitation. *Archives of Physical Medicine and Rehabilitation*, **51**,1–21.

Seelig, J. M., Becker, D. P., Miller, J. D. *et al.* (1981) Traumatic acute subdural hematoma major mortality reductions in comatose patients treated within four hours. *New England Journal of Medicine*, **304**,1245–9.

Selfridge, O. G. (1959) *Pandemonium: a Paradigm for Learning in Mechanisation of Thought Processes*, HMSO, London.

Seligman, M. (1975) *Helplessness: On Depression, Development and Death*, W. H. Freeman, San Francisco.

Semenza, C. (1988) Impairment of localization of body parts following brain damage. *Cortex*, **24**,443–9.

Semenza, C. and Goodglass, H. (1985) Localization of body parts in brain injured subjects. *Neuropsychologia* **23**,161–175.

Servadei, F., Piazza, G., Seracchioli, A. *et al.* (1988) Extradural haematomas: an analysis of changing characteristics of patients admitted from 1980 to 1986. Diagnostic and therapeutic implications in 158 cases. *Brain Injury*, **2**,87–100.

Shaffer, D., Chadwick, O. and Rutter, M. (1975) Psychiatric outcome of localized head injury in children, in CIBA Foundation Symposium, 34, New Series, *Outcome of Severe Damage to the Central Nervous System*, Elsevier, Amsterdam, pp. 191–209.

Shallice, T. (1982) Specific impairment of planning, in *The Neuropsychology of Cognitive Function*. (eds. D. E. Broadbent and L. Weiskrantz), The Royal Society, London, pp. 199–209.

Shallice, T. and Evans, M. E. (1978) The involvement of the frontal lobes in cognitive estimation. *Cortex*, **14**,294–303.

Shapiro, L. B. (1939) Schizophrenia-like psychosis following head injury. *Illinois Medical Journal*. **76**,250–254.

Shaw, L., Brodsky, L. and McMahon, B. T. (1985) Neuropsychiatric intervention in the rehabilitation of head injured patients. *The Psychiatric Journal of the University of Ottawa*. **10**,237–40.

Shaw, R. (1986) Persistent vegetative state: Principles and techniques for seating and positioning. *Journal of Head Trauma Rehabilitation*, **1**,31–7.

Shea, J. B. and Morgan, R. L. (1979) Contextual interference effects on the acquisition, retention and transfer of a motor skill. *Journal of Experimental Psychology: Human Learning and Memory*, **5**,179–87.

Shiffrin, R. M. and Schneider, W. (1977) Controlled and automatic information processing: II. Perceptual learning, automatic attending, and a general theory. *Psychological Review*, **84**,127–90.

Shontz, F. (1967) Behaviour settings may affect rehabilitation clients. *Rehabilitation Record*, **8**,37–40.

Shukla, S., Cook, B. L., Mukherjee, S. *et al.* (1987) Mania following head trauma. *American Journal of Psychiatry*. **144**,93–6.

Shukla, S., Godwin, C., Long L. E. B. *et al.* (1984) Lithium-carbamazepine neurotoxity and risk factors. *American Journal of Psychiatry*. **141**,1604–6.

Sigelman, C. K., Spanhel, C. L. and Vangroff, L. P. (1979) Disability and the concept of life functions. *Rehabilitation Counselling Bulletin*, **23**,103–13.

Silverstone, T. and Turner, P. (1988) *Drug Treatment in Psychiatry*, 4th Edn, Routledge, London and New York.

Simon, H. A. (1955) A behavioural model of rational choice. *Quarterly Journal of Economics*, **69**,99–118.

Sims, A. C. (1985) Head injury, neurosis and accident proneness. *Advances in Psychosomatic Medicine*, **13**,49–70.

Sinanan, K. (1984) Mania as a sequel to road accident. *British Journal of Psychiatry*, **144**,330–1.

Skinner, B. F. (1938) *The Behaviour of Organisms*, Appelton-Century-Crofts, New York.

Skinner, B. F. (1968) *The Technology of Teaching*, Apleton-Century, New York.

Smith, H. W. (1975) *Strategies of Social Research*, Prentice-Hall, New Jersey.

Soderback, I. and Normell, L. A. (1986a) Intellectual function training in adults with acquired brain damage: An occupational therapy method. *Scandinavian Journal of Rehabilitation Medicine*, **18**,139–46.

Soderback, I. and Normell, L. A. (1986b) Intellectual function training in adults with acquired brain damage: Evaluation. *Scandinavian Journal of Rehabilitation Medicine*, **18**,147–53.

Sohlberg, M. M. and Mateer, C. A. (1987) Effectiveness of an attention training program. *Journal of Clinical and Experimental Neuropsychology*, **9**,117–30.

Sohlberg, M. M. and Mateer, C. A. (1989) Training use of compensatory memory books: A three stage behavioral approach. *Journal of Clinical and Experimental Neuropsychology*, **11**,871–91.

Sokolov, E. N. (1969) The modelling properties of the nervous system, in *A handbook of contemporary Soviet Psychology*, (eds M. Cole and I. Maltzman, Basic Books, New York,

Sokolow, J., Silson, J. E. Taylor, E. J. *et al.* (1958) Functional approach to disability evaluation. *The Journal of the American Medical Association*, **167**,1575–84.

Solokov, E. N. (1963) *Perception and the Conditioned Reflex*, Pergamon Press, Oxford.

Sommes, R. (1969) *Personal space*, Prentice-Hall, Englewood Cliff, N. J.

Soroker, N., Groswasser, Z. and Costeff, H. (1989) Practice of prophylactic anticonvulsant treatment in head injury. *Brain Injury*, **3**,137–40.

Spellacy, F. (1978) Neuropsychological discrimination between violent and non-violent men. *Journal of Clinical Psychology*, **34**,49–52.

Spence, S. H., Marzillier, J. S. (1981) Social skills training with adolescent male offenders: Short-term, long-term and generalised effects. *Behaviour Research and Therapy*, **19**,349–68.

Spivack, G., and Shure, M. B. (1974) *Social Adjustment of Young Children: A Cognitive Approach to Solving Real-Life Problems*, Jossey-Bass, San Francisco.

Squire, L. R. (1986) Mechanisms of memory. *Science*, **232**,1612–19.

Squire, L. R. and Slater, P. C. (1975) Forgetting in very long-term memory as assessed by an improved questionnaire technique. *Journal of Experimental Psychology: Human Learning and Memory*, **1**,50–4.

St. Lawrence, J. S. Hansen, D. J., Cutts, T. F. *et al.* (1985) Situation context: Effects on perceptions of assertive and unassertive behaviour. *Behaviour Therapy*, **6**,51–62.

Starkstein, S. E., Boston, J. D. and Robinson, R. G. (1988) Mechanisms of mania after brain injury: 12 case reports and a review of the literature. *Journal of Nervous and Mental Diseases*, **176**,87–100.

Starkstein, S. E., Robinson, R. G., Honig, M. A. *et al.* (1989) Mood changes after right-hemisphere lesions. *British Journal of Psychiatry*, **155**,79–85.

Starr, A. and Phillips, L. (1970) Verbal and motor memory in the amnesic syndrome. *Neuropsychologica*, **8**,75–88.

Stephens, M. A. P., Norris-Baker C. and Willems, E. P. (1983) Patient behaviour monitoring through self-reports. *Archives of Physical Medicine and Rehabilitation,* **64**,67–171.

Stern, J. M., Sazbon, L., Becker, E. and Costoff, H. (1988) Severe behavioural disturbance in families of patients with prolonged coma. *Brain Injury,* **2**,259–62.

Stern, P. H., McDowell, F., Miller, J. M., and Robinson, M. (1970) Effects of Facilitation Exercise Techniques in Stroke Rehabilitation. *Archives of Physical Medicine and Rehabilitation,* **51**,526–31.

Strich, S. J. (1956) Diffuse degeneration of the cerebral white matter in severe dementia following head injury. *Journal of Neurology, Neurosurgery and Psychiatry,* **19**,163–85.

Strub, R. L. and Black F. W. (1985) *The Mental Status Examination in Neurology,* 2nd edn, F. A. Davis and Company, Philadelphia.

Stuss, D. T. and Benson, D. F. (1987) The frontal lobes and control of cognition and memory, in *The Frontal Lobes Revisited,* (ed. E. Perecman), the IRBN Press, New York, New York pp. -.

Stuss, D. T. and Benson, D. F. (1986) *The Frontal Lobes,* Raven Press, New York.

Stuss, D. T., Stethem, L. L., Hugenholtz, H. *et al.* (1989). Reaction time after head injury: Fatigue, divided attention and consistency of performance. *Journal of Neurology, Neurosurgery and Psychiatry,* **52**,742–8.

Sullivan, T., Conine, T. A., Goodman, M. and Mackie, T. (1988) Serial casting to prevent equinus in acute traumatic head injury. *Physiotherapy Canada,* **40**, 346–50.

Suls, J. and Sanders G. S. (1988) Type A behaviour as a general risk factor for physical disorder. *Journal of Behavioural Medicine,* **11**, 101–266.

Sumner, D. (1976) Disturbance of the senses of smell and taste after head injury, in Handbook of Clinical Neurology Vol. 24, (eds P. J. Vinken and G. W. Bruyn), North Holland Publishing, Amsterdam and Oxford, American Elsevier Publishing, New York, pp. 1–26

Sundberg, N. D., Snowden L. R. and Reynold, W. M. (1978) Toward assessment of personal competence in life situations. *Annual Review of Psychology,* **29**, 197–221.

Sunderland, A., Harris, J. E. and Gleave, J. (1984) Memory Failures in everyday life following severe head injury. *Journal of Clinical Neuropsychology,* **6**, 127–42.

Surburg, P. R. (1977) The effect of proprioceptive facilitation patterning upon reaction, response and movement times. *Physical Therapy,* **57**, 513–17.

Sutherland, N. S. (1968) Outlines of a theory of visual pattern recognition in animals and man. *Proceedings of the Royal Society,* **171**, 297–317.

Suzuki, J., Abiko, H., Mizoi K. *et al.* (1987) Protective effects of phenytoin and its enhanced action by combined administration with manitol and vitamin E in cerebral ischemia. *Acta Neurochirugica (Wien),* **88**, 56–64.

Swan, D., Van Wieringen, P. C. W. and Fokkemn, S. D. (1974) Auditory EMG feedback therapy to inhibit undesired motor activity. *Archives of Physical Medicine and Rehabilitation*, **55**, 251–4.

Taylor, A. R. and Bell, T. K. (1966) Slowing of cerebral circulation after concussional head injury. *Lancet*, **ii**, 178–80.

Teasdale, G. and Jennett, B. (1974) Assessment of coma and impaired consciousness: a practical scale. *Lancet*, **ii**, 81–4.

Temkin, N., Mclean, A., Dikmen, S. *et al.* (1988) Development and evaluation of modifications to the sickness impact profile for head injury. *Journal of Clinical Epidemiology*, **41**, 47–57

Teuber, H-L. (1975) Recovery of function after brain injury in man, in CIBA Foundation Symposium 34. New Series. *Outcome of Severe Damage to the Central Nervous System*, Elsevier, Amsterdam, pp. 159–86.

Teuber, H-L. (1969) Neglected aspects of the post traumatic syndrome, in *The Late Effects of Head Injury*, (eds A. E. Walker *et al.*), Charles C. Thomas, Springfield, Illinois, pp. 13–34.

Thompson, R. F. (1983) Neural substrates of simple associative learning: classical conditioning. *Trends in Neuroscience*, 270–5.

Thompson, R. S., Rivara, F. P. and Thompson, D. C. (1989) A case control study of the effectiveness of bicycle safety helmets. *New England Journal of Medicine*, **320**, 1362–7

Thomsen, I. V. (1974) The patient with severe brain injury and his family: a follow-up of 50 patients. *Scandinavian Journal of Rehabilitation Medicine*, **6**, 180–3.

Thomsen, I. V. (1985) Long-term psychological follow-up of patients with severe blunt brain trauma. *Journal of Clinical Experimental Neuropsychology*, **7**, 165.

Thomsen, I. V. (1984) Late outcome of severe blunt head trauma: a 10–15 year second follow-up. *Journal of Neurology, Neurosurgery and Psychiatry*, **47**, 260–268.

Thomsen, I. V. (1981) Neuropsychological treatment and long term follow-up of an aphasic patient with very severe head trauma. *Journal of Clinical Neuropsychology*, **3**, 43–51.

Thorndike, E. L., (1911) *Animal Intelligence*, Macmillan, New York.

Thurstone, L. L. and Thurstone T. G. (1941) *Factorial Studies of Intelligence*. Psychometric Monographs 2, University of Chicago Press, Chicago, Illinois.

Toglia, J. P. (1989) Visual perception of objects: An approach to assessment and intervention. *American Journal of Occupational Therapy*, **43**, 587–95.

Toglia, J. U. and Katinsky, S. (1975) Neuro-otological aspects of closed head injury, in *Handbook of Clinical Neurology*, Vol. 24, (eds P. J. Vinken and G. W. Bruyn), North Holland Publishing, Amsterdam and Oxford, American Elsevier Publishing, New York, pp. 119–140.

Toone, B. (1981) Psychosis in epilepsy, in *Epilepsy and Psychiatry*, (eds E. H. Reynolds and M. R. Trimble), Churchill Livingstone, New York, pp. 113–37.

Trieschmann, R. B. (1980) *Spinal Cord Injuries: Psychological Social and Vocational Adjustment*, Pergamon Press, New York.

Trimble, M. R. (1981) *Neuropsychiatry*, John Wiley and Sons, New York.

Trombly, C. A. (1982) *Occupational Therapy for Physical Dysfunction*, William and Wilkins, Baltimore.

Trower, P. (1987) Social Skills Retraining. *British Medical Journal*, **294**, 663–4.

Trower, P., Bryant, B. M. and Argyle, M. (1978) *Social Skills and Mental Health*, Methuen, London.

Trower, P., O'Mahoney, J. F. and Dryden, W. (1982) Cognitive aspects of social failure: Some implications for social skills training. *British Journal of Guidance Counselling*, **10**, 176–84.

Tucker, J. S. and Riggio, R. E. (1988) The role of social skills in encoding posed and spontaneous facial expressions. *Journal of Non-Verbal Behaviour*, **12**, 87–97.

Tulving, E. (1972) Episodic and semantic memory, in *Organization of Memory*, (eds E Tulving and W. Donaldson), Academic Press, New York, pp. -.

Tulving, E. (1983) *Elements of Episodic Memory*, Clarendon Press, Oxford.

Tunks, E. R. and Dermer, S. W. (1977) Carbamazepine in the dyscontrol syndrome associated with limbic dysfunction. *The Journal of Nervous and Mental Disease*, **164**, 56–63.

Turnbull, J. (1988) Perils (hidden and not so hidden) for the token economy. *The Journal of Head Trauma Rehabilitation*, **3**, 46–52.

Turner, W. A. (1944) Facial palsies in closed head injuries. *Lancet, i*: 756–7.

Tyerman, A. and Humphrey, M. (1984) Changes in self concept following severe head injury. *Journal of Rehabilitation Research*, **7**, 11–23.

Tyerman, A. D. (1984) The problems of personal identity in neurological rehabilitation. *Nursing*, **23**, 679–81.

Ulatowska, H. K., Freedman-Stern, R., Doyel, A. W. *et al.* (1983) Production of narrative discourse in aphasia. *Brain and Language*, **19**, 317–34.

Ullman, P. and Krasner, L. (1969) *A Psychological Approach to Abnormal Behavior*, Prentice-Hall, Englewood Cliffs, New Jersey.

Uzzell, B. P., Dolinskas, C. A., Wiser, R. F. and Langfitt, T. W. (1987) Influence of lesions detected by computed tomography on outcome and neuropsychological recovery after severe head injury. *Neurosurgery*, **20**, 396–402.

Van Deusen, J. and Harlowe, D. (1987) Continued construct validation of the St. Mary's CVA Evaluation: Bilateral awareness scale. *American Journal of Occupational Therapy*, **41**, 242–5.

Van Houton, R., Axelrod, S., Baily, J. S. *et al.* (1988) The right to effective behavioral treatment. *Journal of Applied Behavioral Analysis*, **21**, 381–4.

Van Zomeren, A. H. and Deelman, B.G. (1978) Long-term recovery of visual reaction time after closed head injury. *Journal of Neurology. Neurosurgery and Psychiatry*, **41**, 452–7.

Van Zomeren, A. H. and Van Den Burg, W. (1985) Residual complaints of patients two years after severe head injury. *Journal of Neurology, Neurosurgery and Psychiatry*, **48**, 21–8.

Van Zomeren, A. H., Brouner, W. H., Rothengatter, J. A. and Snoek, J. W. (1988) Fitness to drive a car after recovery from severe head injury. *Archives of Physical Medicine and Rehabilitation*, **69**, 90–6.

Van Zomeren, A. H., Brouwer, W. H. and Deelman, D. G. (1984) Attentional deficits: The riddles of selectivity, speed and alertness, in *Closed Head Injury: Psychological Social and Family Consequences*, (ed D. N. Brooks), Oxford University Press, London,

Varney, N. R. (1988) Prognostic Significance of Anosmia in patients with Closed-Head Trauma. *Journal of Clinical and Experimental Neuropsychology*, **10**, 250–4.

Vauce-Earland, T. (1991) Perception of role assessment tools in the physical disability setting. *American Journal of Occupational Therapy*, **45**, 26–31.

Vigotskii, L. S. (1962) *Thought and Language*, MIT Press, Cambridge.

Vilkki, J. (1988) Problem solving after focal cerebral lesions. *Cortex*, **24**, 119–27.

Vilkki, J. (1989) Hemi-inattention in visual search for parallel lines after focal cerebral lesions. *Journal of Clinical and Experimental Neuropsychology*, **11**, 319–31.

Vilkki, J., Poropudas, K., and Servo, A. (1988) Memory disorder related to coma duration after head injury. *Journal of Neurology, Neurosurgery and Psychiatry*, **51**, 1452–4.

Virkkunnen, M., Nuvtila, A., and Huusko S. (1976) Effect of brain injury on social adaptability. *Acta Psychiatrica Scandavica*, **53**, 168–72.

Vitalo, R. (1971) Teaching improved interpersonal functioning as a preferred mode of treatment. *Journal of Clinical Psychology*, **27**, 166–71.

Vreede, C. F. (1988) The need for a better definition of ADL. *International Journal of Rehabilitation Research*, **11**, 29–35.

Wacker, D. P., Berg, W. K., McMahon, C. *et al.* (1988) An evaluation of labelling-then-doing with moderately handicapped persons: Acquisition and generalization with complex tasks. *Journal of Applied Behavior Analysis*, **21**, 369–80.

Wade, D. T. (1987) Neurological rehabilitation. *International Disabilities Studies*, **9**, 45–7.

Wagenaar, W. A. (1986) My memory: A study of autobiographical memory over six years. *Cognitive Psychology*, **18**, 225–52.

Wahler, R. G. and Fox, J. J. (1981) Setting events in applied behaviour analysis: Toward a conceptual and methodological expansion. *Journal of Applied Behaviour Analysis*, **14**, 327–38.

Wallace, C. J. (1976) Assessment of psychotic behaviour, in *Behavioural Assessment: a Practical Handbook*, (eds M. Hersen and A. S. Bellack), Pergamon Press, New York,

Waller, P. F., Stewart, J. R., Hansen, A. R. *et al.* (1985) The potentiating effects of alcohol on driver injury. *Proceedings of the American Association for Automotive Medicine*, **29**, 1–22.

Warr, P. (1983) Work, jobs and unemployment. *Bulletin of the British Psychological Society*, **36**, 305–9.

Warrington, E., and McCarthy, R. A. (1987) Categories of knowledge. Further fractionations and an attempted integration. *Brain*, **110**, 1273–96.

Warrington, E. K. (1975) The selective impairment of semantic memory. *Quarterly Journal of Experimental Psychology*, **27**, 635–57.

Warrington, E. K. (1981) Neuropsychological studies of the verbal semantic system. *Philosophical Transactions of the Royal society of London, B*, **295**, 411–23.

Warrington, E. K. and Shallice, T. (1984) Category specific semantic impairments. *Brain*, **107**, 829–53.

Watson, R. T., Heilman, K. M., Millar, B. D. and King, F. A. (1974) Neglect after mesencephalic reticular formation lesions. *Neurology*, **24**, 294–8.

Watts, C., Cox, T. and Robinson, J. (1983) Morningness eveningness and diurnal variation in self reported mood. *Journal of Psychology*, **113**, 251–6.

Wechsler, D. (1945) A standardized memory scale for clinical use. *Journal of Psychology*, **19**, 87–95.

Weddell, R., Oddy, M. and Jenkins, D. (1980) Social adjustment after rehabilitation: a two year follow-up of patients with severe brain injury. *Psychological Medicine*, **10**, 257–63.

Wehman, P., Kreutzer, J. S., Stonnington, H. H. *et al.* (1988) Supported employment for persons with traumatic brain injury: A preliminary report. *Journal of Head Trauma Rehabilitation*, **3**, 82–93.

Weinberg, J., Diller L., Gordon, W. A. *et al.* (1977) Visual scanning training effect on reading-related tasks in acquired right brain damage. *Archives of Physical Medicine and Rehabilitation*, **58**, 479–86.

Weinstein, C. J. (1987) Motor learning considerations in stroke rehabilitation, in *The Rehabilitation: The Recovery of Motor Control*, (eds P. W. Duncan and M. B. Badke), Year Book Medical Publishers, Chicago,

Weiskrantz, L. (1986) *Blindsight: A Case Study and Implication*, Oxford University Press, Oxford.

Weiskrantz, L., Warrington, E. K., Sanders, M. D. and Marshall, J. (1974) Visual capacity in the hemianopic field following a restricted occipital ablation. *Brain*, **97**, 709–28.

Welford, A. T. (1959) Evidence of a single-channel decision mechanism limiting performance in a serial reaction task. *Quarterly Journal of Experimental Psychology*, **11**, 193–210.

Wender, P. H. Reimher, F. W. Wood, D. and Ward, M. (1985) A controlled study of methylphenidate in the treatment of attention deficit disorder residual type in adults. *American Journal of Psychiatry*, **142**, 547–52.

West, J. G., Cales, R. H. and Gazzaniga, A. B. (1983) Impact of regionalization: The Orange County Experience. *Archives of Surgery*, **118**, 740–4.

Weston, M. J. and Whitlock, F. A. (1971) The Capgras syndrome following head injury. *British Journal of Psychiatry*, **119**, 25–31.

Whyte, J. (1988) Clinical drug evaluation. *Journal of Head Trauma Rehabilitation*, **3**, 95–9.

Wiley, S. D. (1983) Structural treatment approaches to families in crisis. *American Journal of Physical Medicine*, **62**, 271–86.

Will, B. E., Rosenweig, M. R. and Bennett, E. (1976) Effects of differential environments on recovery from neonatal brain lesions, measured by problem solving scores and brain dimensions. *Physiology and Behaviour*, **16**, 603–11.

Willems, E. P. and Vindberg, S. (1969). Direct observations of patients: The interface of environment and behaviour. *Psychological Aspects of Disability*, **16**, 74–88.

Willems, E. P. (1972) The interface of the hospital environment and patient behaviour. *Archives of Physical Medicine and Rehabilitation*, **53**, 115–22.

Williams, G. H. (1987) Disablement and the social context of daily activity. *International Disability Studies*, **9**, 97–102.

Williams, R. S. (1984) Ability, disability and rehabilitation: A phenomenological description. *Journal of Medical Philosophy*, **9**, 93–112.

Williams, A. F., Preusser, D. F., Bloomberg, R. D. and Lund, A. K. (1987) Seat belt use law enforcement and publicity in Elmira, New York: A reminder campaign. *American Journal of Public Health*, **77**, 1450–1.

Wilson, B. (1987a) The measurement of perceptual impairment. *Clinical Rehabilitation*, **1**, 169–73.

Wilson, B., Cockburn, J., and Baddeley A. D. (1985) *The Rivermead Behavioural Memory Test*, Thames Valley Test Company, 22, Bulsmersle Rd., Reading, Berkshire.

Wilson, B. (1987b) Single-case experimental design in neuropsychological rehabilitation. *Journal of Clinical and Experimental Neuropsychology*, **9**, 527–44.

Wilson, B., Cockburn, J. and Halligan, P. W. (1987) *Behavioural Inattention Test*, Thames Valley Test Company, Titchfield, Hants.

Wilson, B. A. and Moffat, N. (1984) *Clinical Management of Memory Problems*, Croom Helm, London.

Wilson, J. A., Pentland, B., Currie, C. T. and Miller, J. D. (1987) The functional effects of head injury in the elderly. *Brain Injury*, **1**, 183–8.

Wilson-MacDonald, J., Sherman, K. and MacKinnon, J. (1987) Off-the-road motorcycling injuries: 1982–1985. *Injury*, **18**, 196–8.

Wissel, J., Eberersbach, G., Gutjahr, L. and Dahlke, F. (1989) Treating chronic hemiparesis with modified biofeedback. *Archives of Physical Medicine and Rehabilitation*, **70**, 612–17.

Wolf, S. L. (1983) Electromyographic biofeedback applications to stroke patients. A critical review. *Physical Therapy*, **63**, 1448–59.

Wolff, F., Marsnick, N., Tracey, W. and Nichols, R. (1983) *Perceptive Listening*, Holt, Rinehart & Winston, New York.

Wolpert, I. (1924) Die simultanagnosie: Storung der gesamtauffassung. *Z.F.D. Gesamte Neurol. u Psychiatr*, **93**, 397–425.

Woo, S. Matthews J. V., Akeson, W. H. *et al.* (1975) Connective tissue response to immobility. Correlative study of biomechanical measurements of normal and immobilised rabbit knees. *Arthritis and Rheumatism,* **18**, (3) 257–64.

Wood, P. H. N. and Badley, E. M. (1978) Setting disability in perspective. *International Rehabilitation Medicine,* **1**, 32–7.

Wood, R. Ll. (1987) *Brain Injury Rehabilitation: A Neurobehavioural Approach,* Croom Helm, London.

Wood, P. H. N. (1980) Appreciating the consequences of disease – The classification of impairments, disabilities and handicaps. *The WHO Chronicle,* **34**, 376–80.

Wood, R. Ll. and Burgess, P. (1988) Management of Behaviour disorders following brain injury, in *Rehabilitation of the Severely Brain Injured Adult: A Practical Approach,* (eds I. Fussey and G. M. Giles), Croom Helm, London, pp. 43–68.

Wood, R. Ll. and Fussey, I. (1987) Computer based cognitive retraining: a controlled study. *International Disability Studies,* **9**, 149–53.

Wood, R. Ll. and Eames, P. (1981) Application of behaviour modification in the treatment of the traumatically brain-injured adults, in *Applications of Conditioning Theory,* (ed. G. Davey), Methuen, London, pp. 81–101.

Woods, R. T. (1979) Reality orientation and staff attention: A controlled study, *British Journal of Psychiatry,* **34**, 502–7.

World Health Organization (1980) *International Classification of Impairment Disabilities and Handicaps.* World Health Organization, Geneva.

Worrell, J. (1987) Head injuries in pedal cyclists: How much will protection help? *Injury,* **18**, 5–6.

Wright, B. (1980) Person and situation: Adjusting the rehabilitation focus. *Archives of Physical Medicine and Rehabilitation,* **61**, 59–64.

Wright, B. D. and Linacre, J. M. (1989) Observations are always ordinal: Measurements however must be interval. *Archives of Physical Medicine and Rehabilitation,* **70**, 857–60.

Yarnell, P. R. and Rossie, G. V. (1988) Minor whiplash head injury with major debilitation. *Brain Injury,* **2**, 255–8.

Ylvisaker, M. (1985) *Head Injury Rehabilitation: Children and Adolescents,* College Hill Press, San Diego.

Yudofsky, S. C., Silver, J. M. and Schneider, S. E. (1987) Pharmacological treatment of aggression, *Psychiatric Annals,* **17**, 397–407.

Yudofsky, S. C., Silver, J. M., Jackson, W. *et al.* (1986) The overt aggression scale for the objective rating of verbal and physical aggression. *American Journal of Psychiatry,* **143**, 35–9.

Yudofsky, S., Williams, D. and Gorman J. (1981) Propranolol in the treatment of rage and violent behaviour in patients with chronic brain syndromes. *American Journal of Psychiatry,* **138**, 218–20.

Zablotny, C. (1987) Using neuromuscular electrical stimulation to facilitate limb control in the head injured patient. *The Journal of Head Trauma Rehabilitation.* 2:28–33.

Zaidel, S. and Mehrabian, S. (1969) The ability to communicate and infer positive and negative attitudes facially and vocally. *Journal of Experimental Research on Personality,* **3**, 233–41.

Zarksi, J. J., DePompei, R. and Zook, A. (1988) Traumatic brain injury:

Dimensions of family responsivity. *Journal of Head Trauma Rehabilitation*, **3**, 31–41.

Zencius, A. H., Wesolowski, M. D., Burke, W. H. and McQuade, P. (1989) Antecedent control in the treatment of brain injured clients. *Brain Injury*, **3**, 199–205.

Zihl, J. (1981) Recovery of visual functions in patients with cerebral blindness. *Experimental Brain Research*, **24**, 159–69.

Zihl, J. and von Cramon, D. (1979) Restitution of visual function in patients with cerebral blindness. *Journal of Neurology, Neurosurgery and Psychiatry*, **42**, 312–22.

Zihl, J. and von Cramon, D. (1982) Restitution of visual field in patients with damage to the geniculostriate visual pathway. *Human Neurobiology*, **1**, 5–8.

Zoltan, B., Jabri, J., Rykman, D. L. M. and Panikoff, L. B. (1987) *Perceptual Motor Evaluation for Head-Injured and Other Neurologically Impaired Adults*, Santa Clara Valley Medical Center, San José, CA.

Zyanski, S. J. (1978) Coronary-prone behaviour patterns and coronary heart disease: Epidemiological evidence, in *Coronary Prone Behaviour*, (eds T. M. Dembroski *et al.*), Springer-Verlag, New York, pp. 25–41.

Index